Healing Foods For Dummies®

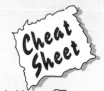

The Healthiest Fats

Fats of quality are an essential part of a healing foods diet. These fats and oils belong in your kitchen.

- ✔ Organic, unsalted butter
- ✔ Extra-virgin olive oil
- ✔ Flaxseed oil
- ✔ Unrefined vegetable oils such as unrefined safflower oil and unrefined sesame oil

Antioxidant Vitamins and Mi...

Antioxidant ...
some of th...
foods. They slow ...
where you'll find them.

- ✔ **Beta-carotene:** Fruits and vegetables that are orange and dark green
- ✔ **Vitamin C:** Citrus, berries, and sweet peppers
- ✔ **Vitamin E:** Cold-pressed, unrefined vegetables oils, whole wheat, kale, lamb, eggs, mackerel, and herring
- ✔ **Selenium:** Shrimp, lobster, scallops, clams, chicken breast, eggs, Brazil nuts, brown rice, and mushrooms

Wholesome Foods to Put on Your Shopping List

Some foods are especially packed with healing nutrients. Be sure to include these winners regularly in your meals.

- ✔ Fatty fish: Salmon and sardines
- ✔ Naturally raised meats and poultry
- ✔ Orange winter squash: Hubbard and acorn
- ✔ Reddish-blue fruit: Berries and grapes
- ✔ Dark leafy greens: Kale and collards
- ✔ Cruciferous vegetables: Cabbage and broccoli
- ✔ Whole grains: Whole wheat and brown rice
- ✔ Legumes: Beans and lentils
- ✔ Seeds: Pumpkin and sunflower
- ✔ Raw nuts: Almonds and walnuts
- ✔ Healing flavorings: Onions, garlic, and chilies

Ten Other Names for Sugar

Be aware that sugar comes in many forms and goes by many names. Many food products contain several kinds, which add up to a considerable amount! Look for these on food labels.

- ✔ Corn syrup
- ✔ Corn sweeteners
- ✔ High fructose corn syrup
- ✔ Dextrose
- ✔ Dextrin
- ✔ Fructose
- ✔ Fruit juice concentrate
- ✔ Malt
- ✔ Invert sugar
- ✔ Evaporated cane juice

Healing Foods For Dummies®

Ten Foods to Buy Organic

Certain foods are known to be grown with especially high levels of pesticides or, like butter and liver, to be a concentrated source of such chemicals. Treat yourself to the organic versions of these foods when you go shopping.

- Strawberries
- Green and red bell peppers
- Spinach
- Peaches
- Celery
- Apples
- Apricots
- Green beans
- Butter
- Liver

Ten Words You Want to See on Food Labels

When shopping for whole foods and food not loaded with chemicals, keep an eye out for words you can trust to mean that the food is natural and of high quality. The only word you can't trust is *natural*, which is used to describe all sorts of foods, good and bad.

- Whole
- Unrefined
- Unprocessed
- Minimally processed
- Raw
- Hormonefree
- Free of antibiotics
- Residuefree
- Free-range
- Organic

IDG BOOKS WORLDWIDE

Copyright © 1999 IDG Books Worldwide, Inc.
All rights reserved.
Cheat Sheet $2.95 value. Item 5198-1.
For more information about IDG Books,
call 1-800-762-2974.

Praise for Healing Foods For Dummies

"This magnificent book provides the reader with a comprehensive and incredibly useful guide to healthy eating. Everyone can benefit from the helpful information that Molly Siple includes on how diet affects a variety of health conditions, as well as her useful tips on food planning and preparation. She has also included many delicious recipes. I highly recommend this book!"

— Susan M. Lark, M.D.,
   author of *The Chemistry of Success*

"Simply browsing through this book is a healing experience in itself. So imagine what is possible for your health and healing when you actually prepare and eat the delicious healing foods so nicely presented in *Healing Foods For Dummies*."

— Christiane Northrup, M.D.,
   author of *Women's Bodies, Women's Wisdom,*
   editor of *Healthy Wisdom for Women*, monthly newsletter

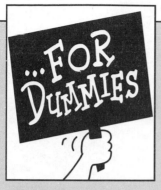
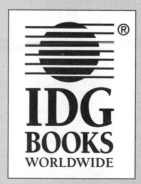

Healing Foods

FOR

DUMMIES®

Healing Foods
FOR
DUMMIES®

by Molly Siple, M.S., R.D.

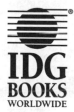

IDG Books Worldwide, Inc.
An International Data Group Company

Foster City, CA ◆ Chicago, IL ◆ Indianapolis, IN ◆ New York, NY

Healing Foods For Dummies®

Published by
IDG Books Worldwide, Inc.
An International Data Group Company
919 E. Hillsdale Blvd.
Suite 400
Foster City, CA 94404
www.idgbooks.com (IDG Books Worldwide Web site)
www.dummies.com (Dummies Press Web site)

Library of Congress Catalog Card No.: 99-66444

ISBN: 0-7645-5198-1

Printed in the United States of America

10 9 8 7 6 5 4 3 2 1

1B/QU/RR/ZZ/IN

Distributed in the United States by IDG Books Worldwide, Inc.

Distributed by CDG Books Canada Inc. for Canada; by Transworld Publishers Limited in the United Kingdom; by IDG Norge Books for Norway; by IDG Sweden Books for Sweden; by IDG Books Australia Publishing Corporation Pty. Ltd. for Australia and New Zealand; by TransQuest Publishers Pte Ltd. for Singapore, Malaysia, Thailand, Indonesia, and Hong Kong; by Gotop Information Inc. for Taiwan; by ICG Muse, Inc. for Japan; by Intersoft for South Africa; by Eyrolles for France; by International Thomson Publishing for Germany, Austria and Switzerland; by Distribuidora Cuspide for Argentina; by LR International for Brazil; by Galileo Libros for Chile; by Ediciones ZETA S.C.R. Ltda. for Peru; by WS Computer Publishing Corporation, Inc., for the Philippines; by Contemporanea de Ediciones for Venezuela; by Express Computer Distributors for the Caribbean and West Indies; by Micronesia Media Distributor, Inc. for Micronesia; by Chips Computadoras S.A. de C.V. for Mexico; by Editorial Norma de Panama S.A. for Panama; by American Bookshops for Finland.

For general information on IDG Books Worldwide's books in the U.S., please call our Consumer Customer Service department at 800-762-2974. For reseller information, including discounts and premium sales, please call our Reseller Customer Service department at 800-434-3422.

For information on where to purchase IDG Books Worldwide's books outside the U.S., please contact our International Sales department at 317-596-5530 or fax 317-596-5692.

For consumer information on foreign language translations, please contact our Customer Service department at 1-800-434-3422, fax 317-596-5692, or e-mail rights@idgbooks.com.

For information on licensing foreign or domestic rights, please phone +1-650-655-3109.

For sales inquiries and special prices for bulk quantities, please contact our Sales department at 650-655-3200 or write to the address above.

For information on using IDG Books Worldwide's books in the classroom or for ordering examination copies, please contact our Educational Sales department at 800-434-2086 or fax 317-596-5499.

For press review copies, author interviews, or other publicity information, please contact our Public Relations department at 650-655-3000 or fax 650-655-3299.

For authorization to photocopy items for corporate, personal, or educational use, please contact Copyright Clearance Center, 222 Rosewood Drive, Danvers, MA 01923, or fax 978-750-4470.

is a registered trademark under exclusive license to IDG Books Worldwide, Inc. from International Data Group, Inc.

About the Author

Molly Siple has a Master of Science in Nutritional Science and is also a registered dietitian. Her other books include two on female health, co-authored with Lissa DeAngelis, *SOS for PMS,* and *Recipes for Change: Gourmet Wholefood Cooking for Health and Vitality at Menopause*, a Julia Child Cookbook Awards nominee. She is an Advisory Board Member for the Oregon Menopause Network. Molly is also a member of the International Association of Culinary Professionals and founded and managed a corporate catering business in New York City. She lectures on nutrition and is a nutrition consultant to food companies. She lives in Los Angeles. Her Web site is www.wellwoman.com.

ABOUT IDG BOOKS WORLDWIDE

Welcome to the world of IDG Books Worldwide.

IDG Books Worldwide, Inc., is a subsidiary of International Data Group, the world's largest publisher of computer-related information and the leading global provider of information services on information technology. IDG was founded more than 30 years ago by Patrick J. McGovern and now employs more than 9,000 people worldwide. IDG publishes more than 290 computer publications in over 75 countries. More than 90 million people read one or more IDG publications each month.

Launched in 1990, IDG Books Worldwide is today the #1 publisher of best-selling computer books in the United States. We are proud to have received eight awards from the Computer Press Association in recognition of editorial excellence and three from Computer Currents' First Annual Readers' Choice Awards. Our best-selling *...For Dummies*® series has more than 50 million copies in print with translations in 31 languages. IDG Books Worldwide, through a joint venture with IDG's Hi-Tech Beijing, became the first U.S. publisher to publish a computer book in the People's Republic of China. In record time, IDG Books Worldwide has become the first choice for millions of readers around the world who want to learn how to better manage their businesses.

Our mission is simple: Every one of our books is designed to bring extra value and skill-building instructions to the reader. Our books are written by experts who understand and care about our readers. The knowledge base of our editorial staff comes from years of experience in publishing, education, and journalism — experience we use to produce books to carry us into the new millennium. In short, we care about books, so we attract the best people. We devote special attention to details such as audience, interior design, use of icons, and illustrations. And because we use an efficient process of authoring, editing, and desktop publishing our books electronically, we can spend more time ensuring superior content and less time on the technicalities of making books.

You can count on our commitment to deliver high-quality books at competitive prices on topics you want to read about. At IDG Books Worldwide, we continue in the IDG tradition of delivering quality for more than 30 years. You'll find no better book on a subject than one from IDG Books Worldwide.

John Kilcullen
Chairman and CEO
IDG Books Worldwide, Inc.

Steven Berkowitz
President and Publisher
IDG Books Worldwide, Inc.

*Eighth Annual
Computer Press
Awards ≥1992*

*Ninth Annual
Computer Press
Awards ≥1993*

*Tenth Annual
Computer Press
Awards ≥1994*

*Eleventh Annual
Computer Press
Awards ≥1995*

Dedication

To my beloved father, Allen G. Siple, who wanted me to write.

Author's Acknowledgments

Huge thank you's go to . . .

- My ever-thoughtful friend and agent, Mari Florence, for seeing the possibility of my writing this book.

- Tammerly Booth, executive editor, for helping me shape the book's content and shepherding the project.

- Pam Mourouzis, Kelly Ewing, and Rowena Rappaport, editors, for your kind suggestions and expert guidance.

- Laura Pensiero for recipe testing and running my recipes through your expert hands.

- My mother, Esma Shaw, who copy-edited my writing with her eagle eye.

- Lissa DeAngelis, my coauthor on earlier books, who introduced me to the world of whole foods cooking and cheered me on.

- Leigh Fortson for your professional assistance in research, and Mark McKenney for your swift Web work.

- And my friends: Dee Yalowitz, for always giving me a New York home; Ann Arlen for reading final chapters; the gang on Mission, Marijane Hebert, April Foster, Jeannie Summers, and Paulette Lee, for my office and for giving me company while I wrote; Wendy Wolosoff for inspiring my new and healing kitchen; and the one and only Victor Watson who built the kitchen, organized my files, did research, brought me food, and gave me fresh lavender every morning.

I am especially grateful to the two expert advisors who contributed to this book, Colette Heimowitz, M.Sc. (Director of Nutrition at the Atkins Center for Complementary Medicine in New York City), and Hugh D. Riordan, M.D., (founder and president of The Center for the Improvement of Human Functioning International in Wichita, Kansas). Thank you, Colette, for your thorough review of the manuscript and your valuable additions to the text. And thank you, Hugh, for helping me make changes where needed and for generously offering advice based on your wealth of knowledge and experience. You both were an essential part of this project.

Publisher's Acknowledgments

We're proud of this book; please register your comments through our IDG Books Worldwide Online Registration Form located at http://my2cents.dummies.com.

Some of the people who helped bring this book to market include the following:

Acquisitions, Editorial, and Media Development

Project Editors: Kelly Ewing, Pamela Mourouzis

Executive Editor: Tammerly Booth

General Reviewers: Colette Heimowitz, M.Sc., and Hugh D. Riordan, M.D.

Recipe Tester: Laura Pensiero

Acquisitions Coordinator: Karen S. Young

Editorial Administrator: Michelle Vukas

Editorial Director: Kristin A. Cocks

Illustrator: Elizabeth Kurtzman

Production

Project Coordinator: Regina Snyder

Layout and Graphics: Amy Adrian, Angela F. Hunckler, Kate Jenkins, Barry Offringa, Jill Piscitelli, Doug Rollison, Brent Savage, Michael A. Sullivan, Brian Torwelle, Maggie Ubertini, Dan Whetstine. Erin Zeltner

Proofreaders: Laura Albert, John Greenough, Paula Lowell, Marianne Santy, Rebecca Senninger, Charles Spencer

Indexer: Sherry Massey

Special Help
Rowena Rappaport, Allison Solomon

General and Administrative

IDG Books Worldwide, Inc.: John Kilcullen, CEO; Steven Berkowitz, President and Publisher

IDG Books Technology Publishing Group: Richard Swadley, Senior Vice President and Publisher; Walter Bruce III, Vice President and Associate Publisher; Joseph Wikert, Associate Publisher; Mary Bednarek, Branded Product Development Director; Mary Corder, Editorial Director; Barry Pruett, Publishing Manager; Michelle Baxter, Publishing Manager

IDG Books Consumer Publishing Group: Roland Elgey, Senior Vice President and Publisher; Kathleen A. Welton, Vice President and Publisher; Kevin Thornton, Acquisitions Manager; Kristin A. Cocks, Editorial Director

IDG Books Internet Publishing Group: Brenda McLaughlin, Senior Vice President and Publisher; Diane Graves Steele, Vice President and Associate Publisher; Sofia Marchant, Online Marketing Manager

IDG Books Production for Dummies Press: Debbie Stailey, Associate Director of Production; Cindy L. Phipps, Manager of Project Coordination, Production Proofreading, and Indexing; Tony Augsburger, Manager of Prepress, Reprints, and Systems; Laura Carpenter, Production Control Manager; Shelley Lea, Supervisor of Graphics and Design; Debbie J. Gates, Production Systems Specialist; Robert Springer, Supervisor of Proofreading; Kathie Schutte, Production Supervisor

Dummies Packaging and Book Design: Patty Page, Manager, Promotions Marketing

◆

The publisher would like to give special thanks to Patrick J. McGovern, without whom this book would not have been possible.

◆

Contents at a Glance

Recipes at a Glance

Snacks

Soups

Cartoons at a Glance

By Rich Tennant

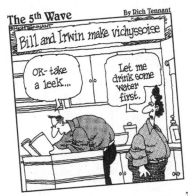

page 7

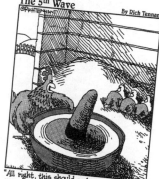

page 47

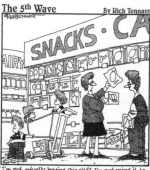

page 27

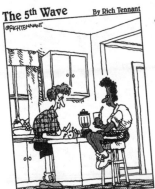

page 281

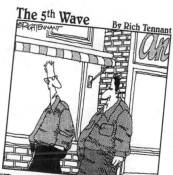

page 161

Fax: 978-546-7747 • E-mail: the5wave@tiac.net

Table of Contents

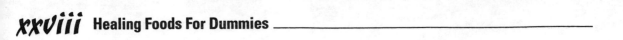

Introduction

*I*f you eat, this book is for you. Every time you choose one food over another, you make a decision that can affect your health. Introducing *Healing Foods For Dummies* — my chance to tell you about all the wondrous natural foods that can help keep you well and speed your recovery when you are sick. Yes, food is a source of pleasure, and eating fancy foods in restaurants can be great fun and has become a form of entertainment. But now I'm inviting you to get to know this other side of food, and its ability to act as a natural medicine.

As a nutritionist, I've witnessed the deterioration in health that poor quality, empty-calorie foods can cause. I've also seen that a change in diet can produce a sometimes dramatic turnaround in how a person feels. Why not take advantage of the healing properties of foods? You have a chance to benefit from every meal. The idea of food being therapeutic is not new. Hippocrates, the father of modern medicine, declared, "Let food be your medicine, and your medicine be your food." He gave a prescription that still holds true today. I invite you to practice this gentle form of self-care.

About This Book

The following chapters give you the full picture of healing foods, the broad brush strokes and the details. You find out about the general differences between natural, whole foods and those that are refined and processed. I show you how to shop for these foods and prepare them in the most health-promoting ways. I'm standing next to you in your kitchen with my apron on!

You also have the chance to discover the hundreds of healing foods and the vitamins, minerals, and many therapeutic phytochemicals they contain. The healing foods are then linked to specific health conditions, with recommendations given for both prevention and treatment. And you have the chance to sample the foods you've been reading about — recipes accompany all the food talk.

The appendixes in the back of the book are also full of information — two extensive guides. One lists healing foods, and the other describes common ailments and the way of eating recommended for each. I also give you a list of mail-order resources for certain healing foods in case you can't find them in your local market.

When can you expect to be feeling better? It depends on the ailment and your general level of health. If you've been abusing your body with junk foods for most meals, a week's worth of better eating could produce results. But to begin to build up a foundation of good health through diet can take three months or longer. You also need to be aware that people's nutritional needs can vary. Some of the dietary recommendations in this book, though they've been proven to be generally effective, may not be beneficial for you. Experiment with these foods and notice how you feel. Your expertise on what works for you is essential information, too.

Conventions Used in This Book

For each recipe in this book, I include preparation and cooking times so that you have an idea of how much time you can expect to spend making each dish. Prep time is how long it may take you to slice the onion or mix the salad dressing, but assumes that all the ingredients are in easy reach and the children and the cat are out of your way. Cooking time refers to the actual boiling, browning, and baking required.

In general, I follow these conventions when giving you recipes:

- All water is filtered.
- All salt is sea salt.
- All oils are cold-pressed and unrefined.
- All butter is unsalted and organic.
- All meat is preferably free of residues of antibiotics and hormones, has been raised under humane conditions, and comes from animals given organic feed.
- All poultry is preferably free of residues of antibiotics, free-range, and raised on organic feed.
- All produce, beans, nuts, seeds, and grains are preferably organic, especially the fruits and vegetables most likely to be treated with pesticides.

Have fun with the recipes! I use simple cooking techniques, like sautéing and baking, and sometimes include less familiar ingredients to give you a taste of something new. I've gone for bright and colorful flavors. Don't expect bland, brown, and green health food! And it's fine to boost the flavors even more by using a heavy hand with the garlic and onions.

What You're Not to Read

When you see the icon Technical Stuff, you don't have to read the text that follows. You can get all the basic info you really need just by reading the regular text. This part gives you the "do this and don't do that" advice. The information under Technical Stuff just tells you why. You can also skip the text in the gray boxes. These sidebars just give you extra information that you don't have to know to understand the topic.

Foolish Assumptions

As I wrote this book, I imagined that in terms of diet, you are already doing some things right but you know there's room for improvement. Probably most of you are feeling pretty well, but maybe not as terrific as you once did, when you were a bit younger (not that you're old now!). Some of you may be working your way through a serious health problem. And others among you may be gorgeous specimens of health and up-to-date on every new food and supplement that hits the market. This book is meant to speak to each one of you.

How This Book Is Organized

I first introduce you to the kinds of food you need for optimal health and then show you how to apply this information to specific health needs. As I introduce each food, I let you in on just how the food affects your body chemistry, fascinating science that I attempt to simplify into small and easily digested bites. Food research is a lively field of study these days, and I include many of the latest discoveries.

Healing Foods For Dummies is packed with information, but the book is organized so that you can open it and just take what you need — the bottom line, what to eat when. Look up a food you're about to cook, read all about fish, or find tips for a specific ailment. Start and stop where you like. Nutrition information can be complicated. Without this book, you may feel overwhelmed and confused by all the dietary advice you're exposed to through the media, from your friends, and even from your mother.

Here's how *Healing Foods For Dummies* is organized.

Part I: Staying Healthy with Good Food

This part introduces you to the basics about healing foods. You find out about the difference between healthy natural ingredients free of chemical additives, and those that are refined and processed. I also introduce you to other approaches to diet and healing with food — the wisdom of eating fresh foods that follow the seasons, and systems of nutrition developed long ago in China and India. Take the best from all of these! Start to form a picture of yourself in very good health. You have a new standard of well-being to have as your goal as you begin to eat more healing foods.

Part II: Setting Up Your Healing Foods Kitchen

Use this part to begin to give yourself a kitchen that supports your health. Get inspiration for reorganizing and outfitting your cooking space so that preparing meals is a pleasure. And make room for the healing ingredients you'll soon be bringing home! Read about the special ingredients you can find in your supermarket, in natural-food stores, and in ethnic food shops. This part also introduces you to the healthiest ways to cook foods and what you can do to *green* your kitchen and make it a healthier place.

Part III: Mother Nature's Best Foods

If you have an idea about what you'd like to cook for dinner but you want to make sure that you're using the healthiest ingredients, start with this part. Each chapter is devoted to certain categories of food. The wealth of information in this part about the special nutrients in certain foods makes it a snap for you to choose ingredients to suit your needs. You discover how to spot healing foods by color, texture, and taste. Start stocking your shelves with quality ingredients. Go on a cooking spree and begin sampling the recipes to make soups, salads, and more. This part gives you an introduction to healing foods that you can bring to the table.

Part IV: Treating Medical Problems with Healing Foods

This part is also about food and healing, but from the other perspective, starting with the ailment. Turn to this part when you want a remedy for an everyday complaint and when you need to treat a more serious medical problem. Find out about the general ways of eating to help prevent serious conditions, such as heart disease and osteoporosis, and about special foods for men, women, and children. Find out about special therapeutic nutrients and where you can find them in foods. Discover the foods and drinks that undermine your health and worsen symptoms. Then cook up some of the recipes, culinary prescriptions for specific conditions. This part helps you put all this food advice into practice in your day-to-day life, whether you cook at home or eat out.

Part V: The Part of Tens

If you want advice that's short but sweet, Part V is for you. This standard section in all ... *For Dummies* books gives you several handy lists, with ten items to a topic. Check it out — ten beautiful ways of serving healing foods, ten eating strategies for elders, and ten reasons to begin eating healing foods today.

Appendixes

This book gives you three additional sections. Appendix A is a symptom guide, a compact A-to-Z reference list for a wide range of medical problems, from acne to yeast infections. You can read about general ways of eating to lower the risk of developing these conditions, along with special foods and nutrients useful in treatment. Following this is Appendix B, an extensive A-to-Z listing of healing foods, from apples to yogurt. With each entry, you find information on the nutrients that the food is especially high in, the benefits of the food and what conditions it especially treats, assorted tips on buying, cooking, and storing, and finally the name of a delicious Healing Foods recipe that features the ingredient for you to sample.

Appendix C gives you mail-order resources for buying foods that you may not easily find in your local markets. I give you sources for organic and hormone-free meats, top-quality wild game, organic grains, beans, nuts, seeds, produce, and health supplies, as well as organizations to call for more information on similar resources.

Icons Used in This Book

Throughout the book, you can find icons that mark the vital information in your healing foods education. Here's a listing of what they mean:

Think of these sections as little menus, consisting of the most nutritious examples of a certain nutrient. I also introduce some more unusual ingredients to encourage you to expand on what you normally eat.

This text uses bigger words and less familiar terms. It gives you a closer look at the chemistry, anatomy, and physiology involved in nutrition. I created these sections to reinforce why a certain food is important to eat, and when I just couldn't resist because I thought the material was so interesting!

Pay attention to these tips and ideas about foods and nutrients. They give you details about what to eat that help you put the nutritional advice on diet into practice.

I use this icon to alert you to foods you need to avoid in certain circumstances or need to handle in a special way, interactions between foods and other substances, and signs to look for that indicate you need to see a physician.

This information consists of general suggestions about cooking and eating that are good to keep mind, useful thoughts that you may soon make your own, forgetting that you ever read it here first.

☺ This little icon in the recipe list at the front of each chapter indicates vegetarian recipes.

Where to Go from Here

You can quickly and easily get started finding out about healing foods, many of which are probably already right in your kitchen! Ever wonder about chilies? If they can bite so in your mouth, how can they be good for you? Turn to Chapter 11 to find out their benefits. When you have the sniffles, turn to Chapter 20 and Appendix A at the back of the book. When you are caring for a child who is under the weather, Chapter 19 is for you. And if you're at a loss for what foods to take with you when you are out and about, take a look at Chapter 22. Or just pick a recipe and spend a few minutes cooking. Tasting nourishing foods and feeling their good effects is the best way to explore the healing power of foods. Turn to any page, walk into your kitchen, put on your apron, and begin.

Be Sure to Read This!

The information in this reference is not intended to substitute for expert medical advice or treatment; it is designed to help you make informed choices. Because each individual is unique, a professional health care provider must diagnose conditions and supervise treatments for each individual medical problem. If an individual is under a doctor's care and receives advice that is contrary to the information provided in this reference, the doctor's advice should be followed, because it is based on the unique characteristics of that individual.

Part I
Staying Healthy with Good Food

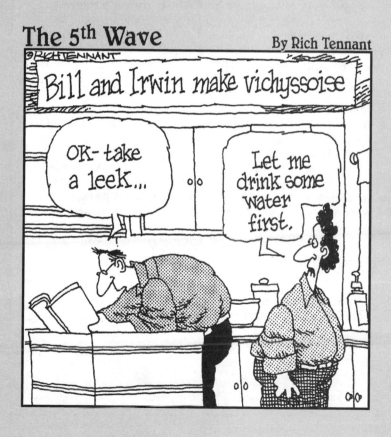

In this part . . .

For the first time in history, people have a very odd relationship with their food — they fear it! If you're like most people, you've been deluged with warnings about this food or that because of the fat, cholesterol, coloring agents, or whatever. You're also probably somewhat aware of what foods are good for you — like broccoli to help prevent cancer. So does that mean you should have it everyday for lunch like a friend of mine does? In this part, you find out about the abundance of healthy foods nature provides and how to keep these in balance.

Eons before the development of modern medicine, cultures around the world evolved various systems of using food, as well as herbs, for healing which worked quite successfully. Two great traditions — Traditional Chinese Medicine and and the Indian system known as Ayurveda, survive today — not to mention the millions of Chinese and Indians who are here because healing foods kept their ancestors alive, and reproducing, despite the presence of disease. In this part, you're introduced to these ancient medicines as well as another approach to diet, eating foods of the season. There's good advice in all these systems of nutrition.

So be my guest. Take a look at Part I. Doing something about your health is just a meal away!

Chapter 1

Food Is Your Friend

● ●

● ●

*N*ourishing foods put a spring in your walk, clear your mind, and balance your emotions. What you eat affects your every waking and sleeping hour. The foods you have eaten over the past few years determined what the tissues of your body, your organs, and your skeleton are made of today. Minerals in seafood, vegetables, and nuts become the very substance of your bones. The vitamin A in a carrot you eat eventually helps form the retina of your eye, which allows you to read this page. Nutrients in food keep your cells humming. Cells are little factories that use vitamins and minerals to produce energy that sustains the many functions of the body. If deliveries don't arrive, the work of the cells slows down, and so do you.

Benefiting from Nature's Best

The earth naturally produces all sorts of healing foods. Fruits, grains, vegetables, beans, nuts, seeds, as well as meats, fish, and poultry contain nutrients that help ensure good health. These ingredients as they are found in nature are called *whole foods*, because they have all their parts. A whole grain that is unrefined retains its nutritious germ and fiber-rich bran. In contrast, a *refined* grain has had its germ and bran taken away. You only get to eat the starchy part that's left. Refined nut and seed oils are also a far cry from the original, having been subjected to a variety of manufacturing processes that destroy nutrients. And processed foods, such as luncheon meats, are not only no longer whole foods, they also often contain preservatives, coloring agents, and artificial flavors.

Native versus modern diets: Dr. Price's amazing findings

Dr. Weston Price, a remarkable researcher who was a trained dentist, assembled an enormous body of research that provides strong evidence that natural, unprocessed, and unrefined foods maintain good health. Dr. Price noticed, in treating the children of his patients, that they had more tooth decay than their parents and that often their teeth were crooked and crowded due to a deformity of the dental arch. He wondered whether poor nutrition was the cause. While the parents had been raised on old-fashioned, more natural foods, the children were receiving a less nutritious diet of more refined foods.

Throughout the 1930s, Dr. Price, aware that the dental health of primitive peoples was usually excellent, set out to visit such cultures to find a nutritional cause of the decline in dental health that he was observing. He traveled the world from northern Scotland to the South Pacific, recording in remarkable photographs the dental health of many native peoples. In some of these cultures, modern foods had already been introduced.

Dr Price's pictures show a dramatic alteration in dental health with the change in diet. Those men and women still eating their native and local foods had movie-star-gorgeous smiles. Tooth decay was extremely rare and even nonexistent among some people. In contrast, those consuming sugar, white flour, canned goods, and refined vegetable oils had diseased, crowded, and missing teeth, and smiles fit for Halloween pumpkins. In addition, those eating refined foods had started to develop many modern degenerative diseases, while among those eating native foods, arthritis, tuberculosis, and cancer were virtually unknown. Such freedom from disease is still a possibility today — by returning to simpler foods.

Another great advantage of eating whole foods is that you're more likely to consume all the nutrients a food actually contains, and in the right proportions. A refined food will be missing some of these. Yes, some products are fortified with nutrients that have been removed. But some compounds that occur naturally in foods haven't even yet been discovered, so there is no way a product will be enriched with these! Far better to go with the original food and benefit from nature's complete package.

Using Native Foods

Traditional cuisines as diverse as Italian, French, Middle Eastern, African, Indian, Asian, and old-fashioned American cooking are based on preparing meals with real food. Cooking in the Caribbean makes the most of root vegetables, and Mexican cooking includes many ways of preparing squashes and beans. Mediterranean cooking relies on olives, fish, and vegetables. In fact, the classic dishes from these cultures are excellent examples of whole foods cooking.

You can use these cooking traditions as your guide for healthy eating. Value is placed on fresh ingredients, grown nearby and eaten in season when the nutrient content is at its peak. Foods are combined in ways that help their digestion and absorption. Cooking juices, rich in vitamins and minerals, are made into sauces and soups. Spices and herbs, all with medicinal properties, are common ingredients. And in this way of cooking, such nonfoods that undermine health as sugar, caffeine, and hydrogenated oils (all covered in the upcoming chapters) are notably lacking. When you base your cooking on traditional cuisines, you benefit from the collective wisdom of countless cooks.

In the following chapters, I include several recipes that stem from native cooking:

- ✔ **From India:** Golden Curried Sweet Potatoes (Chapter 2)
- ✔ **From Greece:** Braised Lamb Shanks with Lentils (Chapter 5)
- ✔ **From Morocco:** North African Roast Chicken with Almonds and Dried Fruits (Chapter 11)
- ✔ **From Istanbul:** Turkish Buckwheat Salad (Chapter 17)
- ✔ **From Cuba:** Banana from Havana (Chapter 20)
- ✔ **From America:** Three-Berry Shortcake (Chapter 25)

Taking a Look at the Modern Western Diet

Despite the debilitating effects of refined and processed foods, the American diet is comprised of large amounts of these. The U.S. Department of Agriculture keeps track of how much Americans eat of various kinds of food. Although the way that the figures are gathered tends to overestimate quantity somewhat, the numbers do give a good indication of the type of food intake year to year. Some of the more processed and refined foods that we ate in 1997 included the following:

- ✔ Sugars and other sweeteners climbed to 155 pounds per person for the year.
- ✔ Consumption of soda rose to about 53 gallons per person, while milk intake declined and fruit juice inched up to about 9 gallons per year. Each person drank over 23 gallons of coffee.
- ✔ Americans ate an average of nearly 60 pounds of frozen potatoes, which usually end up as french fries, which is double the amount recorded in 1970.
- ✔ Fat consumption was 66 pounds per person.
- ✔ The average American ate 28 pounds of cheese and 16 gallons of regular ice cream.

Such eating habits translate into the trend seen today in children of increasing obesity and even heart disease. Children are also developing type 2 adult-onset diabetes, rarely seen in this age group until now. Individuals in their thirties are coming to physicians fatigued in early burn-out with medical problems such as aching joints and digestive problems once more typical of middle age. And degenerative diseases, such as heart disease and osteoporosis, are widespread as compared with the turn of the century when food was less processed and fast food had not yet been invented.

Knowing What Wellness Looks Like

You almost certainly know what disease looks like. But how often do you hear wellness described? This wonderful state of being ideally should include

- Having abundant energy throughout the day
- Waking up in the morning feeling clear-headed and refreshed
- Feeling focused with your feet on the ground
- Having a good memory
- Finding it easy to be cheerful and even optimistic
- Taking stress in stride
- Enjoying freedom from aches and pains
- Avoiding the flu of the season
- Enjoying freedom from degenerative diseases in old age

Take a moment and consider how you envision being healthy and exactly how you'd feel if you were in excellent health. Would you stand up taller and smile more? Would you have more spare time for enjoying life? Whatever images come to mind, why not aim for these? The following chapters can help you reach your goal.

Slow food

Finally, fast food opponents have a voice. Slow food is now on the map. The International Slow Food Movement for the Defence of the Right to Pleasures, founded by Dr. Carlo Petrini and others, was launched Dec. 9, 1989, at the Opera Comique in Paris. The organization is now some 60,000 members strong. Slow Food is dedicated to safeguarding the world's traditional cuisines and cooking wisdom, as well as small-scale agriculture and food production. Bravo! Home-cooking and traditional ways of preparing food are being given the respect they deserve.

Chapter 2

Healing Traditions: Time-Honored Systems of Nutrition

*T*heories abound about what to eat to stay healthy. Of course, some nutrition advice is more valid than others. I remember reading about the martini diet for arthritis, and a girlfriend of mine went on a weight-loss diet that consisted of nothing but wine and apples. She stayed on it for about two days, lost a few pounds, and then gained the weight back.

However, various dietary systems and advice are based on considerable research and have a long history of use. One good general guideline is to eat a variety of foods. Another directive for healthy eating is to consume the foods of the current season, changing your diet throughout the year. Ancient systems of medicine that are practiced in China and India also have fully developed systems of nutrition. Each approach to nutrition has its strengths, and though from diverse origins, they share some common truths. Being aware of these can help you select the healing foods that are best for you.

Eating a Variety of Foods

If you're not careful, you can eat potatoes three times a day — as hash browns for breakfast, as fries for lunch, and as a baked potato for dinner. Typical American meals may look varied, but often the different items in a meal are made of the same basic ingredients. For example, wheat shows up in all sorts of dishes.

Eating a wide assortment of foods helps assure that you'll be consuming a variety of nutrients, all of which you need for optimal health. None function independently. You need several different vitamins (A, B, and C) to help you manage stress. Many minerals (calcium, magnesium, and so on) are required to build bones. And you need both vitamins and minerals (B vitamins and magnesium) to convert food into energy.

Eating Foods of the Season

Another approach to healthy eating is to choose foods that are currently in season and grow in the general area where you live. This way of eating was the norm for most of history, before the days of long-distance transportation and refrigeration. Cooks prepared meals using ingredients that were by necessity of the season and region.

Choose local produce

Produce grown locally is usually fresher and is likely to be higher in nutrients. In addition, local produce need not be treated with preservatives to keep it from spoiling during transport or storage. Fruits and vegetables grown close to home are also automatically of the season.

You probably already have some favorite dishes that you turn to as you feel the seasons change. Summer temperatures inspire salads. A chill in the air calls for soup. Here is a recipe to keep on hand for when the time is right.

Support your local farmers market!

If you've never visited a farmers market, you're in for a treat! Expect to find an abundance of colorful produce that is in season, as well as unusual varieties of usual fruits and vegetables, homebaked breads, really fresh nuts, perhaps some local cheese, free-range chickens, and fresh-caught fish. (I once bought a gorgeous rainbow trout, just pulled from a stream the day before, at the farmers market in the heart of New York City.)

Prices are sometimes a little higher than in grocery stores, but because the food is very fresh and usually of excellent quality, you'll probably be eating all of it and not throwing any away. You're also likely to find organic produce.

Look in your neighborhood paper for the days of your local farmers market, which takes place usually only once or twice a week, or call your local Chamber of Commerce.

Wintry Squash Soup

Winter is the time to savor golden squash — butternut, acorn, and calabazas, which you can find in Latin food markets. These vegetables are orange because they're high in beta-carotene, the antioxidant nutrient that also lowers cancer risk. Compared with other legumes, chickpeas are especially high in zinc, an immune booster that helps ward off winter colds.

Preparation time: *30 minutes*

Cooking time: *2 hours, 45 minutes*

Yield: *6 servings*

1 cup dry chickpeas, or 2 15-ounce cans, rinsed and drained

2 quarts filtered water

1 pound butternut squash, ends trimmed, halved lengthwise

2 tablespoons extra-virgin olive oil

1 large Spanish onion, finely diced

4 cups organic chicken broth or vegetable broth

2 tablespoons tomato paste

Salt and freshly ground black pepper to taste

Pinch of cayenne

1 Soak the chickpeas overnight. Bring the filtered water to boil in a large saucepan. Add the chickpeas, lower heat to medium, and cook, covered, until beans are soft, 1½ to 2 hours — the beans should be tender with the skin still intact. Drain and set aside.

2 Preheat oven to 375°. Place the squash, cut-side down, on a baking sheet and bake until tender, about 45 minutes. Let cool slightly. Using a spoon, scrape out and discard the seeds and fiber. Scrape the pulp from the skin. Set aside.

3 While the squash is baking, heat the oil in a large saucepan over medium-high heat. Sauté the onion, stirring occasionally, until translucent, 5 to 7 minutes. Let onion cool.

4 In a food processor, puree in batches the squash, onion, broth, and half the chickpeas. Return puree to saucepan with the remaining whole chickpeas. Stir in the tomato paste, salt and pepper, and cayenne. If necessary, add up to another ½ cup of broth to thin to desired consistency. Bring to a simmer.

5 Warm soup on medium-low heat for 10 minutes to blend flavors and pour into mugs for a hearty start to a winter's meal.

In sync with the seasons

Did you know that your physical needs for certain foods change with the seasons? Consider this: When you're skiing and feeling chilled on the slopes, you probably don't hunger for seviche, the raw seafood salad served everywhere in Mexico. Conversely, when you're sweltering on a sandy beach in the Caribbean, you don't want buckwheat kasha with mushroom gravy for lunch.

You crave certain foods at different times for specific reasons. Happily, nature provides these foods as the seasons change.

- ✔ **Spring foods:** Spring is a time for cleansing and renewing the body, just as the plant world itself is being reborn, with fledgling leaves on the trees and new crops in the fields. Young lettuce, asparagus, and spring peas abound — green foods rich in chlorophyll, a nutrient that cleanses the body. Other fruit, such as apples, oranges, and grapefruit, can also help purify the system. During this season, the diet is shifting from one high in protein and fat to a less heavy diet in which vegetables, fruit, grains, and legumes predominate.

- ✔ **Summer foods:** In this season of higher temperatures, the body requires more fluids and a lighter diet. Nature responds with an abundance of juicy fruits and vegetables, such as melons, peaches, tomatoes, and cooling cucumbers. In summer, raw foods taste good. Lunch can be a bowl of cold gazpacho soup. Chicken salad for dinner seems right.

- ✔ **Autumn foods:** As the harvest begins, people enjoy the last of summer produce, and then the menu shifts to squashes and root vegetables, which are less watery than summer foods and have more substance. To be edible, these foods need to be cooked. Again, there is harmony because as the air cools and days shorten, cooked foods are more appealing. At this time, nuts, seeds, grains, and legumes are harvested, adding protein and fats to meals.

- ✔ **Winter foods:** When temperatures drop, it is a time for resting and recouping energy. The body needs substantial fuel. The focus is on whole grains, squashes, and root vegetables, such as potatoes and beets — all sources of complex carbohydrates. These foods store well while the earth is dormant. You may also feel inclined to include more meat, dairy, poultry, and mineral-rich fish in your meals at this time.

For further reading about eating foods of the season, take a look at the classic *Staying Healthy with the Seasons,* by Elson M. Haas, M.D. (Celestial Arts, Berkeley, California, 1981).

Healing Foods in Traditional Chinese Medicine

Traditional Chinese Medicine (TCM) is the world's oldest, continuously practiced professional medicine. More than 30,000 volumes documenting the practice of TCM predate 1900. Traditional Chinese Medicine is not simply a folk medicine.

TCM makes use of a wide assortment of foods, as well as numerous herbs and acupuncture, to prevent and treat disease. To get an idea of how this special Chinese form of nutritional therapy works, it's helpful to know something about its basic concepts:

- ✔ **The body, with its various systems and organs, is more like a landscape than a machine, which is the image in Western medicine of how the body works.** In TCM, the flow of fluids and energy in the body are spoken of as seas, reservoirs, rivers, and channels. Images are from nature. A coated tongue might be described as covered with moss.

- ✔ **In diagnosing a patient's condition, a TCM physician assesses patterns — that is, the relationship between symptoms.** Relationship is the ultimate truth, not the cause, such as a specific bacteria or virus.

- ✔ **Each patient is a unique individual, with a unique pattern of disharmony.** Patients with the same disease may require different treatments.

- ✔ **Factors that cause disease are wind, heat, cold, dryness, and dampness.** These are the five climates that occur internally. Conditions of health and disease are described in terms of weather.

- ✔ **The purpose of nutritional therapy is to maintain good health by nourishing the blood, vital fluids, and *chi*, or life force.** Diet therapy is also used to treat chronic and acute conditions.

The use of food as medicine in TCM can be traced back as far as 3000 BC. In China and Taiwan, using food as medicine is so integrated into the culture that certain restaurants specialize in serving dishes for medicinal purposes. Cooking ingredients and medicinal herbs are carefully chosen according to classic, healing recipes. Foods used medicinally include garlic, barley, wheat, black and red dates, adzuki beans (small, dried, russet-colored beans with a sweet taste) and seaweeds, such as kombu (a popular Japanese seaweed, which is dried and sold in grayish black sheets). (Chapter 6 tells you more about seaweed.) Customers describe their ailments and are prescribed a menu. Some bring their own herbs, which the cook works into the dishes being prepared. Herbs are usually brewed as teas or added to soups.

Even if you know just a little about the Chinese way of healing with food, you can apply some of this ancient wisdom in your cooking. You just need to become familiar with the following two concepts: the notion of yin/yang and the five-phase theory. (I love seeing foods with new eyes. If I am sick, I sometimes reach for my yin/yang and five-phase charts to figure out what to eat.)

Comparing yin and yang

In Chinese philosophy, *yin* and *yang* are two opposing yet complementary principles. Yin is that which is negative and dark; yang is that which is positive and bright. Yin is also said to be female and yang male, which sounds like a gender bias, but actually has deeper roots. The harmony of the universe depends upon the interaction of these two eternal principles. Disease occurs when there is an imbalance between them. Table 2-1 shows you the different qualities categorized in terms of these two principles.

Table 2-1	Complementary Principles of Yin and Yang
Yin Qualities	*Yang Qualities*
cold	hot
watery	dry
heavy	light
interior	exterior
hidden	revealed
descending	ascending
substantive	active
contracting	expanding

To keep from forever mixing up which is yin and which is yang, which I used to do, I thought up these word associations: Yin goes in, and expanding yang goes bang!

Every food group has a predominant yin or yang quality, as does each individual food. Furthermore, among the many yin foods are those that are less yin and consequently are more yang, and vice versa. For example, fish and meat are categorized as yin, but meat is more yin. Fruit and fruit juice are both yang, but fruit juice is more yang. It's all relative. Some of the differences are subtle, but some are not. Salty foods are at the far end of the yin spectrum, and sugary foods and alcohol are at the far end of the yang spectrum.

You may never master the subtleties of yin/yang theory, but being aware of what kind of foods are especially yin or yang is useful in composing a healthy diet. Knowing about yin and yang foods can help you avoid extremes. Following is how Chinese medicine categorizes foods:

- ✔ Yin foods include eggs, meat, poultry, fish, and vegetables that grow downward, such as carrots and turnips. The yin flavors are bitter, salty, and sour.

- ✔ Yang foods are fruits, vegetables that grow upward and outward, sugar, coffee, and alcohol. Yang flavors are spicy and sweet.

- ✔ Grains and beans are relatively neutral foods.

How a food is cooked can make it more yin or more yang.

Most yin   *Most yang*

Raw   Steaming   Sautéing   Baking   Frying   Broiling

Raw foods are very yin because they promote the loss of body fluids and heat, but not because they are eaten chilled. Yang foods are warming because they stimulate circulation and generate body heat. Foods prepared with a lot of fat are also more yang. The American diet is full of yang foods such as fried chicken, chili, sugary breakfast cereal, jelly donuts, and coffee. No wonder we like to salt our food! Salting makes it more yin. (Another theory of why we like so much salt on our food is that, as a population, we are so deficient in trace minerals, salt is exceptionally satisfying.)

Yin and yang also are expressed in certain physical characteristics and behavior (see Table 2-2). Which best describes you? Or are you in perfect balance?

Table 2-2	Yin and Yang Characteristics
Yin Characteristics	*Yang Characteristics*
Speak in a soft, weak voice	Speak loudly and project your voice
Have a low level of energy	Have high energy
Tend to be lethargic	Are hyperactive
Often feel cold	Usually feel warm
Hypotensive	Hypertensive
Have a pale complexion	Have a flushed, ruddy complexion

Like cures like

Various treatments in Chinese medicine are based on the principle that like cures like. For example, leafy green vegetables, such as kale and collard greens, are considered good for the lungs because the lacy structure of the leaves of these vegetables resembles the lung's intricate system of arteries and vessels.

If you suspect that you are overly yin, you need the stimulating effects of warming spices, vegetable soups and stews, and grilled foods. Tex-Mex cooking and curries are in order, as is sautéed garlic shrimp washed down with a fruit juice sangria or a tall glass of beer. Living on raw vegetable salads is not for you, even if someone devoted to raw foods tells you so.

On the other hand, if you decide that you are overly yang, treat yourself to a cup of soothing and naturally salty miso soup to restore your energy balance. Miso soup is easy to make and even easier to order in a Japanese restaurant, where most of the mineral-rich foods served tend to be yin. You might also enjoy a Greek salad made with feta cheese, another salty and delicious yin food.

The five-phase theory

The *five-phase theory* is a bit more complicated than yin/yang, but it does have an inherent logic. Like TCM anatomy, it refers to natural elements and makes sense in terms of how the natural world works. The five phases are wood, fire, earth, metal, and water. Their relationship is usually diagrammed as a circle.

The circle of the five phases is not a static chart, but a representation of the dynamic relationship among the five elements. Each phase of this unending cycle is said to nourish and promote the activities of the next phase. For example, wood nourishes fire by fueling it. Water nourishes wood because trees need water to survive. Conversely, each phase controls or checks the phase located opposite to it in the circle. Water controls fire by putting it out. Metal checks wood by cutting through it.

Besides the specific element each phase is associated with, these phases can also be described in terms of color, taste, the season, emotions, and actions (see Table 2-3).

Ways of preparing food that increase chi

The energy that you personally put into your cooking transfers to the food. Stirring, tossing, whipping, fluffing, and beating *by hand* are all actions that increase chi. So, too, are chopping and slicing — even the type of cut matters. The roll cut (see figure) especially boosts chi. (Start with a carrot, slice off a piece on the diagonal, roll the carrot a quarter turn, and slice again on the diagonal. This gives you a complex little geometric shape with many surfaces that can absorb cooking heat and flavors.) To rev up the chi in food that's been frozen, stir in a fresh ingredient as you cook it, such as freshly chopped parsley.

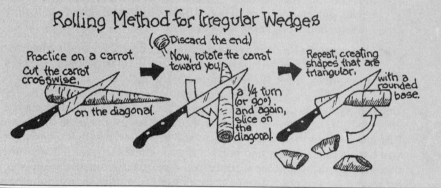

Rolling Method for Irregular Wedges

Practice on a carrot. Cut the carrot crosswise, on the diagonal.

(Discard the end) Now, rotate the carrot toward you, a 1/4 turn (or 90°) and again, slice on the diagonal.

Repeat, creating shapes that are triangular, with a rounded base.

Table 2-3		The Five Phases and How They Show Up			
Phase	**Color**	**Taste**	**Season**	**Emotion**	**Action**
Wood	Blue, green	Sour	Spring	Anger	Planning, making decisions
Fire	Red	Bitter	Summer	Joy	Initiating action
Earth	Yellow, orange	Sweet	Indian summer	Pensiveness	Imagining
Metal	White	Pungent	Autumn	Grief	Keeping rhythmic order
Water	Black	Salty	Winter	Fear	Preserving by willpower

In addition to the categories in Table 2-3, all foods and beverages are associated with one of the five phases. Read through these lists and try to sense the particular element that they embody. (Some are more obvious than others!)

- ✔ **Wood foods:** Barley, lima beans, lettuce, broccoli, lemon, alfalfa seeds, saffron, cashews, sour cream, soft-shell crabs, chicken, beef liver, and vinegar

- ✔ **Fire foods:** Popcorn, red lentils, asparagus, tomato, apricot, persimmon, strawberry, sesame and sunflower seeds, pistachios, shrimp, lamb, beer, wine, coffee, and chocolate (wouldn't you know?)

- ✔ **Earth foods:** Millet, yam, chickpeas, butternut squash, artichoke, apples, bananas, pumpkin seeds, vanilla, almonds, milk, yogurt, salmon, tuna, quail, rabbit, honey, and maple syrup

- ✔ **Metal foods:** Rice, Great Northern and soybeans, cabbage, cucumber, garlic, ginger, onion, radish, pear, peach, dill, horseradish, walnuts, cheese, flounder, turkey, and beef

- ✔ **Water foods:** Buckwheat, kidney beans, beets, seaweed, mushrooms, blackberries and blueberries, chestnuts, caviar, octopus, oysters, sardines, duck, pork, pickles, and salt

Yes, this system is complex, and I haven't even told you about how the different principles are applied to treat specific diseases. But even if you know only this much about the theory, you can still experiment with it. For example, if you have a dinner party and you want your guests to have a lively time, feed them fire foods, which are stimulating — spicy popcorn and sunflower seeds for munchies and chocolate cake for dessert — rather than a quieting slice of pumpkin pie, an earth food.

In turn, you can use an earth food to comfort yourself if you're feeling sad or grieving, which are water emotions. Remember, earth dams water. Munch on a baked yam. Or to treat digestive problems, a disharmony in the earth realm, give yourself earth foods, such as the squash and chickpea soup in this chapter, as well as fire foods, like lamb and apricots, which nourish earth.

To find out more about Chinese medicine and nutrition, take a look at *Between Heaven and Earth,* a guide to Chinese medicine by Harriet Beinfield, L.Ac., and Efrem Korngold, L.Ac. OMD, Ballantine Books, 1992.

The Ancient Wisdom of Ayurveda

Ayurveda, a Sanskrit word meaning "science of life," is a system of medicine native to India and preserved by Hindus. This early science was first recorded in the Vedas, the world's oldest body of literature. Ayurveda has been practiced in daily life for more than 5,000 years. In this section, you find out how this ancient wisdom might apply to you and read about the types of foods you need for health, according to Ayurvedic theories of nutrition.

Healing food, Indian-style

Healthy food, according to Ayurveda, is that which is

✔ Grown close to home

✔ Fresh, because the longer it is uprooted, the less energy it has

✔ The least processed, refined, and otherwise transformed so that it carries with it more of its memories of the cosmos

✔ Cooked with love

As in Traditional Chinese Medicine, earlier in this chapter, in Ayurveda, health is about balance of body, mind, and consciousness. According to the Ayurvedic system, this is achieved when there is a balance of the *doshas* — a Sanskrit word referring to the basic principles thought to govern all the biological and psychological functions, as well as disease.

There are three doshas — *vata, pitta,* and *kapha* — and each has unique characteristics. (These are the basic Sanskrit buzzwords you need to know if you plan to tell your friends about Ayurveda.)

✔ **Vata** partakes of the qualities of air and ether or space. It is a principle of movement and involves the subtle energy within the body that governs physical change. Vata involves small movements, such as breathing, blinking of the eyelids, and the beating of the heart. Vata governs nervousness, anxiety, and muscle spasms.

✔ **Pitta** partakes of fire and water. It refers to the heat energy of the body and involves metabolism and the absorption of food and nutrients, body temperature, the luster of the eyes, and intelligence, understanding, and anger.

✔ **Kapha** has the qualities of earth and water. Kapha governs the physical structure of the body, provides vigor and strength, and supports immunity. Memory, emotional attachment, forgiveness, and love are also governed by kapha.

Each person embodies a different combination of these *doshas,* which is the same as the Western concept of one's constitution. The mix is determined both genetically and by the changing environment. When diagnosing a patient, an Ayurvedic doctor first assesses which of the doshas dominate and which are deficient. Then various treatments may be prescribed, including cleansing, emotional release, herbs, and a change in diet. As in Chinese medicine, no one cure fits all. Each treatment is custom-designed.

Certain physical characteristics and behaviors are typical of each dosha. Table 2-4 shows you just a few examples, which can cover a wide range of topics. See whether you can figure out your basic dosha type.

Table 2-4	Characteristics and Behaviors of Each Dosha		
	Vata	*Pitta*	*Kapha*
Frame	Thin	Moderate	Thick
Weight	Low	Moderate	Heavy
Appetite	Variable, scant	Good, excessive	Slow but steady
Taste	Sweet, sour, salty	Sweet, bitter, astringent	Pungent, bitter, astringent
Thirst	Varying	Excessive	Scant
Physical activity	Very active	Moderate	Lethargic
Speech	Fast cutting, sharp	Monotonous	Slow
Economic status	Poor, buys trifles	Moderate, buys luxuries	Rich, saves, buys food

In addition, each dosha is associated with the risk of certain diseases. Individuals with vata constitutions are prone to gas, lower back pain, sciatica, arthritis, *neuralgia* (a painful condition caused by pressure on nerves and other factors), and paralysis. Pitta types can develop skin disorders, bile and liver disorders, gallbladder disease, peptic ulcers, and inflammatory diseases, such as gastritis. Someone who is kapha may come down with sinusitis, tonsillitis, bronchitis, lung congestion, or stomach disorders.

Ayurveda categorizes foods according to their capability to aggravate or balance a dosha. For example, if you think you are overly kapha, you don't want to eat an abundance of kapha-aggravating foods. You want to eat foods that balance kapha. The following gives various lists of foods you can refer to when you want to boost or dampen a particular dosha.

- ✔ **Vata-aggravating foods:** Raw vegetables, tomatoes, white potatoes, broccoli, peas, dried fruit, watermelon, apples, barley, corn, rye, lamb, pork, most beans, and ice cream

- ✔ **Vata-balancing foods:** Cooked vegetables, carrots, asparagus, sweet potatoes and yams, sweet fruits, banana, mango, rice, wheat, beef, poultry, seafood, lentils, nuts, seeds, spices, and oils

- ✔ **Pitta-aggravating foods:** Pungent vegetables, garlic, onions, radishes, hot peppers, beets, sour fruits, cranberries, grapefruit, buckwheat, brown rice, beef, pork, lamb, seafood, lentils, most nuts and seeds, some spices, and cheese

✔ **Pitta-balancing foods:** Sweet fruits, grapes, oranges, pears, sweet and bitter vegetables, cabbage, leafy greens, mushrooms, oats, white rice, wheat, white meat chicken and turkey, venison, beans, unsalted butter, and olive oil

✔ **Kapha-aggravating foods:** Sweet and sour fruits, pineapple, lemons, sweet and juicy vegetables, cucumber, zucchini, oats, rice, wheat, beef, lamb, pork, seafood, all nuts, most sweeteners, dairy, oils, and salt

✔ **Kapha-balancing foods:** Apples, berries, pears, dried figs, raisins, pungent and bitter vegetables, eggplant, lettuce, white potatoes, barley, corn, rye, dark meat chicken and turkey, shrimp, most legumes, raw honey, and all spices

Using these different groupings of food, you can invent recipes that suit your nature. That's what I did when I made up this dish.

Golden Curried Sweet Potatoes

For someone with an airy, vata nature such as myself, this dish is the ultimate comfort food. The sweet yams and yogurt contribute earthy kapha energy, which is grounding, while the many spices add the fiery qualities of pitta. On a day when you are feeling spaced-out, this dish may be just what you need.

Preparation time: 10 minutes

Cooking time: 15 minutes

Yield: 6 servings

3 tablespoons organic, unsalted butter

2 medium onions, diced

1-inch length fresh ginger root, minced

1 clove garlic, minced

3 tablespoons organic, unsalted butter

2 green cardamom seeds

2 teaspoons ground cumin

1 teaspoon ground coriander

1 teaspoon ground turmeric

1 teaspoon ground cinnamon

1 teaspoon chili powder

3 medium sweet potatoes (about 1 pound), peeled, halved lengthwise, and cut into ¼-inch thick slices

1¼ cups filtered water

½ cup plain yogurt

1 Heat the butter in a large sauté pan. Add the onion and cook over low heat until the onion begins to color, about 10 minutes. Add the ginger and garlic and cook another 2 to 3 minutes, stirring often.

(continued)

2 Add all the spices, stir, and continue to cook the mixture for a few seconds.

3 Add the sweet potatoes and water. Cook, covered, until tender, about 15 minutes. Remove from heat. Using a slotted spoon, transfer the cooked sweet potatoes to a bowl. Leave the sauce in the pan, allowing it to cool slightly.

4 Add the yogurt to the sauce and combine. Pour over the sweet potatoes and gently stir to combine. Season with salt and serve.

Note: Curry powder has its uses, but not in this dish. The mix of individual spices listed produces a unique depth of flavor.

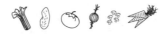

The Ayurvedic system of nutrition has many more layers and correlations. To find out more, an excellent book to start with is Dr. Vasant D. Lad's *Ayurveda, The Science of Self-Healing*, Lotus Light Publications, 1984.

Part II

Setting Up Your Healing Foods Kitchen

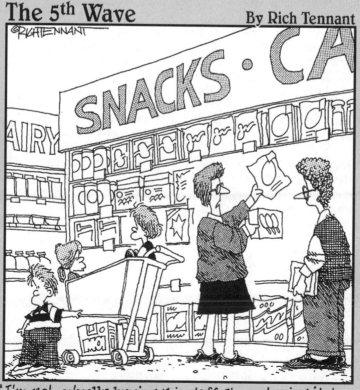

The 5th Wave · By Rich Tennant

"I'm not actually buying this stuff, I'm just using it to hide the fruit, legumes, and greens until we get checked out."

In this part . . .

As you give up processed and preserved foods for healthier versions, you'll need to change your kitchen some to suit the fresh and more fragile ingredients you'll be buying. Time to throw out some items and do a little reorganizing of your shelves. You may also need some new appliances to help you cook in healthier ways. And while you're at it, why not make sure that all the products you use to clean your kitchen are also as healthy and nontoxic as possible? This part guides you through these changes.

I also give you general guidelines for shopping so that you can begin filling your kitchen with healing foods. I stroll with you down market aisles and point out good brands to buy. I put on my glasses and read to you from labels and start putting organic foods into your shopping cart. The result of all these changes can be a kitchen that really suits you, a place where you can work efficiently, which is in itself health-promoting because it reduces stress.

As you start to refine the details of your kitchen, it can become a very special place, even if it has old appliances and a funny linoleum floor. If you are so inclined, you can even connect with something sacred about this place where you prepare food. The Greeks felt that the hearth was important enough that they even designated a goddess, Hestia, to preside over its sacred fire. Invite the goddess into your hearth space.

Now roll your sleeves up and get ready to transform your kitchen into a smooth-running and healing place.

Chapter 3

The Conscious Kitchen

*H*ow you cook your food and the setting in which you do this can affect your health. Your kitchen can be a place of healing if it is well-appointed and arranged to your liking, bringing you a sense of peace and reducing daily stress. You can also choose cookware, cleaning products, and cooking methods with your health in mind. This chapter begins by taking a look at the healthiest ways of cooking certain foods.

Cooking in Healthy Ways

You can turn healing foods into less-than-healthy dishes just by the way you cook them. It pays to understand how different cooking techniques affect the nutritional value of various foods.

✔ **Steaming** is great for vegetables. The vegetables sit on a steaming rack set into a pot, and vitamins and minerals are better preserved than if the vegetables were cooked in water. The standard method for cooking grains, in a pot with a little liquid, is also a form of steaming. The grain absorbs the cooking liquid, and no nutrients are lost from either.

✔ **Boiling** vegetables results in nutrients escaping into the cooking liquid. Add this cooking liquid to soup, and you can still benefit from these nutrients. However, tough leafy greens such as collards can stand up to being cooked in liquid. These vegetables are so high in nutrients that they still retain a lot. Boiling also works for beans because you can discard the cooking water, which contains gaseous compounds.

✔ **Poaching** foods such as fish, poultry, vegetables, and fruit in a small amount of liquid collects nutrients into the relatively small amount of liquid used and also keeps the food moist. You can reduce this liquid to make a nutrient-rich sauce.

✔ **Stewing** foods such as meats and poultry over a period of time breaks down these foods so that you can easily digest their protein and absorb the nutrients. And all the juices become the broth.

✔ **Sautéing** at low temperatures in a small amount of butter or oil is a gentle way to cook chops, chicken parts, and seafood. You can easily control temperatures and prevent the meat from charring and forming toxic compounds.

✔ **Stir-frying,** which uses only a small amount of fat, is a method of quick cooking that preserves nutrients. Use it for preparing meats, poultry, seafood, and vegetables.

✔ **Baking** requires no fat, and nutrients are retained. Nutritious juices that do escape can be turned into gravy. Baking is a good way to cook such foods as meats, poultry, and root vegetables like carrots and beets.

✔ **Grilling** adds intense flavor to slimming foods such as vegetables, fish, and chicken breasts without requiring the addition of fat. But grilling is a mixed blessing. Cooking fatty foods over charcoal or wood chips can generate carcinogenic compounds that can end up in your food (see the sidebar "How risky is grilling?".

Practicing healthy cooking

Follow these healthy cooking tips when you prepare dinner:

✔ **To clean vegetables and ready them for cooking, first wash them and then cut them into pieces** — not the other way around, which allows nutrients to be washed away.

✔ **If you're boiling potatoes, boil them in their skins, which holds in the nutrients.** Then peel the potatoes and slice or mash away!

✔ **Cook green vegetables for a minimum amount of time.** Cooking green vegetables until they are a drab gray-green is a sign that they've lost magnesium.

✔ **Grill lowfat foods such as fish and chicken without the skin.** Use grills with drip pans and set the grill as many inches as possible away from coals. Cook over woods that produce less smoke, such as hickory, oak, and maple, rather than pine or fashionable mesquite.

✔ **To use a minimum of amount of fat in cooking, use a preseasoned pan.**
To preseason a sauté pan, first scour the pan with salt. Next, coat the
pan with a light film of oil, and then, using an absorbent towel, rub the
pan to remove excess oil and cover bare spots.

✔ **Certain ways of cooking with fat can ruin a perfectly acceptable food.**
Pan-frying and deep-frying, in which cooking oils are heated to very high
temperatures, have no place in healing foods cooking. At high temperatures, compounds in fat begin to break down into toxic substances. (You
can read more about fats and oils in Chapter 10.) A good alternative is to
sauté at lower temperatures in a small amount of unrefined oil or butter.

Once you decide on what you want to cook, you next need to choose a cooking technique that suits the particular food and keeps it nutritious. The
following two recipes make use of cooking techniques that are sensitive to
the type of foods being prepared and also respect the cooking requirements
of the fats in these dishes, keeping them intact and safe to eat.

Poached Salmon and Cucumbers

Cold-poached salmon is commonly garnished with slices of raw cucumber. (Sometimes
the fish is fancied up with rows of these meant to resemble fish scales.) For a change, in
this dish the cucumbers are poached with dill and served hot. Salmon is an abundant
source of fragile essential fatty acids, which are protected in this low-heat method of
cooking. The cucumbers are slimming — a cup of cucumber has only 14 calories but
supplies lots to chew on. The sorrel, an herb that has a pleasant sour taste, or lemon
adds a nice tartness that balances the sweet cucumber.

Preparation time: 10 minutes

Cooking time: 20 minutes

Yield: 4 servings

1 cucumber, peeled and sliced into ¼-inch rounds

1 stem fresh dill, finely chopped, or ½ teaspoon dried dill

1 cup apple juice

1 tablespoon apple cider vinegar

4 salmon filets, 6 ounces each

Sea salt and freshly ground black pepper to taste

Filtered water

1 cup sorrel, or juice of half a lemon

1 In a small saucepan, put the cucumber, dill, apple juice, and vinegar. Over medium heat,
cook the cucumber, covered, until tender, about 10 minutes. Set aside and keep warm.

(continued)

2 Select a shallow saucepan wide enough to hold the salmon filets in 1 layer. Season the filets with salt and pepper and put them in the saucepan. Cover them with filtered water and top with sorrel leaves or add lemon juice and a pinch of pepper. Bring to a boil, lower the heat to a simmer, and poach for about 7 to 8 minutes, or until cooked.

3 Using a slotted spatula, carefully transfer the poached salmon, along with the wilted leaves of sorrel as a garnish, to individual warmed serving plates. Serve with the cucumbers alongside or as a band over the top of the filets.

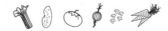

Green Beans with Sautéed Shallots

In healthy cooking, different fats require different cooking methods. Butter that is stable at high temperatures and doesn't break down into toxic compounds is fine for sautéing, while delicate flaxseed oil shouldn't go near direct heat. Drizzle this oil on hot foods already dished up so that it's warmed only by borrowed heat.

Preparation time: *10 minutes*

Cooking time: *12 minutes*

Yield: *4 servings*

1 teaspoon organic, unsalted butter

2 shallots, finely chopped

¾ pound green beans, ends trimmed

2 tablespoons flaxseed oil

Juice of half a lemon

Sea salt and freshly ground black pepper to taste

1 In a small sauté pan, melt the butter over medium heat and add the shallots. Cook, stirring continuously, until slightly brown, about 2 minutes. Set aside.

2 In a medium saucepan fitted with a steamer, place the green beans. Cook, covered, until beans are tender, about 8 to 10 minutes. (If the beans are overcooked, their emerald color will be lost.)

3 Transfer the cooked green beans to a heated serving bowl. Drizzle with flaxseed oil. Add the reserved shallots and sprinkle with lemon juice. Season with sea salt and pepper. Toss to coat green beans evenly with the flavorings. Serve at once.

How risky is grilling?

When you grill, the fat melts, drips down onto the charcoal or wood chips, sizzles as it heats to super-hot temperatures, and then begins to undergo chemical changes that produce a substance called *benzopyrene*. In animal studies, benzopyrene has proven to be carcinogenic. As smoke from the coals rises, the benzopyrene is carried with it and deposits on your chops!

How much of a risk is grilling food? Very slight, say some experts, if you eat grilled foods only occasionally. However, eating barbecued foods regularly coupled with the vast array of chemicals you are exposed to daily may change the odds. If you want to add a charred, smoky flavor to food, a healthier alternative is smoking meat, a process that generates fewer toxins.

Microwaving your food

Many studies have investigated whether microwaving food destroys vitamins and minerals and, for the most part, have found little evidence that any significant loss occurs. However, the effect of microwaving on protein is more controversial. Several studies have investigated the effect of microwaving on both cow milk and human milk, protein-rich foods. (In many intensive care nurseries, breast milk is often frozen and later thawed in a microwave oven.) Researchers have found evidence that changes can occur in protein compounds that play a role in immunity.

A microwave oven is best suited to quick-heating foods at low temperatures, just what is needed to cook vegetables. If you want to cook main dishes and casseroles, it's best to use a conventional oven, which you can rely on to cook food evenly throughout the dish. Besides, the final product tastes so much better.

Microwaving food is so simple to do that it's easy to forget that important guidelines must be followed:

- ✔ **Be sure to use ovenproof containers with glass tops, rather than plastic containers.** Many studies document that toxic chemicals from plastics migrate into food. In addition, don't let plastic film touch food during cooking.

- ✔ **Never microwave in containers like yogurt cups.** The chemicals from the cups can enter the food.

✔ **Never thaw food in the microwave if the food is still in its foam tray packaging.** The packaging will break down and enter the food.

✔ **Never microwave food in a waxed bag.** According to one study, 60 percent of the wax on the bag migrated into the food.

✔ **Don't microwave food in vintage ceramic dinnerware made before 1950.** Dangerously large amounts of lead, a toxic mineral, can leach out and enter the food.

✔ **If you microwave meat, use a thermometer probe to test the internal temperature.** Making sure that the meat is thoroughly cooked helps ensure that any bacteria present is killed. Microwave ovens are generally unable to uniformly heat foods such as a whole chicken.

Choosing Healthy Cookware

The kind of cookware you use to prepare food can make a difference in its nutritional value. Build up a collection of pots and pans that are stainless steel-lined aluminum or copper and include some cast-iron sauté pans, too. (However, avoid all-aluminum cookware to limit your exposure to this mineral, which can interfere with kidney function and possibly the composition of bone.) You also need a fold-up steamer that fits into pots, baking dishes, a juicer, a blender (see Figure 3-1), and possibly a spice mill. A slow cooker (see Figure 3-2) can also be useful. I like using a *tawasha,* a natural fiber brush for scrubbing vegetables, and lots of glass storage jars to hold staples that I buy in bulk.

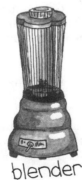

Figure 3-1:
Blender.

blender

When you burn dinner

Whether you char what you're cooking on purpose — for example, if you're preparing trendy "blackened" Cajun-style catfish — or you accidentally overcook what's in the skillet, the health effects are the same. Charring can alter animal proteins, producing carcinogenic compounds called *heterocyclic amines.* Whatever the cooking technique — grilling, frying, or roasting — these compounds can form when meat burns until it's black.

Figure 3-2:
Slow
cooker.

slow cooker

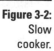
Plastic cutting boards were once thought to be more sanitary than ones made of wood. Now new research shows that wooden ones are far safer. A plastic surface harbors germs, even after it is washed, but a wood cutting board after being washed shows no sign of bacteria even after being left overnight.

Giving Yourself a Healthy Place to Cook

If you really want to make changes in how you prepare food, don't just cook with healthy foods. Make sure that your kitchen is a healing place as well. Working in a kitchen that doesn't suit you can be stressful, and stress is known to weaken the immune system. Fix up your kitchen so that it suits you. Simplify storage. Give yourself good lighting and fresh air. Also, use nontoxic cleaning agents and avoid those that contain chemicals linked to various ailments. Bring a fresh clarity and cleanliness to your work space. Walking into your kitchen should be a pleasure, and an invitation to start cooking!

Your environment is an expression of where you're at. Making your kitchen as comfortable as possible can lessen stress and give you breathing room to cook daily meals. Once your kitchen is comfortable to work in, you may even eat more meals at home, which are probably healthier than the ones you eat out. Whether you happen to be building a new kitchen, remodeling an old one, or just wishing that you could fiddle with the kitchen you're stuck with, here are some pointers to keep in mind.

- ✔ **Decide whether you want an open or closed kitchen.** Do you like to be onstage when you cook, or are you more the inspired-genius type who prefers to work in solitude, putting your masterpiece on view only when it's finished? If you like an audience, plan an open kitchen combined with a sitting and dining area. You can also divide the cooking and eating space with a counter. Friends and family can sit luncheonette-style on stools and talk and eat as you prep. Or for privacy, have a separate kitchen, keep the door closed, and on the door knob, hang a "do not disturb" sign.

- ✔ **Consider your height when you are planning counters.** You want to have a straight back while working so that your chest and lungs can expand and you inhale more oxygen when you breathe. (Taking deep breaths helps reduce stress and generates energy.) Also consider arm reach and stride when you position appliances. Don't let the architect, carpenter, or noncooking members of your family make these decisions for you!

   To have the experience of being in a spacious kitchen, you need to be able to step back from wherever you are working and not bump into any-thing — for example, when you're standing at the sink washing dishes. You may miss the furniture behind you by only a few inches, but that doesn't matter. What you experience is roominess.

- ✔ **Give yourself ample storage space.** Because a healing foods diet emphasizes fresh, unprocessed, and preservativefree ingredients, such as vegetables, unrefined oils, and whole grains, you need ample refriger-ator space for keeping these chilled to extend their shelf life. At the same time, you need less cabinet space for canned and packaged foods. I have an old stand-up freezer in which I keep a few staples, such as my chicken broth and frozen blueberries, plus a large, new refrigerator with the freezer at the bottom. Its drawers for produce and all the shelves are closer to chest height, making fresh food easier to find and reach.

   Clutter is tiring. A good rule for storage of cookware and dinnerware is to keep what you use regularly close at hand, and the gravy boat you use only on Thanksgiving far, far away on an upper shelf. This may sound obvious, but take a look at your own cabinets. Over time, platters, pitch-ers, and odd bowls migrate to just where you don't want them.

- ✔ **Make sure that your kitchen has proper lighting.** I have a dear friend who likes to cook in the dark. Her kitchen is like a night club, moody and lit only with a few down lights. I like plenty of light, both general and task lighting so that I can really see what I'm doing — one less reason to feel stressed while cooking. If you decide that you don't have proper lighting, adding a lamp or two or having first-rate lighting properly installed is a great investment.

Choose your light bulbs with care

The kind of light bulb you use affects how you feel. Full-spectrum lighting, which is close to natural sunlight, is health-enhancing. The rays of natural light, including ultraviolet light in small quantity, stimulate a myriad of body functions. You can find full-spectrum light bulbs in hardware stores and specialty lighting shops or mail-order bulbs from Ott Light Systems, 28 Parker Way, Santa Barbara, CA 93101; 800-234-3724.

Full-spectrum light, which includes ultraviolet light, activates the synthesis of vitamin D, needed for the absorption of calcium. Furthermore, in studies the UV component of sunlight has been shown to reduce blood pressure and cholesterol and to treat symptoms of psoriasis. Being exposed to large amounts of UV light is thought to increase the risk of cancer, but UV light in trace amounts is an essential nutrient.

Most light bulbs give off a predominance of yellow, red, and infrared light. Research has shown that animals do not thrive in this light. Fluorescent bulbs lack the blue-violet portion of the spectrum. Exposed to fluorescent light, you may feel fatigue, and, according to one study, fluorescent light increases levels of stress hormones. Fluorescent light is even banned in some hospitals in Europe.

Cleaning Your Kitchen

A grotty kitchen is a downer, an uninviting room that drains your energy, not to mention that it's not sanitary and may harbor bacteria. Treat yourself to a sparkling-clean kitchen, a space that inspires healthy cooking. Wash the shelves, mop the floor, and get up your courage to look behind the refrigerator.

The cleansers, degreasers, disinfectants, and polishes in your broom closet most likely contain an assortment of potentially harmful chemicals, including benzene, xylene, naphthalene, phenol, and carbon-based compounds (VOCs) that release from cleaning agents as gasses. (By the way, most labels don't list ingredients.) Being exposed to an assortment of these chemicals has been linked to such side effects as headaches, nausea, fatigue, dizziness, and skin irritation, which can show up within hours of exposure. If you're sick, you may be especially vulnerable.

Long-term exposure has been linked to higher risks of respiratory illness, suppression of the immune system, cancer, birth defects, and damage to the nervous system. Symptoms such as hyperactivity and poor learning ability can manifest before more obvious physical illness develops.

One easy way to limit the accumulation of airborne toxic chemicals in your kitchen is to keep it well ventilated. Open the windows. Turn on the fan.

Shopping for greener cleaners

As you make efforts to eat healthier foods, perhaps adding more organic foods to your diet, why not keep going and clean your kitchen with nontoxic cleaning agents? You'll be sure that you're avoiding any possible side effects of toxic chemicals that show up in cleaning products, and you won't be introducing these chemicals into the environment. You win; the earth wins.

Many companies offer safe, nonpolluting cleaning products. In stores, you'll find Bon Ami Polishing Cleanser, a nonchlorinated scouring powder that also is nonabrasive. Murphy's Oil Soap and Ecover are vegetable-oil detergents, recommended if you have hard water. Seventh Generation and Planet brands offer full lines of nontoxic household cleaning products. Visit their Web sites at www.seventhgen.com and www.planetinc.com, respectively. And the Earthrite line of cleaning products is widely available, sold in natural-foods store and also in chains such as Pathmark and Shop Rite.

Here are two mail-order sources for toxinfree cleaning agents:

⊷ The Clean Environment Co., P.O. Box 4444, Lincoln, NE 68504; 402-464-0988; www.ecomall.com; e-mail: envirocycle@aol.com

⊷ Morganics, 13610 N. Scottsdale Rd., Suite 10, Scottsdale, AZ 85254; 800-820-9235; www.morganics.com

Avoid cleaning products that display these warnings on the labels: DANGER, POISON, WARNING, TOXIC, FLAMMABLE, or CORROSIVE.

Chapter 4

Shopping for Healing Foods

● ●

In This Chapter

▶ Finding healing foods in your supermarket
▶ Exploring natural-food stores
▶ Deciding to go organic

● ●

*N*o matter how much you know about which foods are healing and why, you won't benefit from all this wisdom until you actually go out and buy such foods, cook them, and eat them. It's time to go shopping! Explore your old haunts with new eyes and go into food shops where you have never ventured before. You may find the prices for quality foods a bit higher than you are accustomed to paying, but you're spending your money well. Even if you splurge, your grocery bills will be lower than your doctor bills if you choose to ignore the importance of food in maintaining your health. Quality food is not a luxury!

Shopping in Good Places

I toured my local markets to research the healing foods for sale in various kinds of stores, from natural-foods supermarkets to little ethnic food shops. Granted, I have a lot of resources to choose from, living in health-conscious, multi-ethnic Los Angeles. However, even in the standard supermarket, you can find quite an assortment of healing foods if you know where to look.

Taking a fresh look at your supermarket

Your supermarket is a fine source for such natural and whole foods as fruits, vegetables, and fresh herbs; whole grains, such as brown rice; many kinds of dried beans, lentils, and peas; and bottles of filtered water. You may also find wild rice, raw nuts and seeds, 100 percent rye pumpernickel bread, soba buckwheat noodles, corn tortillas, fresh soybeans, and fresh-made fruit and vegetable juices. Even organic fruits and vegetables are beginning to sneak into produce sections of many supermarkets. And you may find naturally raised chicken.

Table 4-1 lists products I spotted in a tour of my neighborhood supermarkets. I chose certain brands because they were free of additives, others because they were unrefined or organic and because they didn't contain caffeine, hydrogenated oils, or added sugars.

Table 4-1	Healing Foods in Your Supermarket
If You 're Shopping For . . .	*Check Out This (These) Brand(s) . . .*
Breakfast cereal (organic)	General Mills
Breakfast cereal (whole grain)	Quaker Oats, Weetabix, Familia, McCanns, Roman Meal
Brown rice	Carolina
Buckwheat	Wolff's
Dairy foods	Horizon, Alta Dena
Eggs	EggLand's Best, Naturally Nested, Saunders
Extra-virgin olive oil	Bertolli, Colavita
Fruit juice	R.W. Knudsen, Martinelli's, Sunsweet
Fruit spreads	Smucker's, Polanar, Dickinson's
Herbal and green teas	Lipton, Good Earth, Bigelow
Maple syrup	Maple Grove Farms
Pilaf packaged mixes	Near East
Raisins (preservativefree)	Sun-Maid, Dole
Raw nuts	Diamond, Flanagan Farms
Spaghetti sauce	Newman's Own, Five Brothers
Whole-wheat bread and bagels	Oroweat, the Baker, Matthews
Whole-wheat crackers	ak-mak Bakeries, Carr's

Getting to know your natural-food store

You probably have a *natural-food store* in your area. These food stores are popping up in many cities and towns as the demand for healthy food increases. You may have in your area a branch of one of the several new and innovative chains of natural-food stores. Look for these store names: Wild Oats, Bread & Circus, Fresh Fields, Bread of Life, Merchant of Vino, Wellspring Grocery, and Whole Foods. Trader Joe's is another rapidly expanding market with branches now on both coasts. Its products are a mix of gourmet and natural.

You will find that the great majority of foods for sale are natural, whole, organic, unadulterated with chemical additives, and minimally processed. Browsing the aisles you are sure to find unusual soups, interesting packaged pilafs, whole-grain breakfast cereals galore, a wide selection of nuts and seeds, raw honey, naturally raised chicken and meats, and on and on.

The respected companies shown in Table 4-2 are committed to providing healthy and often organic foods. In general, these products are minimally processed, additivefree, and do not contain hydrogenated oils or refined sugar. Several of these companies produce many more products than those indicated here.

Table 4-2	Foods to Try
Type of Food	*Trusted Brand(s)*
Baby food	Earth's Best, Healthy Times, Organic Baby
Baking powder (aluminumfree)	Rumford, Featherweight
Beans	Bob's Red Mill, Arrowhead Mills
Blackstrap molasses (unsulphured)	Plantation, Tree of Life, Wholesome Foods
Breadcrumbs (whole grain)	Jaclyn's Food Products
Breakfast cereal	Arrowhead Mills, Barbara's, Erewhon, Health Valley, Kashi, Mother's
Breakfast meats	Shelton's Poultry, Season
Canned goods	Hain, Health Valley, Westbrae
Coffee substitutes	Bambu, Cafix, Teeccino, Roma, Pero
Condiments	Westbrae, Hain, Spectrum Naturals, Tree of Life
Cookies	Ener-g, Glennies, Jennies, Midel, Pamela's

(continued)

Table 4-2 *(continued)*

Type of Food	Trusted Brand(s)
Crackers (whole grain)	Hain, Health Valley, Old Stone Mill, Ryvita, Tree of Life, Wasa
Dairy products	Organic Valley, Alta Dena, Stoneyfield Farm, Horizon, Redwood Hill Farm, Brown Cow Farm, Juniper Valley, Cow Organic
Deli meats	Golden Farms, Pederson's, Citterio
Dried fruit (unsulphured)	Timbercrest Farms, Pavich Family Farms, Made in Nature
Eggs	Organic Valley, Veg-a-Fed, Happy Hen
Frozen entrees	Cascadian Farms, Amy's, Health's Wealth, Ling Ling, Legume, Thai Chef
Fruit preserves	Cascadian Farms, Sorrell Ridge
Glutenfree baking mixes	Sylvan Border Farms
Grains	Arrowhead Mills, Bob's Red Mill, Eden Foods, Lundberg Family Farms
Herbal teas	Celestial Seasonings, Traditional Medicinals, Alvita, Stash, Long Life Teas
Honey (raw)	Manuka, Sweet William of Earlville, Champlain Valley
Juice	R.W. Knudsen, Cascadian Farms, Martinelli, Santa Cruz Organic, Naked Juice, Ferraro's, Tree of Life
Mayonnaise	Spectrum Natural, Hain
Meats	Coleman Natural Meats, Kohler Farms, Larsen Beef, Maverick Ranch Lite Beef
Maple syrup	Shady Maple Farms, Spring Tree, Northern Comfort, W & E Allen
Nut butters	Maranatha Natural Foods, Sahadi
Non-irradiated seasonings	The Spice Hunter, Joes, Frontier Herb, Herbamare
Oils	Barlean's Organic Oils, Flora, Omega Nutrition, Spectrum, Loriva, Tree of Life

Type of Food	Trusted Brand(s)
Pasta (whole grain)	Ancient Harvest, Bionature, Eddie's, Organica di Sicilia, VitaSpelt, Tree of Life
Pickles (organic)	Cascadian Farms
Poultry	Foster Farms, Holly Farms, Rocky, Shelton's
Salad dressings	Newman's Own, Annie's Naturals, Michelle's Cardine
Sauces	Tree of Life
Soups	Imagine Foods, Pacific Foods of Oregon, Health Valley, WestBrae, Bronner, Hain
Tomato products	Muir Glen, Millina,
Whole-grain bread and waffles	Baldwin Hill, French Meadow, Vans, Rudi's, Matthews, Shiloh Farms, Alvarado

Reading Labels: Checking for Additives

Over 2,000 additives are approved for use in the manufacture of food products. Most are added to preserve the food, make it easier to prepare, or to enhance the appearance of the food to make it more appealing to a potential customer. Relatively little is known about the health hazards of most of these chemicals, especially their long-term effects. Animal studies indicate that when several additives are present in the animal feed, as they are in the foods you eat, health is undermined more than when additives are ingested one at a time. Not enough is known about which additives may be carcinogenic or toxic to the nerves and brain. You can sidestep the issue by simply increasing the amount of natural, unprocessed foods in your diet.

A suspected neurotoxin is monosodium glutamate (MSG), a flavor enhancer, which is also present in such substances as hydrolyzed vegetable protein (HVP). Aspartic acid, found in aspartame marketed under the name NutraSweet, can also cause an MSG-type reaction. Some individuals are sensitive to sulfites, a common additive. Reactions can range from diarrhea and nausea to acute asthma attacks, loss of consciousness, and anaphylactic shock, an allergylike reaction. You will find the highest levels of sulfites on dried fruit, in fruit juices made from concentrates, dehydrated potatoes, molasses (unless otherwise specified), and possibly some canned foods served in restaurants. (Figure 4-1 shows some other places where you might find sulfites.)

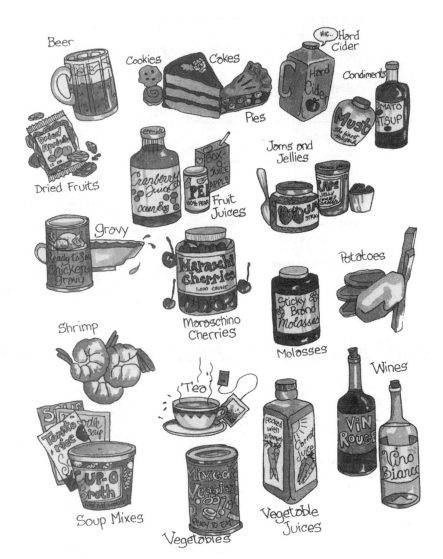

Buying Organic Foods

Of the many healing foods, those that are organic are the healthiest of all. Organic fruits and vegetables are grown without the use of synthetic pesticides, herbicides, or fertilizers. Also, they are not treated with fumigants, waxes, or artificial colors to make the produce look more attractive. I highly recommend incorporating organic foods into your diet, as I have done over the last few years, because of what these foods *do not* contain. Pesticides, herbicides, fungicides, waxes, and chemical additives, as well as hormones and drugs, are present in significant amounts in the normal (nonorganic) food supply. Taken together, this mix of chemicals is quite a stew! Some information is known about the health effects of these substances when one substance is consumed at a time, and what may be tolerable levels of this consumption for the human body. However, much less is known about how these compounds affect the body when several are consumed over a long period of time.

In a market's produce section, you may find bins of fruits or vegetables labeled "In transition" or "Transitional." These terms indicate that the food was grown on land during the three-year waiting period when prohibited chemicals are no longer in use, but organic certification has not yet been granted.

To find out more about organic foods and farming, contact the Organic Trade Association, P.O. Box 1078, Greenfield, MA 01302. You can phone them at 413-774-7511 or check their Web site at www.ota.com. Membership and publications are available.

The health hazards of pesticides

After World War II, farmers began to grow their crops with liberal amounts of chemical pesticides. Since 1945, the amount used has increased 3,300 percent. According to the most recent figures from the Environmental Protection Agency (EPA), 771 million pounds of active ingredients were used in agriculture in the United States in 1995. The EPA has approved some 350 active pesticide ingredients, with at least 70 classified as possibly or probably cancerous to humans. Some pesticides, such as those made from *organophosphates* (an easily absorbed, extremely toxic compound containing phosphorus), are damaging to the nervous system and are associated with a higher incidence of such conditions as Parkinson's Disease. Other pesticides can cause birth defects, miscarriages, disorders of the immune system, and behavioral changes.

Over this same period, the incidence of diseases such as cancer has been on the rise. While it is difficult to prove that the consumption of pesticides leads directly to these diseases, animal studies and human studies focusing on farmers and farm workers who handle pesticides document significantly higher rates of health problems. In contrast, according to a Danish study published in 1994, organic farmers and individuals who consumed organic foods were found to have twice the sperm count of men who did not eat organic foods.

You can obtain information about toxins in foods from these organizations:

- Pesticide Hotline. U.S. Environmental Protection Agency, NPTN, Oregon State University, 333 Weniger Hall, Corvallis, OR 97331; 800-858-7378 6:30 a.m. to 4:30 p.m. (PST) seven days a week.

- Pesticide Action Network, North American Regional Center, 965 Mission St., Suite 514, San Francisco, CA 94103; 415-981-1771.

Going Organic

When some people learn about possible toxins in their food supply, they are astounded at the statistics and take the plunge, immediately switching all their food purchases to organic. Others, like myself, first put a toe in, testing the waters, and then slowly make changes. Either way is fine.

To reduce the amount of pesticides that you may be consuming, you can start by avoiding the following items, also known as the dirty dozen, designated by the Environmental Working Group to be the most contaminated of nonorganic foods. The worst offenders lead the list: Strawberries, green and red bell peppers, spinach, U.S.-grown cherries, peaches, Mexican-grown cantaloupe, celery, apples, apricots, green beans, grapes from Chile, and cucumbers. Here's an organic foods shopping list that includes these items, as well as other foods likely to contain toxins. (Also see Chapter 7 to read about organic meats and poultry.)

- **Fruit:** Apples, blackberries, blueberries, boysenberries, cantaloupe, cherries, cranberries, grapes, peaches, pears, plums, raspberries, and strawberries
- **Vegetables:** Asparagus, beets, bell peppers, bok choy (see Figure 4-2), broccoli, cabbage, carrots, cauliflower, celery, collard greens, cucumbers, kale, leeks, iceberg lettuce, mustard greens, scallions, parsley, parsnips, garden peas, hot peppers, potatoes, radishes, soy beans, summer and winter squash, sweet potatoes, tomatoes, and turnip greens
- **Grains and beans:** Rice from India and lentils
- **Nuts and seeds:** Peanuts, cashews, and sesame seeds

Yes, you can find wine that is organic. The following vineyards produce organic wines: Fetzger, Frey, Konrad, Coturri, Bonterra, Organic Wine Works, and Headlands.

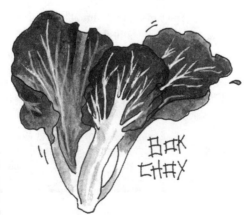

Figure 4-2:
Bok choy.

Part III
Mother Nature's Best Foods

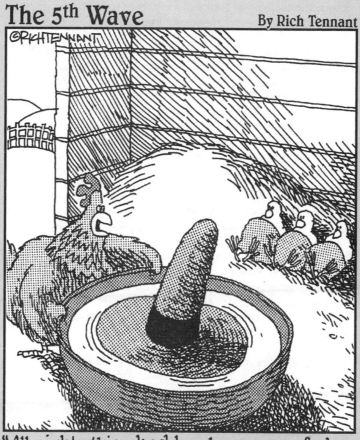

The 5th Wave   By Rich Tennant

"All right, this should make everyone feel a
little better. It's a bowl of my own, homemade
chicken farmer soup. Sip it down carefully and
watch for bones."

In this part . . .

If you've been shopping for food for years, you probably feel like an expert. What more is there to know? Plenty, if you want to make sure that you are buying the highest quality and healthiest foods. In this part, I tell you about the major categories of food from fruits to flavorings, with eggs, beans, meats, and veggies in between.

I'm sending you into the store to buy whole foods free of additives and preservatives. You want to buy foods an ancestor of yours would have recognized as edible. Not protein powder, but lamb chops. I introduce you to lots of foods that may be new to you, such as quinoa and nopales, and ask you to expand your vegetable repertoire beyond potatoes and string beans. You find out about the medicinal properties of common kitchen spices and herbs, the mainstay of many traditional home remedies.

This part also tells you all about the nutritional treasures in foods fresh from nature, the vitamins and minerals as well as the array of newly discovered phytonutrients. These compounds have powerful disease-fighting properties. You'll start to see the products in your supermarket in a new light! What not to buy is also covered. You wield a great deal of power when you shop. You send a message to manufacturers about the kind of food you really want and you send a message to your body that you plan to take good care of it.

Read on and get ready to write a healthy foods shopping list!

Chapter 5

Rediscovering Whole Grains and Bringing Back Beans

- -

In This Chapter

▶ Differentiating between whole and refined grains

▶ Reviving classic whole grains

▶ Determining whether you're gluten-sensitive

▶ Bragging about beans

▶ Rethinking soy's benefits

▶ Combining grains and beans

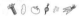
- -

Grains and beans have been staples of the human diet for thousands of years. These foods have sustained civilizations throughout history and were some of the first crops cultivated in the early days of agriculture. Today, in the Western diet, what passes for acceptable grain and flour are impoverished versions of the originals. And beans, once a primary source of protein, have been demoted to side-dish status. This chapter takes a fresh look at these two valuable sources of nourishment.

Praising Whole Grains

Grains that you eat are the seeds of grasses. Each kernel is a little package of nourishment bursting with protein, healthy fat, starch, vitamins, and minerals. Of course, I'm referring to *whole* grains, such as whole wheat and brown rice. The health benefits of whole grains are well documented. According to an article published in the *American Journal of Clinical Nutrition* in 1999, various studies show that eating whole grains reduces the risk of coronary heart disease, diabetes, hypertension, and some types of cancer. However, there's a world of difference between whole grains and the refined and processed grains used in typical American meals.

Refining flour versus leaving well enough alone

One cup of flour made from refined wheat contains smaller amounts of most of the B vitamins and significantly lower levels of many minerals as compared to 1 cup of whole-wheat flour. (See Table 5-1.) In addition, 25 to 30 percent of the protein content of the grain, and as much as 97 percent of the fiber, is lost. Both kinds of flour have the same number of calories.

Yes, manufacturers do "enrich" refined flour. You see this term used on labels for flour and grain products such as pasta and breakfast cereals. But of the more than 20 nutrients that are removed or are greatly reduced when the original grain is processed, only five are returned — thiamin, riboflavin, niacin, folic acid, and iron — and the amount added often fails to reach the original levels.

Take wheat, for example. Whole wheat is a great source of B vitamins, which are important for liver function and the health of the nervous system; vitamin E, a potent antioxidant that also promotes heart health; magnesium, which helps sustain a steady heartbeat; zinc, which provides energy; fiber, which facilitates healthy bowel function; essential fatty acids, which transport oxygen to the cells; and more than 16 other major and trace minerals that are involved in all sorts of activities throughout the body.

When flour is made from whole wheat, all these nutrients remain in the final product. The reason is that the entire kernel of wheat is milled, and all three of its primary parts — the germ, the bran, and the endosperm (see Figure 5-1) — are ground into flour.

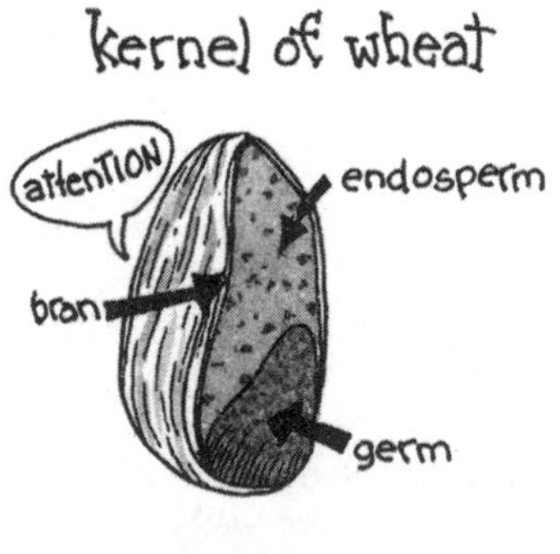

Figure 5-1:
All three primary parts of a kernel of wheat are important.

✔ The *germ,* which is the portion of the grain that sprouts when the grain is planted, contains fat-soluble vitamins E and K, essential oils, a range of minerals, and some protein.

✔ The *bran,* which is the outer covering of the kernel, consists of fiber, plus some protein, B vitamins, and minerals, particularly iron.

✔ The *endosperm* makes up the bulk of each grain and is mostly starch.

Guess what happens when whole wheat is refined to make flour? The germ and bran are removed! (The wheat is also bleached to make the flour white.) This process eliminates the risk that the oils in the wheat will turn rancid, lengthening the shelf life of the flour and any baked goods made from it. This is just what a manufacturer wants, but the person eating such food is short-changed. Flour that is missing the germ and the bran is also missing vitamins, minerals, and fiber. (See Table 5-1 for a comparison.)

Table 5-1	Comparing the Nutritional Value of Flour	
Nutrient	*1 Cup Enriched Wheat Flour*	*1 Cup Whole-Wheat Flour*
Vitamins (in milligrams and micrograms)		
Thiamin, mg	0.48	0.66
Riboflavin, mg	0.28	0.14
Niacin, mg	3.9	5.2
Vitamin B5, mg	0.51	1.32
Vitamin B6, mg	0.066	0.41
Folic acid, mcg	24	65
Biotin, mcg	1.1	6
Minerals (in milligrams and micrograms)		
Calcium, mg	18	49
Copper, mg	0.21	0.6
Iron, mg	3.2	4
Magnesium, mg	28	136
Phosphorus, mg	96	446
Potassium, mg	105	444
Selenium, mcg	21.7	77.4
Zinc, mg	0.77	2.88

Rice undergoes the same nutrient-depleting process. Manufacturers produce white rice by removing the hull and polishing the rice, a process that reduces the generous amount of B vitamins and fiber that the grain originally contains. Like wheat flour, white rice is usually enriched, but again, B vitamin levels are only partially restored. In addition, the process strips away many minerals that support health and prevent degenerative disease. One cup of brown rice contains 172 mg of magnesium, a mineral essential for bone health and the prevention of osteoporosis, whereas 1 cup of enriched white rice contains only 13 mg. When you shop, always choose whole grains over refined, and when you eat out, if you have the option, again choose whole grains. I find that some Chinese and Thai restaurants have begun to offer brown rice. I also invite you to experiment with whole grains in your own cooking.

Another advantage of eating whole grains is that you digest them more slowly than their refined versions. Whole grains enter your system gradually and raise your level of blood sugar very little in comparison with refined grains and white flour. When your blood sugar is in control like this, you are less likely to develop heart disease and diabetes, not to mention gaining weight.

Shopping for common whole grains

When shopping for grains, look for the word *whole,* which means that all three nutritious parts of the kernel are present in the product. Only a whole grain is a *complex* carbohydrate, the original with all its parts. A refined grain is just a *carbohydrate,* and it's less nutritious. You sometimes hear and see "complex carbohydrate" used loosely, referring to a food made from refined grain and flour. Now you know the difference!

Consult this list of grains and flours before you go shopping. I tell you how to spot the whole-grain versions and what to look for on labels. You're most likely to find these whole grains in natural-food stores, which often sell them in bulk at a very good price. Also look for whole-grain croissants and breakfast pastries, which are new on the market.

> ✔ **Wheat:** Wheat is usually sold as a flour. The whole-grain versions are called *crushed, cracked,* or *whole wheat,* depending upon how the wheat is cut. (The crushed version, bulghur wheat, is used to make the Middle Eastern dish tabbouleh.) Many whole-grain mixes for wheat pancakes, muffins, and cakes are now on the market, as well as a variety of baked goods, including bagels and English muffins.

> Don't assume that a loaf of bread is whole wheat because it has a nice, rich brown color. Some companies use white flour and add molasses to color it and make it look more wholesome. Inspect the ingredient list on the label to find out what's actually in there!

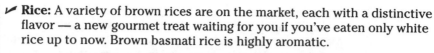

✔ **Rice:** A variety of brown rices are on the market, each with a distinctive flavor — a new gourmet treat waiting for you if you've eaten only white rice up to now. Brown basmati rice is highly aromatic.

A good mail-order source for rice is Indian Harvest Specialtifoods, Inc., P.O. Box 428, Bemidji, MN 56619-0428; 800-294-2433; Web site www.indianharvest.com. This company sells many types of exotic rice and other grains.

✔ **Oats:** In the 1980s, this grain became a media superstar, as research indicated that eating oats and oat bran regularly may help lower your cholesterol levels and benefit your heart. Oat bran began to show up in muffins, cookies, and meatloaf as people eagerly sought this path to long life. The oat message has now been modified, and this traditional grain takes its place within an overall heart-wise diet. (See Chapter 15 for more on eating for a healthy heart.)

Oatmeal is a whole grain. It's made up of whole oats that are rolled and flattened, which shortens the cooking time. Instant oatmeal is a processed grain — the flakes of oatmeal are chopped into smaller pieces. This process exposes oils that are normally in oats to heat and oxygen, which can turn the oils rancid. This rancid oil contains toxic compounds that can increase the risk of heart disease and cancer. Sniff oats before cooking them to check for rancidity, especially in the summertime.

If you have plenty of time in the morning or you're staunchly Scottish, another option is to cook yourself a pot of whole oats, which takes about 45 minutes. Then set your teeth into this chewy, richly flavored porridge.

✔ **Barley:** Whole-grain barley is referred to as *hulled barley*. In processing, only the outer husk is removed, making hulled barley the most nutritious form of the grain. *Scotch barley* is hulled and coarsely ground. These grains have an oval shape. You can find both types in health-food stores. The type in the supermarket is *pearled barley,* which has a round shape. It has been hulled and then steamed and polished. Pearled barley cooks more quickly, but contains fewer nutrients than whole barley.

✔ **Wild rice:** This grain, which is not a rice, has a luxurious, nutty flavor and chewy texture and supplies riboflavin, phosphorus, and magnesium. It's pricy, but it's quite affordable when you mix it with other grains such as brown rice in pilafs.

✔ **Pasta:** Many commercial pastas are made from semolina flour, which sounds special. Semolina is unique in that it is made from hard durum wheat, but semolina is a refined flour composed of only the nutrient-poor, starchy center of the grain.

A variety of whole-grain pastas are now on the market that are made from whole-wheat flour, corn, and brown rice. Some pastas also contain flour made from the Jerusalem artichoke, an iron-rich vegetable that's a variety of sunflower. An excellent brand is De Bole's.

- **Couscous:** Couscous is a starchy staple of North African cooking. It looks like a grain, but it's actually made from pasta flour formed into tiny pieces. Couscous in American markets is made from semolina, refined wheat flour. However, in natural-food stores, you can find whole-grain couscous, a richly flavored, nutty, whole-wheat version.

- **Millet:** Various minor grains grown around the world are known as millet. This mild-flavored grain, and the flour made from it, is a staple in Asia and Africa because of its high nutritional value. Millet is a great source of riboflavin, niacin, calcium, iron, and phosphorus. It's a good source of protein, and because the body converts it slowly to energy after you eat it, millet promotes stable blood sugar levels.

- **Buckwheat:** Buckwheat is not actually a grain, nor is it a wheat. Buckwheat is the seed of a thistle. This tawny brown, three-sided seed is a hearty and warming starch, a restorative food well-suited for the cold climates in which it grows. Buckwheat is a staple in Eastern Europe and Russia, where it's eaten in its roasted form, *kasha*. Unroasted buckwheat that is crushed is buckwheat groats, and Japanese soba noodles are made from buckwheat. (Try Turkish Buckwheat Salad in Chapter 17.)

  Buckwheat consists of a remarkable 15 to 20 percent of protein, containing all eight essential amino acids, plus fiber, B-complex vitamins, vitamin E, potassium, and some calcium, manganese, and phosphorus. It is unique among grains in that it provides flavonoids, which are vitaminlike compounds that strengthen capillary walls, thereby lessening menstrual cramping and reducing the development of varicose veins.

Has gluten got you?

Gluten is a protein in flour that gives dough its elastic quality. It's part of the reason bread rises. Wheat is high in gluten, but rye, oat, and barley also contain varied amounts.

Some individuals, especially as they age, develop a sensitivity to grains and baked goods that contain gluten. Enjoying a lovely croissant made with wheat flour can result in intestinal distress, fatigue, and brain fog.

To find out whether you are sensitive to gluten, try eating a big plate of wheat pancakes after a good night's sleep, but skip beverages that contain caffeine (including decaffeinated coffee, tea, and colas), which could give you an energy kick. Notice whether you start to feel tired and fuzzy-headed a few minutes after eating, and if you experience gas and bloating, all signs that your body is reacting to the gluten. Then, the next morning, have pancakes or waffles (see Appendix C for recommended brands) made with rice flour and compare the results.

Buckwheat, quinoa, amaranthe, and rice are the low-gluten grains.

If you've never tasted dishes made with whole grains, you need to do so! Their flavor has more depth and substance. I found that as I switched to whole-grain foods, their refined counterparts started to taste flat and uninteresting.

Exploring ancient American grains that are making a comeback

Some grains that were staples of earlier civilizations, and then long forgotten, are been reintroduced into American cooking. They have names that sound like romantic foreign destinations. Here are some of the common ones:

- ✔ **Amaranthe:** A staple of the Aztecs and Mayans, this grain is an excellent source of protein. It also provides magnesium, iron, copper, and fiber.

- ✔ **Quinoa:** This whole grain (see Figure 5-2) is native to Central America and was a staple in North America for 4,000 years. Quinoa (pronounced "KEEN-wa") is high in protein, calcium, and iron, with a variety of B vitamins and other minerals.

- ✔ **Kamut:** The name of this whole grain originates from the ancient Egyptian word for wheat. Kamut is a variety of high-protein wheat that has never been hybridized and is nutritionally superior to its modern-day counterparts. In natural-food stores, you can find kamut used in cereals, crackers, and pasta. The grain itself is not available on the market.

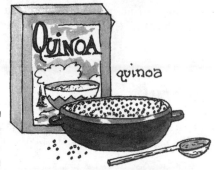

Figure 5-2:
Quinoa.

Applauding Legumes

Beans, peas, and lentils belong to a single class of foods termed *legumes* or *pulses.* You probably eat beans once in a while — baked beans with spare ribs, beans in chili, and so on. But in general, legumes make up only a small part of typical American meals, served as side dishes at best. Yet legumes are one of the most nutritious forms of food the earth offers. More than 70 varieties exist. Legumes have been part of the human diet for more than 10,000 years. They are part of every traditional cuisine around the world and are considered as essential as grains.

A source of lowfat protein

Beans offer a nonmeat source of high-quality protein. If you're looking for the perfect diet food, beans are the answer! A cup of cooked kidney beans provides 16 g of protein and only 1 g of fat. In contrast, 2 ounces of broiled ground beef provides 14 g of protein but 10 g of fat, and 2 ounces of cheddar cheese contains 14 g of protein and 18 g of fat. You can add cooked beans to soups, salads, and stews.

If you're a part-time vegetarian, cook up some tasty beans for a main course — a most satisfying entrée. (Try the Sunday Supper White Bean Soup that appears later in this chapter, for example.) However, if you're a full-time vegetarian, you need to take care to combine your beans with grains. Each supplies some of the essential amino acids from which your body makes protein, but neither grain nor beans provide the full range. Only when you combine grains and beans do you get all you need. If some amino acids are missing, certain vital proteins cannot be made, which can drastically undermine health. However, it's not that hard to consume what you need. You can eat your grains in one meal and your beans in another, within the same day, and still benefit from this combination.

Standard, canned, barbecued beans are normally swimming in a sugary sauce that supplies plenty of calories. They have all the nutritional shortcomings of any sugar-coated food.

Fiber in every mouthful

By eating beans, you increase your intake of fiber: what your great-grandmother called "roughage" — that is, bulk. Two types of fiber exist (beans, lentils, and peas contain both types):

- ✔ **Insoluble:** Your body does not digest this type of fiber, such as the stringy bits in celery. Insoluble fiber is well recognized for its usefulness in preventing constipation as well as reducing the risk of such intestinal ailments as diverticulosis and colon cancer. Beans are only second to wheat bran in the amount of insoluble fiber they provide: about 9 g of fiber per cup of cooked beans, which is more than 25 percent of your daily goal. The recommended daily intake of fiber is between 20 and 35 grams.

✔ **Soluble:** This type of fiber is partially digested. Recently, soluble fiber has gained attention for its ability to lower blood cholesterol levels, in particular LDL (the "bad" cholesterol). Soluble fiber helps stabilize blood sugar, which is a problem for people who have hypoglycemia and diabetes. It also provides a satisfying feeling of fullness that can ease your hunger pangs when you're dieting. The fiber in beans is predominantly soluble.

Packed with nutrients

Beans supply B vitamins, such as thiamin for memory, calcium and boron for bones, iron for energy, potassium for reducing high blood pressure, and zinc for immunity. They are an excellent source of folic acid, which is essential for cell division and is required by women during pregnancy. Beans also contain protease inhibitors, which are known to prevent the development of cancerous cells. Unlike many vegetables, beans still retain most of their nutrients even after long cooking.

Canned beans are nearly as nutritious as dried beans, although the canned version has somewhat less of the B vitamin and folic acid, as well as extra sodium, which you can partially remove by rinsing. For flavor, nothing beats dried beans that you soak and cook yourself. However, bottled beans, which are starting to appear on the market, are an acceptable alternative. You can make the following recipe for this satisfying soup with beans that are dried, canned, or bottled.

Sunday Supper White Bean Soup

This nourishing puree of bean soup is a substantial little meal. Beans supply protein equivalent to that supplied by meat when they are combined with a grain such as the whole-wheat croutons in this recipe.

Preparation time: 15 minutes

Cooking time: 20 minutes (does not include cooking the beans)

Yield: 8 servings

(continued)

1½ cups dried Great Northern beans (or 3 14-ounce cans, drained)

4 cups chicken stock, preferably organic or hormonefree

3 medium carrots, sliced into rounds

1 yellow onion, peeled and quartered

1 large clove garlic, crushed

1 tablespoon fresh thyme, or 1 teaspoon dried

½ cup buttermilk or regular whole milk*

Sea salt and freshly ground black pepper to taste

Prepared croutons**

Freshly grated Parmesan cheese

Parsley

1 Cook the dried, bottled, or canned beans as directed on the package and then drain them.

2 In the meantime, put the chicken stock, carrot, onion, garlic, and thyme in a medium saucepan. Cook, uncovered, on medium heat until the onion softens, about 15 minutes. Remove from heat.

3 Using a pair of tongs, transfer only the onion and garlic to a food processor, leaving the carrot in the broth. Transfer the beans to the food processor. Add ½ cup water. Puree until smooth.

4 Transfer the bean puree to a large bowl. Whisk the chicken stock and then the milk into the puree.

5 Return the soup to the saucepan. Simmer briefly to heat the soup. Season to taste with sea salt and pepper. Ladle into individual soup bowls and garnish with croutons, cheese, and parsley.

Suggested accompaniments: *Sardine Tapenade in Chapter 8.*

*The texture and flavor of this soup are excellent, with or without the milk. However, if you're preparing the nondairy version, make sure to use the croutons, sautéed in butter or oil, because fat carries flavor.

**Save stale whole-grain bread and cut it into ½-inch cubes. Sauté them in butter or, better yet, basil-scented olive oil. The richer flavor of whole-grain croutons is just right for this soup.

Shopping for beans, peas, and lentils

Follow these tips when you're shopping for beans, peas, and lentils:

- ✔ **Green beans:** Eating green beans provides you with the same range of nutrients as does eating other beans, but to a lesser extent, because green beans are less dense. They also contain some beta-carotene and vitamin C.

✔ **Fava beans:** You occasionally find fava beans sold fresh in gourmet stores, but dried fava beans are readily available in Italian and Hispanic markets, where they are called *habas*. Fava beans (see Figure 5-3) are an excellent source of vitamin B5, which you need for energy, a healthy digestive tract, and to withstand stress.

✔ **Soybeans:** Fresh soybeans are a nutritious whole food, providing lots of protein, large amounts of iron, potassium, and calcium, and healthful unsaturated fats. Supermarkets now sell bags of frozen soybeans, and they're served as appetizers in Japanese restaurants. Tofu, or bean curd, is a custardlike substance made from curdled soy milk. You can find it in the dairy section of your supermarket, labeled like mini-mattresses: soft, medium, and firm. Fermented soy foods include *tempeh,* a somewhat chewy, fermented soy cake; and *miso,* fermented bean paste. Miso has a wonderful, earthy flavor, and is the basis for miso soup, served in every Japanese restaurant. (Enjoy a Puree of Green Soybean Soup in Chapter 17.)

✔ **Bean sprouts:** Sprouting beans increases their nutrient content many fold, as each bean prepares to become a bean stalk. Sprouted mung beans are common ingredients in Asian cooking, showing up in Thai salads as well as in Chinese fried rice dishes. They are high in vitamin C. Eaten raw, these vital, living foods, which are full of nutrients and enzymes, help counteract chronic fatigue and help boost immunity. Sprouted mung beans are commonly found in supermarkets, while a wider variety of fresh sprouts are sold at natural-food stores and farmers markets. Sprouts can contain a lot of mold, so allergy sufferers should probably skip eating sprouts, especially during allergy season.

✔ **Peas:** Trendy chefs have rediscovered the enchanting emerald green of just-picked peas and now capture their color in delicious fresh pea soup. Peas have been elevated to gourmet status, but for most cooks, they remain a homey staple, supplying basic nutrition to everyday meals. Peas are a good source of protein and fiber. You most likely eat the bright green, flash-frozen version, which is fine; processing does not significantly destroy the nutrients. These nutrients include the antioxidant vitamins A and C, plus the B vitamins thiamin and folic acid, which support the health of your nervous system.

Split peas, either yellow or green, are a variety grown specifically for drying. In processing, they are split along a natural seam. They're exceptionally high in protein, with ½ cup of cooked split peas providing nearly 20 percent of your recommended daily needs. They also contain potassium, which is thought to reduce the risk of strokes.

Snow peas are lower in protein than split peas, but are an excellent source of calcium. They're one of the many plant food sources of this mineral, which is essential for bone health.

✔ **Lentils:** Lentils (see Figure 5-4) come in a variety of colors — red, green, yellow, and brown — all with about the same nutritional value. They supply B vitamins, in particular niacin, which can lower high blood pressure. They are an excellent source of fiber and are thought to lower the risk of colon cancer.

Lentils are also a good source of calcium, iron, and zinc. However, they do contain phytic acid, which can bind with these minerals and prevent their absorption. Eating a food that contains vitamin C, such as a raw green pepper or a fresh slice of orange, along with a serving of lentils increases the amount of iron absorbed. Lentils may also cause problems if you have gout, because they promote the depositing of uric acid crystals in joints. In soup or as a side dish, lentils make good eating. In the following recipe, they're served with lamb.

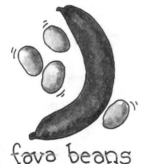

Figure 5-3:
Fava beans.

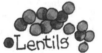

Figure 5-4:
Lentils.

Making beans socially acceptable

If you're like most people, you tend to avoid eating beans because they're difficult to digest and they cause gas. Beans contain raffinose and other sugars. Breaking down these sugars requires the digestive enzyme alpha-galactosidase. Unfortunately, you don't have this enzyme! Within your bowels, friendly bacteria to which you play host feed on these sugars and ferment them. A natural byproduct of this process is hydrogen and carbon dioxide gases.

Many folk remedies and cooking procedures exist for reducing gas. Their effects are subtle in comparison to the benefits of supplementing with the missing enzyme, alpha-galactosidase (sold under the brand name Beano), found in natural-food stores.

Braised Lamb Shanks and Lentils

Many traditional cuisines combine the two protein foods, meat and legumes, to create foods of substance. In the Middle East, for example, lentils are paired with lamb. By cutting back on the meat and increasing the lentils, you can enjoy a protein dish that's lower in fat but still has all the roasted meat flavor.

Preparation time: *5 minutes*

Cooking time: *2 hours, 50 minutes*

Yield: *4 servings*

4 lamb shanks, preferably organic and residuefree trimmed of fat

Whole-wheat flour

Sea salt and freshly ground pepper to taste

2 tablespoons organic unsalted butter

2 tablespoons extra-virgin olive oil

2 garlic cloves, crushed

1 bay leaf

1 tablespoon oregano, or 2 fresh sprigs

1 cinnamon stick

2 to 3 cups beef broth

1 cup green lentils, sorted and washed

1 onion stuck with 8 cloves

2½ cups filtered water

¼ cup finely chopped fresh parsley

1 Dust the lamb shanks lightly with whole-wheat flour. Rub with sea salt and pepper.

2 In a large saucepan, over medium-high heat, melt the butter and add the oil. Sear the lamb shanks in the butter mixture until they're browned on all sides, about 8 to 10 minutes.

3 Add the garlic, bay leaf, oregano, cinnamon stick, and broth. Add enough beef broth to bring liquid halfway up the sides of the lamb shanks, about 2 to 3 cups, depending on the size of the pot. Cover and simmer for 1 hour.

4 In a large pot, put the lentils, onion, and water. Simmer, covered, until they are tender but still have their form, about 45 minutes. Stir occasionally and add boiling water as needed. Drain the lentils and mix with the parsley.

5 Preheat oven to 350°. Spoon the lentils into a large baking dish and arrange the lamb shanks on top.

6 Bake, covered, for 25 minutes. Remove the cover and continue baking until the lamb shanks are tender and the flavors are blended, about 20 to 30 additional minutes. Add more liquid, ⅓ cup at a time, if necessary, during cooking.

7 Serve immediately with carrots and a green salad garnished with feta cheese.

Chapter 6

Getting Bushels of Health Benefits from Fruits and Vegetables

The Dietary Guidelines for Americans recommend that you eat five servings of fruits and vegetables a day. To someone in the habit of eating fruits and vegetables and who appreciates how delicious these foods can be, eating five servings a day is not a stretch. However, if you skip breakfast, grab a ham and cheese sandwich for lunch, and rely on a fast-food hamburger for dinner, you may have consumed barely one serving's worth. Catsup on your hamburger doesn't count!

Before you start reprimanding yourself for your low intake, consider this: According to a 1990 analysis of the National Health and Nutrition Examination Survey, conducted by the Council for Responsible Nutrition, fewer than 10 percent of Americans actually eat the recommended two servings of fruit and three servings of vegetables a day. Furthermore, five servings a day is just the minimum recommended, based on a diet of 1,600 calories a day, a modest amount. If you consume 2,200 calories a day, you need to eat seven servings of fruits and vegetables, and for 2,800 calories a day, nine servings are recommended.

For optimal health, eat fruits and vegetables in their most unprocessed, *whole* form — the general premise of this book. Take advantage of the fresh, whole foods available in the produce section of your supermarket, which is a treasure trove of healing nutrients.

Looking at the Health Benefits of Fruits and Vegetables

Fruits and vegetables contain vitamins and minerals that are essential for health. Once inside your body, vitamins and minerals don't just sit around giving off good vibes. They go to work, participating in thousands of critical chemical reactions that generate energy, build tissue, and generally run the goings on in your body. Many scientific studies testify to the health-protective effects of fruits and vegetables. Table 6-1 lists just a few of the essential body functions and organs each nutrient supports, along with the fruits and vegetables that contain good amounts of that nutrient.

Table 6-1	Essential Nutrients and How They Work for You		
Nutrient	**Functions Benefited**	**Fruit Sources**	**Vegetable Sources**
Vitamin A	Eyesight	Apricots	Butternut squash
	Immunity	Cantaloupe	Carrots
	Tissue repair	Mangoes	Sweet potatoes
Thiamin	Heart	Avocados	Green peas
	Metabolism	Grapes	Jerusalem artichokes
	Nerves	Pineapple	Potatoes
Riboflavin	Immunity	Apples	Acorn squash
	Energy	Berries	Mushrooms
	Blood	Figs	Sweet potatoes
Niacin	Digestion	Dates	Asparagus
	Energy	Figs	Avocados
	Skin	Prunes	Potatoes
Vitamin B5	Adrenals	Figs	Artichokes
	Hormones	Plantains	Corn
	Metabolism	Oranges	Mushrooms
Vitamin B6	Immunity	Bananas	Bok choy

Nutrient	Functions Benefited	Fruit Sources	Vegetable Sources
	Metabolism	Mangoes	Broccoli
	Muscles	Watermelon	Spinach
Folic acid	Blood	Avocados	Asparagus
	Metabolism	Boysenberries	Beets
	DNA synthesis	Cantaloupe	Turnip greens
Vitamin C	Adrenals	Guavas	Broccoli
	Immunity	Kiwis	Brussels sprouts
	Tissue repair	Papayas	Sweet peppers
Vitamin E	Blood	Avocados	Asparagus
	Heart	Cucumbers	Cucumbers
	Hormones	Mangoes	Kale
Boron	Bones	Apples	Dandelion greens
	Hormones	Apricots	Potatoes
	Joints	Figs	Spinach
Calcium	Bones	Figs	Collard greens
	Muscles	Cherimoyas	Kale
	Teeth	Papayas	Okra
Chromium	Blood sugar	Apples	Asparagus
	Energy	Grapes	Beets
	Heart	Prunes	Mushrooms
Copper	Blood	Figs	Collard greens
	Energy	Grapes	Potatoes
	Tissue repair	Pears	Shiitake mushrooms
Iodine	Energy		Potatoes
	Growth		Spinach
	Thyroid		Seaweed

(continued)

Table 6-1 *(continued)*

Nutrient	Functions Benefited	Fruit Sources	Vegetable Sources
Iron	Blood	Figs	Beets
	Energy	Peaches	Leeks
	Metabolism	Raisins	Parsley
Magnesium	Bones	Avocados	Beets
	Heart	Figs	Broccoli
	Muscles	Plantains	Spinach
Manganese	Bones	Bananas	Collards
	Energy	Blackberries	Okra
	Nerves	Pineapple	Peas
Phosphorus	Bones	Apricots	Artichokes
	Energy	Peaches	Corn
	Muscles	Raisins	Potatoes
Potassium	Heart	Papayas	Beet greens
	Kidneys	Plantains	Potatoes
	Nerves	Raisins	Swiss chard
Selenium	Heart	Oranges	Cabbage
	Reproduction	Pears	Carrots
	Skin	Pineapple	Mushrooms
Zinc	Digestion	Avocados	Corn
	Reproduction	Cantaloupe	Mushrooms
	Tissue	Figs	Seaweed

Antioxidants in the spotlight

In recent years, one group of vitamins has achieved celebrity status, stealing headlines and showing up on the evening news — antioxidants. Antioxidants stop the action of free radicals, which damage cell walls and tissues. Free radicals have been singled out as a fundamental cause of aging.

A free radical is a molecular fragment with a single unpaired electron, which darts about and readily reacts with other molecules. When a free radical's single electron comes in contact with a pair of electrons, it steals one away and joins with this electron to form a stable molecule. But this reaction produces a new unpaired electron, triggering a chain reaction that disrupts normal biological functioning. The normal chemical processes of the body produce some free radicals, but other sources include air pollutants such as cigarette smoke, solvents, radiation, overheated and rancid fats and oils, and pesticides.

Beta-carotene, vitamin C, vitamin E, and selenium are considered the four primary antioxidants. Take a look at what foods contain them and make a point of including more of these foods in your meals.

- ✔ **Beta-carotene:** Sweet potatoes, carrots, butternut squash, acorn squash, pumpkin, spinach, kale, red peppers, cantaloupe, mangoes, apricots, plantains (see Figure 6-1), and papayas (see Figure 6-2)

- ✔ **Vitamin C:** Papayas, kiwis, citrus, mangoes, cantaloupe, watermelon, strawberries, sweet peppers, broccoli, brussel sprouts, kohlrabi, mustard greens, and kale, and tomatoes

- ✔ **Vitamin E:** Whole wheat, millet, cornmeal, bulgur wheat, cold-pressed and refined oils, almonds, Brazil nuts, hazelnuts, sunflower seeds, flax seeds, shrimp, haddock, mackerel, herring, salmon, eggs, round steak, liver, lamb, sweet potatoes, kale, and cucumber

- ✔ **Selenium:** Brazil nuts, shellfish, cod, tuna, salmon, flounder, sole, perch, chicken breasts, liver, beef, lamb, pork, carrots, cabbage, mushrooms (see Figure 6-3), cauliflower, potatoes, green beans, garlic, seaweed, whole wheat, brown rice, bulgur, and blackstrap molasses

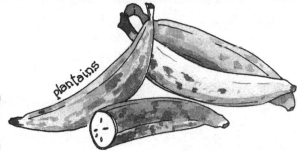

Figure 6-1:
Plantains.

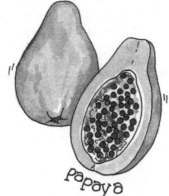

Figure 6-2:
Papayas.

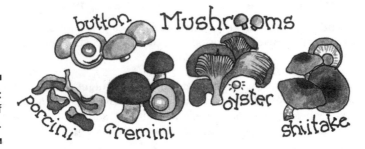

Figure 6-3:
A variety of
mushrooms.

These foods are great sources of antioxidants and belong in your meals every day of the week. Having adequate levels in your body helps protect your skin from sun damage, lessens the severity of arthritis, reduces the risk of cataracts and heart disease, and can slow the onset of senility.

The body also produces a type of antioxidant antioxidant *enzymes,* located within a cell to protect the cell's internal structures. For your body to synthesize these enzymes, you need a ready supply of certain minerals — copper, iron, manganese, selenium, and zinc.

- **Copper:** Organ meats, seafood, nuts, legumes, blackstrap molasses, and raisins

- **Iron:** Meats, eggs, fish, poultry, cherries, blackstrap molasses, green leafy vegetables, and dried fruit

- **Manganese:** Whole grains, green leafy vegetables, legumes, nuts, pineapple, and egg yolk

- **Selenium:** Tuna, herring, whole grains, and sesame seeds

- **Zinc:** Oysters, herring, pumpkin seeds, sunflower seeds, seafood, meats, mushrooms, soybeans, and eggs

You need good amounts of *all* antioxidants, because each patrols certain turf. They also protect each other from damage. For this reason, you need to make a special effort to eat a range of fruits and vegetables to ensure that you're getting all the antioxidants and their partner minerals.

Other substances in foods function as antioxidants as well. *Pycnogenol* is a potent antioxidant found in grapeseed oil. *Co-enzyme Q10* is present in nuts (such as walnuts, pistachios, and peanuts), sesame seeds, mackerel, and sardines. Watermelon, asparagus, avocado (see Figure 6-4), other common fruits and vegetables, and some meats contain *glutathione.* Other substances that have antioxidant activity are *indoles,* present in broccoli; *quercitin,* in onions; and *lycopene,* in tomatoes. All are phytonutrients, and you can read the following section for more about these healing compounds.

Avocados

Figure 6-4: Avocados.

Hass   Fuerte

The fabulous phytonutrients

Plants contain many compounds that protect them against such foes as bacteria, fungus, and bad weather. Scientists have long been aware of these compounds, but only recently have discovered that these substances can also help prevent disease in humans. The general term for these compounds is *phytonutrients* or *phytochemicals* (*phyto* comes from the Greek word for plant).

Thousands of phytonutrients are found in virtually all plant foods. Many of these compounds also give a fruit or vegetable its characteristic color, flavor, and scent. When you eat fresh, whole fruits and vegetables (as well as grains, beans, nuts, and seeds) rather than the refined or processed versions, you can be sure that you're consuming all the phytonutrients the food originally contained.

The following sections present some of the phytonutrients that have recently made news.

Carotenoids

Fruits and vegetables contain at least 500 known carotenoids, all members of a single family of phytonutrients. Carotenoids are also pigments — red, orange, and yellow. Carotenoids work together to provide the most dramatic benefits, a good reason to eat a variety of fruits and vegetables that can supply you with several kinds. Beta-carotene, a precursor to vitamin A and a carotenoid, is a useful vitamin supplement, but you still need the variety found in nature.

- **Beta-carotene:** Beta-carotene is an orange pigment and a potent antioxidant. It's prevalent in deep-orange foods such as apricots, broccoli, carrots, mangoes, oranges, pumpkin, sweet potatoes, and winter squash (see Figure 6-5). Green vegetables like kale are also an excellent source of beta-carotene, although the presence of this orange-colored nutrient is not evident. The chlorophyll covers it up. Because of its antioxidant activity, beta-carotene can help slow the effects of aging and protects against cataracts, stroke, angina, and heart disease. Beta-carotene also boosts immunity and fights off bacterial and viral infection. Check out Chapter 15 for a good carrot recipe.

Your body can more easily absorb the beta-carotene in a food if it has been lightly cooked.

- **Lutein and zeaxanthin:** Lutein and zeaxanthin are the carotenoids present in green foods, especially in dark, leafy greens. Southern cooking serves up ample helpings of these greens — collard greens, mustard greens, turnip greens, and kale, which has especially high amounts. However, spinach has even higher amounts of these two carotenoids. Studies show that eating these leafy green vegetables protects against various forms of cancer. These nutrients are retained in cooking and freezing. Other sources include red peppers, okra, romaine lettuce, parsley, dill, celery, and egg yolks.

The darker the green of the leaf, the more cancer-protective carotenoids it contains.

New research shows that a diet that provides lutein and zeaxanthin lowers the risk of age-related macular degeneration (AMD), a common cause of poor eyesight in older people. The yellow coloring in the *macula* (the circular area on the retina) is composed of these two pigments.

- **Lycopene:** Lycopene, another carotenoid, is a red pigment and an antioxidant. Along with its other carotenoid family members, lycopene slows aging, helps reduce the risk of heart disease, and is cancer-protective. Lycopene is heat stable and is not destroyed in canning. Foods that contain lycopene include red bell peppers, pink grapefruit, guava, apricots, watermelon, and tomatoes (see Figure 6-6). This next recipe gives you the chance to enjoy tomatoes broiled, the way the British serve them.

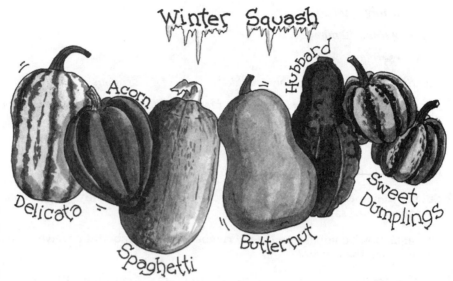

Figure 6-5:
Winter
squash.

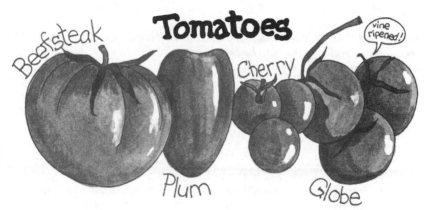

Figure 6-6:
Tomatoes.

English Breakfast Broiled Tomatoes

In London hotels, broiled tomatoes, a source of lycopene, are served for breakfast, along with eggs, kippers, sausages, beans, and fried bread. Try them at home with turkey sausage and whole-grain English muffins for simpler, healthier fare. Research shows that you benefit the most from tomatoes when you eat them cooked and with a little fat, as in this recipe.

(continued)

Preparation time: 10 minutes

Cooking time: 10 minutes

Yield: 4 servings

4 medium tomatoes, preferably organic	*1½ teaspoons dried thyme*
Sea salt and freshly ground black pepper to taste	*2 tablespoons unsalted melted butter or extra-virgin olive oil*
½ cup whole-grain bread crumbs*	*2 tablespoons flaxseed oil*

1 Preheat the broiler.

2 Cut the tomatoes in half crosswise. Place cut-side up in a lightly buttered baking dish. Season with sea salt and pepper.

3 In a small bowl, combine the bread crumbs, thyme, and butter or olive oil. Spread the mixture over the tomatoes.

4 Broil the tomatoes until softened and the tops are golden, about 10 minutes, 5 inches from the source of heat. Drizzle with flaxseed oil and season with salt and pepper. Serve immediately.

*You can make these tomatoes with the usual bread crumbs made from white bread, but this recipe gives you an excuse to begin buying the healthier whole-grain version. Look for Jaclyn's brand in natural-food stores.

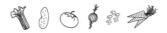

Flavonoids

Flavonoids are found in the pulp and pith of fruits and vegetables, so to benefit from these phytonutrients, you need to eat these foods in their whole form. The highest concentration is found in the fuzzy center of lemons. Other produce that contains flavonoids include onions and apples; beverages that contain them include green tea, black tea, and dark beer.

Flavonoids reduce inflammation and susceptibility to allergies and viruses. They also help protect against heart disease and stroke, helping to reduce the stickiness of blood platelets. And they help balance hormones. (Look at Chapter 17 on female health for more on this role of flavonoids, as well as phyto-estrogens, which also help normalize hormone levels.)

Flavonoids belong to a class of phytonutrients called *polyphenols,* which have been shown to lower cholesterol levels and reduce blood pressure. Polyphenols are present in red grapes and red wine, strawberries, blueberries, sweet potatoes, and artichokes. To sample some flavonoids, try the Fruity Flavonoid Syrup in Chapter 20.

When you eat a variety of colors, you consume a variety of nutrients

This wonderfully visual maxim makes sense in that many of the phytonutrients are also pigments, which determine the color of foods. When you shop, search out the yellow-orange vegetables and fruit for vitamin A, green vegetables for magnesium, and purplish red fruits for flavonoids. Assembling this palette also makes it easy to create gorgeous vegetable salads and fruit desserts.

Making Sure That You Eat a Variety of Fruits and Vegetables

Your health depends on taking in a wide range of vitamins and minerals. One of the best ways to ensure that you're giving your body what it needs is to eat a variety of fruits and vegetables. You may think that you're already eating quite a mix, but if you are typical of most Americans, you probably are not. In 1993, the U.S. consumption of potatoes was 132.7 pounds per person. Other standard vegetables were iceberg lettuce, tomatoes, onions, cucumbers, celery, carrots, corn, broccoli, and green cabbage. This is a start, but variety is limited. Of the fruits and vegetables on the following lists, which ones are you really eating regularly?

- **Fruit:** Apples, apricots, bananas, blackberries, blueberries, cantaloupe, cherimoyas (see Figure 6-7), currants, dates, grapefruit, grapes, kiwi, lemons, limes, mangoes, oranges, papaya, peaches, pears, pineapple, plantains, plums, raspberries, strawberries, tangerines, and watermelon

- **Vegetables:** Artichokes, asparagus, avocado, beets, broccoli, carrots, cabbage, cauliflower, celery, Chinese cabbage, collard greens, corn, green beans, jicama (see Figure 6-8), kale, lettuce (see Figure 6-9), mushrooms, onions, peas, peppers, potatoes, spinach (see Figure 6-9), sweet potatoes, tomatoes, turnip greens, watercress (see Figure 6-9), winter squash, and yams

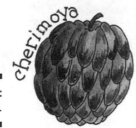

Figure 6-7:
Cherimoya.

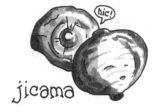

Figure 6-8:
Jicama.

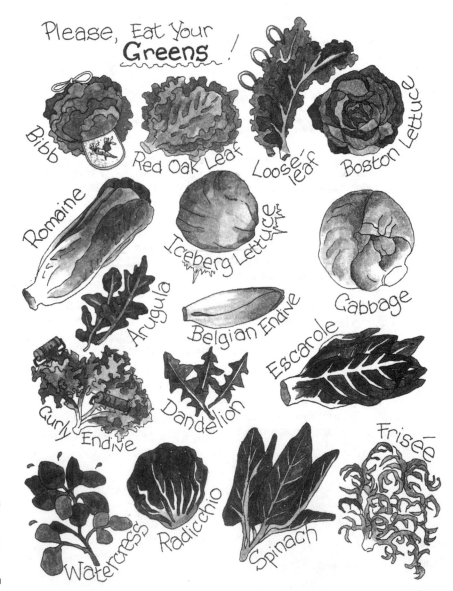

Figure 6-9:
Favorite
salad
greens.

If you are not particularly a vegetable eater, you may be surprised at how tasty vegetables can be when you cook them in novel and imaginative ways. Try these baked vegetables, a far cry from vegetables boiled in water!

Savory Baked Vegetables

Root vegetables take well to baking. Here they are seasoned with savory spices. This recipe calls for carrots and turnips, but you can also give potatoes, beets, and celery root a try. Walnuts and walnut oil add healing fats.

Preparation time: *15 minutes*

Cooking time: *55 minutes*

Yield: *4 servings*

4 carrots

4 turnips

¼ teaspoon grated nutmeg

⅛ teaspoon ground allspice

¼ cup walnut pieces

Sea salt and freshly ground black pepper to taste

8 shallots, in skins

1 tablespoon melted butter

1 tablespoon walnut oil

1 Preheat oven to 400°F.

2 With a sharp knife, cut the carrots and turnips lengthwise into quarters and then cut the quarter slices into 3-inch lengths.

3 In a small bowl, combine the nutmeg, allspice, walnuts, and sea salt and pepper.

4 Place the carrots, turnips, and shallots in a roasting pan and sprinkle with the spice-nut mixture. Drizzle with melted butter. With a spoon, turn the vegetables to coat them with the flavorings and butter.

5 Cover the roasting pan with foil and place in the preheated oven. Bake for 45 to 55 minutes, stirring occasionally, until the vegetables are brown and tender. Add the walnuts during the last 20 minutes of cooking.

6 Drizzle the cooked vegetables with walnut oil and serve immediately.

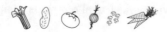

You can incorporate more fruit into your meals by adding such ingredients as prunes and apricots to meat stews or apples and pears to salads and by using spiced fruit as a condiment. Start with this tropical fruit salsa.

Mango Salsa Cha Cha Cha

This Caribbean version of Latin salsa starts with tropical fruit and ends with spices and hot pepper. Every ingredient in this condiment has a health benefit, strengthening immunity, stimulating circulation, and fighting cancer. And because of the wonderful flavors, this salsa can also keep you in good spirits!

Preparation time: 10 minutes

Cooking time: 1 hour

Yield: About 2 cups

1 mango, cut into small chunks	1 tablespoon finely chopped fresh ginger
¼ cup red onion, finely chopped	Juice of 1 lime or small lemon*
4 sprigs cilantro, leaves removed and finely chopped	¼ teaspoon hot pepper flakes

1 Place all the ingredients in a small bowl and gently combine them by using a wooden spoon.

2 To combine the flavors, refrigerate the salsa for 1 hour before serving. Serve with sautéed or grilled poultry, fish, or meat.

*I'm privileged to have three Meyer lemon trees in my backyard. These lemons are nearly as sweet as oranges. I tested this recipe by using a Meyer lemon, which added a lovely, soft flavor. Look for them in specialty produce stores.

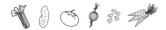

Some people hate chewing on a bunch of "grass" and scowl when they find lettuce on their hamburger. Even if you enjoy salads and relish a steamed artichoke or poached pears, increasing your intake of such foods may sound difficult. To help you do this, I've put together the following tips:

- **Treat yourself to the most luscious and appealing fruits,** such as fresh mangoes in season, fresh pineapple, figs, raspberries, or whatever catches your fancy, even if you have to pay a little more. You may simply be bored with your frugal offerings of apples and pears throughout the winter.

- **Poach a mix of dried apricots, apples, prunes, and figs** when the fresh harvest is meager and enjoy a bowlful of these flavors.

✔ **Keep frozen fruit, packaged fruit, or your own fruit on hand.** Freeze peaches and defrost them for dessert, garnished with fresh mint. Freeze a peeled banana and nibble on this like a Popsicle when the weather turns hot. For a variation, before freezing the peeled banana, you can also roll it in crushed nuts, gently pressing these into the fruit.

✔ **Enjoy fruit made into a sauce for pancakes.** (See Chapter 20, Fruity Flavonoid Syrup, for how to cook this sauce.)

✔ **Buy bags of precut mixed lettuces to jump-start salad making and eliminate excuses.** But only if the greens are organic. The usual packaged precut lettuces are treated with preservatives. Select mixes that contain a variety of greens — not just iceburg lettuce with a little grated carrot.

✔ **Give yourself a cheese and veggie pita-pocket sandwich** that has a shape well designed to hold a mixture of vegetables, such as avocado, cucumber, tomato, red onion, sprouts, and fresh herbs.

✔ **Double up on vegetables** when cooking them and steam several kinds together.

✔ **Discover the pleasures of vegetarian lasagna,** heavy on the eggplant, zucchini, and tomato and light on the cheese.

✔ **Bake several whole apples, beets, and sweet potatoes together** to save cooking time and then enjoy them with meals or as sweet snacks.

✔ **Buy baby carrots, which are very sweet, preferably organic, and eat them like candy.** Crunchy snacks like these are particularly satisfying.

"Peaches for sale, fresh corn"

Once when I was staying at my friend Beverly's house in upstate New York, we were in the front yard and tourists stopped us to find out where they could buy the fresh peaches and fresh corn they saw a sign for down the road. It was late November, and the farm stand that sold fresh produce in summer was long gone. I smugly thought, "These city slickers have forgotten that fruits and vegetables are seasonal!"

Of course, it's hard to remember that nature can only produce certain foods at certain times, because grocery stores now sell such a huge diversity of produce, carted in from other climates, year-round. The advantage of such availability is that you can eat more of a variety more months of the year. But to benefit most from fruits and vegetables ripened to perfection, with optimal flavor and nutrients, you need to eat these foods when they are in season.

✔ **Fall:** Persimmons, pomegranates, artichoke, squash, potatoes, and apples

✔ **Winter:** Celery root, rutabaga, and turnips

✔ **Spring:** Strawberries, asparagus, avocados, green beans, and fresh peas

✔ **Summer:** Peaches, nectarines, corn, zucchini, tomatoes, and melon

Fortunately, what's in season is often also the cheapest!

Onions and Garlic: Mediterranean Medicine

Onions, and their botanical cousin garlic, have a special status, in that they show up in probably more recipes than any other vegetables. They both have a long history of use as medicinals, and their benefits are now verified by modern science.

Garlic and onions, as well as shallots, leeks, scallions, and chives, contain the active compound *allicin.* This phytonutrient significantly lowers cholesterol, reduces the stickiness of blood, and widens blood vessels, helping to prevent heart disease and stroke. Allicin also enhances immunity, warding off bacterial and fungal infections as well as viruses. Cancerous cells are also a target; allicin helps deactivate carcinogenic substances.

Before you use garlic in cooking, be sure to crush it first and set it aside for 10 to 15 minutes to allow its healing properties to develop. Crushing releases the allicin and makes it available to you. Baked whole garlic, a darling of gourmet chefs, can't deliver this phytonutrient.

Onions are also packed with one of the most potent flavonoids, quercetin, which has the ability to reduce inflammation and counteract bacterial and viral infection. Quercetin is also an anticancer agent. Garlic helps fight cancer because it contains *saponins,* which inhibit DNA's ability to initiate replication of cancerous cells. Here's a delicious way to enjoy these healing foods.

Leafy Greens with Garlic

The flavors of garlic and onions stand up to the strong taste of dark leafy greens such as kale, turning these down-home vegetables into gourmet foods. Greens supply calcium and magnesium, both needed to maintain strong bones.

Preparation time: *10 minutes*

Cooking time: *25 minutes*

Yield: *4 servings*

2 cloves garlic

1 pound kale with stems under ¼ inch thick, washed with tough stems removed

1 tablespoon extra-virgin olive oil

4 shallots, peeled and finely chopped

¼ cup filtered water

Sea salt to taste

(continued)

1 Using the flat side of a knife, crush the garlic cloves and set aside for 15 minutes.

2 Cut the kale leaves down the middle and then crosswise into 1-inch strips.

3 In a large pot, heat the oil over medium heat. Add the garlic and shallots. Cook, stirring with a wooden spoon, for 15 seconds, to keep garlic and shallots from browning.

4 Add the water and sea salt. Bring mixture to boil. Add the greens, tossing to mix well. Cover the pot.

5 Steam the greens until they are just tender but retain a bright green color, about 5 to 7 minutes. Uncover the pot and continue cooking, stirring, until most of the water has evaporated and the greens are quite tender, about 3 minutes. Serve with roasted chicken and Wild Western Cornbread (see Chapter 19).

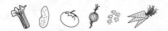

Snacking on Seaweeds: Veggies of the Sea

You may never have eaten seaweed, but I highly recommend it both as a gourmet food and as a terrific source of nutrients. Oceans are great repositories of minerals. Salty seawater contains calcium, magnesium, potassium, phosphorus, iron, sodium, and iodine. These minerals become part of the plants that grow in this water, making seaweed an exceptionally rich source of minerals.

Seaweed also provides B vitamins, including vitamin B12, which is predominantly found in animal foods. If you're a vegetarian, you may need this vitamin.

The following three sea vegetables, which are widely available in their dried form in Asian markets and specialty foods stores, have a mild, easy-to-like flavor. You can add any of these seaweeds to a soup or stew to increase its nutritional value, and no one will be the wiser.

- ✔ **Arama** in its natural state is a brown seaweed with large, tough leaves. To prepare it for market, producers parboil it, shred it, and then dry it. Like other seaweed, arama is usually sold in cellophane packages. The final product is long, black strands that look something like noodles (see Figure 6-10).

- ✔ **Dulse** is a seaweed with a European heritage, common to the British Isles and found in Canada and Maine. You can buy little containers of powdered dulse, which you can add to sandwiches or cooked dishes for a mineral boost.

✔ **Nori** is sold in paper-thin sheets and is used to wrap sushi (see Figure 6-10). To enjoy nori as a condiment or garnish, toast a sheet directly over heat for a few seconds. When it turns from black to green, it's ready to eat.

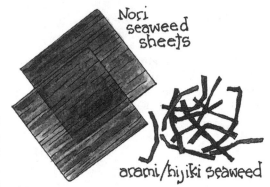

Figure 6-10:
Two types of
seaweed.

Taking Precautions When You Buy Nonorganic Produce

In Chapter 4, I explain why organic fruits and vegetables are healthier than conventionally raised produce. You really should be buying organic produce whenever you can, but when you don't, you can still remove a lot of the chemicals used in farming by following these procedures.

✔ **Before peeling and cutting most fruits and vegetables, wash and scrub them.** The exception to this rule is that you need to chop vegetables that have irregular surfaces, such as broccoli and cauliflower, before washing. You have several options of cleaning agents you can use. These may not remove all foreign substances, but can eliminate a significant amount.

   • Add a drop of mild dishwashing detergent to a pot of water and plunge produce into this solution. Rinse thoroughly with clean water.

   • You can also use a solution of white vinegar and water, 1 ounce to 1 quart of water, and soak the produce for 20 minutes.

- Add commercial grapefruit seed extract, sold in natural-food stores, to water and use this solution for rinsing.

- Rinse with the product Organiclean, which removes pesticides, chemicals, dirt, and other inorganic pollutants. Call 1-888-VEG-WASH or go to its Web site at www.organiclean.com.

Some chemicals are absorbed into the interior tissues of a plant and cannot be washed away.

✔ **Remove the outer leaves of lettuces and cabbage.**

✔ **Trim the top and leaves of celery.**

✔ **Peel all waxed fruits and vegetables.**

Chapter 7

Including Meats, Poultry, and Game in Your Diet

*M*eats and poultry certainly can have a place in a healthy diet. These foods are rich in B vitamins, which are essential for the production of energy and necessary for the normal functioning of the nervous system. Having healthy eyes, hair, and skin depends on adequate levels of the B vitamins.

Animal foods are also an excellent source of readily absorbable iron, which makes it possible for the blood to transport oxygen. Meats also contain zinc, a mineral with numerous functions, including the healing of wounds and burns. These foods are, of course, also an excellent source of protein — raw material for building body tissue.

That said, whether to eat meat and poultry is a highly charged subject these days. You may be concerned about residues of drugs and added hormones in these foods. The decision whether to eat animal foods is not as easy as it once was. And what constitutes top-quality meat and poultry is being redefined.

This chapter gives you the lowdown on all this and more, helping you determine how meat and poultry can fit into your own diet.

Getting Your Daily Protein from Animal Sources

How much protein from animal sources do you gobble up each day? Moderate portions are now the rule. The average person needs a total of about 65 g of protein a day. From animal sources, this is equivalent to one egg, one chicken leg, plus one hamburger patty the size of the palm of your hand. However, grains, beans, and other plant foods also supply protein, so if you're getting protein from plant foods, you need even less from animal sources.

The FDA's Food Guide Pyramid also recommends dainty portions of animal foods — two 3-ounce servings a day. This serving is the size of a pack of play-ing cards. One way to make the most of a small portion of meat is to top a salad with slices of meat, as in the following recipe.

Broiled Steak Salad with Roasted Red Peppers

A healthy diet can still include red meat if you consume it in smaller quantities than is customary in American cooking. A small amount of grilled steak is ample when served as the topping for a green salad, such as the one in this recipe.

Preparation time: *15 minutes*

Cooking time: *10 minutes*

Yield: *4 servings*

2 large sweet red peppers

½ medium head romaine lettuce

2 tablespoons extra-virgin olive oil

1 tablespoon balsamic vinegar

1 teaspoon soy sauce

2 cloves garlic, minced

Sea salt and freshly ground pepper to taste

1 tablespoon capers

1 pound beef sirloin, preferably organic and residuefree

1 Roast the red peppers by piercing each pepper with a fork and holding it directly over a burner. As sections crisp and darken, rotate the pepper until all sides are charred. Place them in a medium bowl and cover tightly, allowing them to steam off their skins for 15 minutes. Uncover and slip off the skins, cut the peppers in half vertically, and remove the core and seeds. Then cut the peppers into strips and set aside.

2 Tear the romaine lettuce into bite-sized pieces and set aside.

3 In a small bowl, whisk together the olive oil, vinegar, soy sauce, minced garlic, and capers. Season with salt and pepper.

4 In a large bowl, toss the romaine, roasted peppers, and dressing. Set aside.

5 Preheat the broiler.

6 Rub the steak with the remaining clove of garlic, halved. Put the meat on a grid fitted into a shallow baking pan. For a 1½-inch-thick steak, position the pan so that the steak is 3 inches from the heat source. Cook, about 7 minutes for rare and about 8 minutes for medium, total cooking time. Remove from the broiler and place on a wooden cutting board. Slice the steak across the grain (see Figure 7-1).

7 Arrange the dressed salad greens on individual serving plates and top with steak slices. Serve with fresh-baked whole-grain French bread and a glass of red wine.

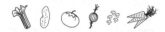

Cutting Across the Grain

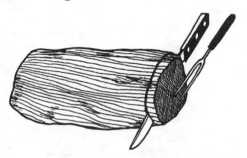

Figure 7-1: Cut across the grain to avoid shredding meat.

If you're like most Americans, you eat much more than 65 grams of protein a day. As much as 100 grams is common, High intake of animal protein, along with the fat it contains, has been linked to heart disease, and high protein consumption can be associated with osteoporosis. A higher intake of red meat in particular has been associated with a greater risk of colon, prostate, and possibly breast cancer. People with certain body types do better when they eat a lot of meat and other protein foods, but there is a healthy way to do this. Use grains and beans as a source of some of your daily protein, and eat more poultry and fish and less red meat. It's also smart to know how different cuts of meat compare in terms of fat. For more on this, take a look at the following section.

Bidding a Fond Farewell to Marbled Meat and Lamb Roast Trimmings

Fat is a flavor carrier, so lean meat isn't as tasty as a fat-streaked center cut. But it's prudent to cut back on animal fats, which are saturated and solid at room temperature, because research shows that eating these fats can raise your cholesterol levels and clog your arteries, leading to heart disease.

Table 7-1 shows you how various meats and poultry compare in terms of calories, total fat, saturated fat, and cholesterol.

Table 7-1	Comparing Types of Meat and Poultry			
3-Ounce Portion	*Calories*	*Total Fat*	*Saturated Fat*	*Cholesterol*
Beef round	164	6.6 g	2.8 g	69 mg
Chicken dark meat	174	8.3 g	2.3 g	79 mg
Chicken light meat	147	3.8 g	1.1 g	72 mg
Lamb leg	162	6.6 g	2.4 g	76 mg
Pork loin chop	171	6.9 g	2.5 g	70 mg
Turkey dark meat	158	6.1 g	2.1 g	72 mg
Turkey light meat	133	2.7 g	.9 g	59 mg

If you're a calorie counter, be forewarned that these standard figures for fat content refer to portion samples that have been cooked and trimmed of fat with great precision. When you cook these meats, you may cut away some excess fat, but bits remain here and there. And the chicken and turkey figures refer to poultry without skin.

Selecting the Kindest Cuts of Meat

One easy way to cut fat from your diet is to buy the leanest cuts of meat. The leanest beef is labeled Select grade, followed by Choice, and then Prime, which has the most marbling. (If the grade is not listed, it can be any of these, so make sure to ask the butcher.)

Eating meat in the good old days

Meat was a regular part of the early human diet. By the time hunter-gatherer societies appeared 40,000 to 10,000 years ago, researchers estimate that the diet consisted of about 33 percent protein, much of which came from animal foods. And in the twentieth century, many native peoples thrived on diets in which animal foods predominated. As recently as the 1930s, Indians living in the far north of Canada in the winter months had a diet almost entirely limited to wild animals.

If eating a lot of animal foods was good enough for them, why not you?

- First, animals in the wild were far leaner and contained more of the healthful polyunsaturated fats and less saturated fat than today's commercially raised meats.

- Second, people ate virtually the entire animal, including the organs, which are extremely high in nutrients. The adrenal glands provide vitamin C, and the tissues near the eye are very high in vitamin A. Scottish haggis, a mixture of organ meats, oatmeal, and spices fitted into the lining of a sheep's stomach and cooked, was considered fine fare — noble sustenance for Scottish clansmen and warriors. We prefer to eat cuts of muscle tissue such as steaks, which are high in protein but not as rich in nutrients.

- Third, we don't need as much protein and fat because we have a more sedentary lifestyle — unless you spend your days kayaking as you hunt seal for dinner.

The following cuts are lower in fat:

- **Beef:** Sirloin, top loin, round steak
- **Pork:** Tenderloin, boneless sirloin chop, boneless loin roast, boneless top loin chop, pork loin chop

None of these cuts has more fat than a typical chicken leg. But common beef cuts, such as tenderloin, have twice as much fat as beef round. Pork boneless rib roast has twice the fat of pork tenderloin — which is a pricey cut that's not commonly eaten.

Milwaukee Pork Chops with Cabbage

If you're hungry for meat, pork is a good choice because it's lower in saturated fat than beef. In this recipe, you prepare it with lots of vegetables. Enjoy this casserole with mashed Yukon Gold potatoes, and you have a splendid meal with meat and vegetables in proper proportion.

(continued)

Preparation time: *15 minutes*

Cooking time: *1 hour, 20 minutes*

Yield: *4 servings*

2 teaspoons extra-virgin olive oil or unrefined safflower oil

4 center-cut pork chops, trimmed of fat

Sea salt and freshly ground black pepper to taste

2 tablespoons apple cider vinegar

12-ounce bottle nonalcoholic beer (mild flavored)

1 cup apple juice

½ pound red cabbage, thinly sliced

2 cloves garlic, minced

½ teaspoon dried sage

1 apple, peeled if not organic, coarsely grated

1 medium white potato, coarsely grated

1 Preheat oven to 350°.

2 Heat the oil in a large pan over medium-high heat. Add the pork chops, seasoned with salt and pepper, and cook until well-browned, about 4 minutes per side. Remove the chops and set aside.

3 Add the vinegar, beer, and apple juice to the skillet. With a spatula, and over medium heat, loosen the browned bits of food on the bottom of the pan. Set aside.

4 In a casserole with a tight-fitting lid, put ⅓ of the cabbage, garlic, and sage. Then arrange a layer of pork chops. Cover with the grated apple, followed by a layer of ½ the remaining cabbage and then a layer of the potato. Top with the remaining cabbage.

5 Pour in the vinegar, beer, and apple juice.

6 Cover the casserole and bake for 45 minutes. Uncover and continue to bake for 15 to 20 minutes.

7 Remove from oven. On a heated serving platter, arrange the cabbage mixture and top with the pork chops. Season with sea salt and pepper to taste. Serve immediately with grainy mustard and pickles.

Note: *Some pork carries the parasite trichinosis, so pork traditionally is served only well done. But researchers have discovered that the parasite is killed at 137°. The USDA now recommends that pork be cooked to an internal temperature of 160°, or "medium." The meat will have traces of pink and still be juicy.*

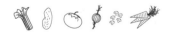

Deli delights

If you want a meat sandwich, the healthiest way to make one is to slice some meat off a roast and go from there. Most luncheon meats are a poor substitute. Those made from ground chicken or turkey, which may contain skin and a variety of poultry parts in the mixture, can have fivefold the fat content. And if you buy the many lowfat versions now on the market, there's still the added sodium, the sugars sometimes added to sweeten the meat (as in honey-roasted), and the nitrates used as preservatives, which can convert to carcinogenic compounds.

But you have other options: uncured ham and salami, chicken bologna, breast of turkey free of chemicals, prosciutto without nitrates and more. Several brands (see Chapter 4) now offer such items, made of meat from naturally raised animals and free of nitrates, nitrites, sugar, and artificial flavors. Look for these deli meats at your local natural-food store, and if they don't carry such items, suggest that they do!

Because such meats do not contain artificial preservatives, they stay fresh for only up to three days. So if you don't plan to quickly use what you've bought, you'll need to freeze the meat until you are ready to eat it.

Light and dark meat poultry also vary significantly in fat content, as Table 7-1 shows. A chicken leg contains more fat than a chicken breast; the thigh contains twice as much as the leg; and the back is even fattier than the thigh.

If you want juicier chicken, cook it with the skin on. The skin holds the moisture in the meat, just like a lid on a pot keeps water inside from boiling away. Don't worry; fat from the skin does not migrate into the meat. Just remove the skin before eating the chicken.

Shopping for Clean Protein

Conventionally raised cattle are treated more like meat products than animals, even before they are brought to slaughter. They are routinely injected with antibiotics, and they're sprayed with insecticides. Growth hormones to shorten the time it takes to ready them for market are injected into the animals or added to the feed. And the cattle are fed in crowded and stressful feedyards.

Would you eat your car's oil filter?

Even if you opt for conventionally raised meat and poultry, the one cut of meat that you must eat in its most natural and unadulterated form is liver. Like the filter in your car engine, the liver filters the blood. For this reason, liver tissue has far higher levels of accumulated toxins than other cuts of meat. Unless you want a concentrated dose of all these chemicals for dinner, only eat liver from animals that were raised without hormones or antibiotics and, even better, raised on organic feed.

If you don't have a source of organic liver, a way to remove a significant amount of toxins from the meat is to cut the liver in strips and soak them in whole milk overnight. Then rinse the meat before cooking it and throw away the milk. Calves' liver is preferable to beef liver.

The war over what practices are permissible in the raising of animals for consumption is being waged internationally. When countries refuse to let certain animal products into their markets because of health concerns, should you also use caution and not bring those foods into your home? Here are some of the issues:

- ✔ **Cattle are fed growth-stimulating hormones to bring them to market at a targeted weight well before their naturally raised brethren.** Scientists question whether eating meat that contains residues of these hormones interferes with your own hormone function.

- ✔ **Cattle may be fed the female hormone estrogen to fatten them for market.** Consuming this estrogen, coupled with the many estrogenlike compounds you may absorb from a variety of environmental toxins, may be enough to upset your hormone balance. Elevated levels of estrogen are associated with breast cancer.

- ✔ **Cattle and poultry routinely receive antibiotics, either given by injection or incorporated into their feed in small doses.** The drugs are meant to prevent diseases that readily develop in the factory settings in which the animals are raised. But there's concern that consuming these same antibiotics in meats may lower your resistance to bacterial infection. People who are at risk include women on birth control pills, people taking prescription medications, and people who have immune deficiencies.

- ✔ **Cattle raisers have developed the practice of adding meat products to cattle feed.** This practice has caused alarm because cattle are herbivores, not carnivores, by nature. In addition, cows in England were fed diseased organ meat, triggering the outbreak of "mad cow disease," which impairs the central nervous system.

> ✔ **On the environmental front, raising animal protein requires enormous amounts of land and water as compared to raising plant sources of protein.** People question whether the planet can sustain the production of animal foods to feed the rapidly growing population.

Much is at stake (pardon the pun!), both financially and in terms of health. One way to play it safe, before the results of further research have been tallied, is to begin buying what is known as *clean protein*.

Meats and poultry that have been to some degree naturally raised are beginning to show up in many supermarkets as demand for these products grows. The store at which you shop may already carry free-range chicken or beef without added hormones. Being familiar with the meanings of the different terms helps you search out higher-quality foods (and if your butcher needs educating, you can be the one to provide the information!):

✔ **Natural:** The USDA definition of natural refers only to how the meat is processed. A meat product labeled natural contains no artificial preservatives, colorings, or flavors.

  In some markets, the label natural means much more: At the time of slaughter, the animal contained no traces of artificial growth hormones or antibiotics. However, in some brands, the animals may have received these chemicals at some point in their lives. But any claims that a chicken is free of hormones has little meaning. Giving hormones to chickens is illegal.

✔ **Residuefree:** This term means the same thing as *natural*. A residuefree chicken, for example, has no traces of antibiotics.

✔ **Nitratefree:** Curing bacon requires the use of nitrates, which are potentially carcinogenic. Natural-food stores carry brands of nitratefree, uncured bacon, which is as tasty as cured bacon.

✔ **Organic:** Until national standards for organic meat go into effect, meat cannot be labeled organic. You can, however, ask at your store's meat counter for brands from companies that are known to raise animals on organic feed. Such feed is free of pesticides and herbicides. Some producers also prohibit chlorinated drinking water.

✔ **Free-range:** Meat labeled free range comes from animals that roamed and grazed freely, living in stressfree conditions. Such meat is tender. A stressed animal produces adrenaline, the major stress hormone, which turns into sugar that darkens and toughens the meat. Free-range meat is also lower in fat.

✔ **Humanely raised:** Meat labeled humanely raised comes from animals that lived in spacious barns or paddocks, not in Dickensian factory conditions.

✔ **Kosher:** *Kosher* refers to how an animal was killed (salt is used to remove the blood), but this label gives no information about what the animals were fed or whether they received drugs or hormones.

Veal: Not a pretty picture

Think twice before you buy veal or order veal scaloppini in a restaurant, for health reasons *and* humane reasons. Commercial veal, the meat of calves, can contain a variety of medications. The reason is that these creatures live their lives until slaughter chained in tiny crates — breeding grounds for disease. The calves are also kept anemic so that the final product is pale and light-colored. "Milk-fed" veal does not mean that their mothers suckle the calves!

Pacific Pastures brand of veal, approved by the Humane Farming Association, offers flavorful, pink-colored meat from calves raised naturally.

Although these terms can tell you a lot about what you're buying, the safest bet is to buy reputable brands. Certain companies define themselves by how clean their products are. Look for these brands:

✔ **Beeler's, producers of naturally raised pork:** Bee Lor Inc., 235 Oak Street, Brunsville, IA 51008; 712-533-6042; beelers95@aol.com

✔ **Coleman Natural Beef:** 5140 Race Ct., Denver, CO 80216; 800-442-8666

✔ **Fresh Australian Range Lamb:** For information on ordering, contact the Australian Meat & Live-Stock Corporation, 750 Lexington Avenue, 17th floor, New York, NY 10022; 212-486-2405; www.amlc.com

✔ **Jamar Foods:** Distributor of meats and poultry raised naturally, without chemicals, pesticides, or hormones (beef, pork, lamb, buffalo, organic ostrich, chicken, turkey, duck); Floral Park, NY 11001; 800-597-8325; fax 516-488-3432

✔ **Petaluma Poultry Processors, producers of Rocky the Range Chicken and Rocky Junior:** 2700 Lakeville Hwy., Petaluma, CA 94954; 707-763-1904

✔ **Shelton's, producers of chicken and turkey:** 204 North Loranne Ave., Pomona, CA 91767; 714-623-4361

Winning with Game

Add variety to your diet by eating some game once in a while — quail, pheasant, wood pigeon or squab, rabbit, venison, buffalo, or ostrich. Upper-end supermarkets and some natural-food stores stock these foods, and they even show up at farmers markets. If you have a gourmet supermarket or butcher in your city, you may be able to special-order elk, wild boar, and alligator. (I once needed 2 quarts of elk broth to do some professional recipe testing, and Bristol Farms in Los Angeles obliged with the elk. They even had buffalo, on sale!) And if you have a sudden craving for emu (a large, flightless bird that runs very fast and is native to Australia), you can contact the American Emu Association at 214-559-2321.

You can substitute rabbit for chicken in any recipe. You can also make a very acceptable curry dish by using buffalo — I speak from experience!

Game is an excellent source of nutrients and lower in fat than most meats. Take a look at these comparisons.

- ✔ Most 3-ounce servings of cooked game contain 130 to 175 calories and only 2 to 5 g of fat, which is generally lower than in standard meats.

- ✔ Game contains about the same amount of cholesterol as other meats.

- ✔ Game contains a higher percentage of polyunsaturated fats, especially the omega-3 fatty acids, than most red meats because of the wild foods the animals eat. The omega-3s support the health of tissues throughout the body.

- ✔ Compared to other meats, game birds contain significantly more thiamin, vitamin B6, vitamin B12, calcium, phosphorous, potassium, and iron.

- ✔ The breast meat of one breed of duck, White Pekin, is lower in fat than chicken breast if you don't eat the skin — but who can resist?

Commercially produced game may be given hormones and drugs just like herds of cattle and sheep are. Your butcher should be able to tell you how the game you're buying was raised.

Deciding Not to Eat Meat

As of 1995, more than 12 million Americans ate a vegetarian diet — double the number of ten years prior. A vegetarian diet can provide ample protein, as well as healthy fats and carbohydrates. In fact, most vegetables have about an ideal ratio of protein, carbohydrates, and fat, so it is possible to have rosy cheeks and plenty of stamina without eating meat. But living on salads and pizza isn't the way to go. Certain guidelines are important to follow.

- ✔ **Plan your meals carefully.** Plan your meals with considerable care to ensure that you receive the full range of essential amino acids that make up protein. Your meals also need to supply the right mix of fats and all the various vitamins and minerals that support health. (Take a look at Chapter 5, about combining beans and grains to make a complete protein.)

✔ **Remember that cheese isn't a main course.** Vegetarians who are hungry for fat often substitute dairy foods full of saturated fat for the meat and poultry they're not eating. To satisfy your need for fat, increase your intake of nuts, seeds, and healthful unrefined oils instead. Then use cheese as a flavorful condiment.

For example, for lunch, have a whole-grain pita pocket filled with vegetables and spicy hummus (see the recipe Chickpeas in Disguise in Chapter 24) or a bowl of chili with whole-grain garlic bread and a green salad. For dinner, savor lasagna laced with walnuts and ricotta, or have a plateful of New Orleans-style red beans and rice, with okra (see the recipe Quick and Easy Cajun Okra in Chapter 18) on the side.

You can always be a vegetarian for just a few days a week. Load up on vegetables, fruit, whole grains, and beans on some days, and on the other days have your meat or poultry of choice. This sort of semi-vegetarian diet is characteristic of native diets in Mediterranean countries where degenerative diseases are far less common than in the United States. In Asia, too, the same association has been found. In areas where individuals typically ate only small amounts of meat and virtually no dairy foods, the incidence of heart disease and cancer were relatively low.

A little bit of meat can go a long way when you skewer it. Combine this with several vegetable and bean side dishes and you have a feast, with only a modest amount of meat. Try this lamb dish for starters.

Greek Lemon Lamb

A spear holding chunks of broiled lamb is the perfect complement to the many vegetable-based side dishes typical of traditional Greek cooking. Begin with a bowl of lentil soup and serve the kebabs with Turkish Buckwheat Salad (see Chapter 17), cucumbers in yogurt, and stuffed grape leaves. You can enjoy the flavors of the savory lamb, while vegetables, grains, and legumes make up the majority of the meal.

Preparation time: *10 minutes*

Cooking time: *1 hour for marinating, plus 10 minutes for broiling*

Yield: *8 servings of 1 skewer each*

8 skewers, wood or metal, at least 10 inches long

¼ cup dry white wine

Grated zest and juice of 1 organic lemon

2 tablespoons extra-virgin olive oil

3 cloves garlic, minced

6 dried bay leaves

2 tablespoons fresh, finely chopped oregano

¼ teaspoon freshly ground black pepper

1½ pounds boned leg of lamb, well trimmed, cut into 32 1½-inch cubes

1 large onion, cut into 8 wedges

1 Combine the wine, lemon zest and juice, oil, garlic, bay leaves, oregano, and pepper in a shallow glass dish. Mix well.

2 Add the lamb to the marinade and stir to coat each piece evenly. Cover the dish and refrigerate for at least 1 hour. Stir the lamb once while marinating.

3 Preheat the broiler. Line the broiler pan with foil and insert the broiler rack.

4 On each skewer, in this order, thread 4 chunks of lamb, 1 marinated bay leaf, and 1 wedge of onion.

5 Place the lamb skewers on the rack in the broiler pan, positioned 3 to 5 inches from the source of heat. Broil for about 10 minutes, turning the skewers frequently.

6 Transfer to a warm serving platter and garnish with lemon wedges.

Chapter 8

Saving a Place for Seafood

· ·

In This Chapter

▶ Boning up on minerals and vitamins in seafood

▶ Praising fatty fish

▶ Cracking open the benefits of shellfish

▶ Avoiding tainted fish

▶ Choosing quality seafood

Recipes in This Chapter

▶ Sardine Tapenade
▶ Flounder with Flavor

· ·

*F*ish and shellfish are healing foods; fish and shellfish are corrupted foods. It all depends upon what type of seafood you're talking about. The quality varies depending on the waters the fish inhabits. How seafood is handled after harvesting — and how you decide to cook it — also affects how healthy it is for you.

Seafood is an excellent source of minerals and vitamins. Fish that are native to cold waters are especially high in essential fatty acids that are healing and heart-healthy. However, fish and shellfish can also carry natural toxins and microbes, as well as industrial pollutants and toxic metals. Seafood spoils easily once it's out of the water. And when seafood is deep-fried, it turns into junk food because of the cooking fats it absorbs.

All this may sound like reason enough to swear off fish for the rest of your life. However, these worries about seafood are no reason to avoid it. You just need to find out which fish are safest to eat and the best ways to handle and prepare them.

In this chapter, I tell you all the basics you need to know to make fish and shellfish a part of your healing foods diet. You find out about the many nutrients these foods contain and why they are good for you. Then I give you simple guidelines for buying whole fish and filets. You also become savvy about how to avoid eating tainted or spoiled seafood.

As part of a healing foods diet, high-quality fish and shellfish belong on your menu two or three times a week.

Giving High Marks to Seafood for Nutrition

Food from the sea is a more reliable source of minerals than food grown on the land because as farmland is overworked, minerals are depleted from the soil. The oceans, however, are still an abundant source of many major and trace minerals. Seafood such as cod, ocean perch, and lobster, to name just a few, supply calcium, copper, iodine, iron, magnesium, manganese, phosphorous, potassium, and zinc. In canned salmon and canned sardines, the bones are edible, making canned fish a particularly good source of calcium. These many minerals contributes to the structure of bones, nourishes the blood, and participates in thousands of chemical reactions throughout the body.

Seafood also contains a range of B vitamins, and the oilier fish, such as salmon and tuna, are good sources of the two fat-soluble vitamins, vitamin A, and vitamin D. Herring and mackerel also contain vitamin E. When you choose to make a meal of seafood, your calories are well spent.

Speaking of calories, fish is not a fattening food, with many types of fish — such as turbot, bluefish, striped bass, pompano, and oysters — being relatively low in fat. In addition, fish is low in saturated fats, which are associated with heart disease, and high in the healthier polyunsaturated fats, such as the omega-3 essential fatty acids.

Fishing for your omega-3s

Omega-3 fatty acids are not the kind of fats that thicken your waistline. They are workhorses. Omega-3 fatty acids are found in abundance in the tissues of the brain, the nervous system, the eyes, and the sex and adrenal glands. They transport oxygen, remove cholesterol from arteries, prevent blood clots from forming, and lower blood pressure. And omega-3 fatty acids are anti-inflammatory. Studies show that fish oils reduce the swelling and pain associated with joint diseases such as arthritis and rheumatoid arthritis. In animal studies, omega-3s have even been associated with a reduced incidence of cancer.

The fattier a fish, the more omega-3 essential fatty acids it contains. Fish that are high in omega-3s are cold-water creatures that depend on these fats to keep from freezing. Although fish are able to manufacture these fats, they take in a significant amount through diet. Because fat is a flavor carrier, these fish cook up into tasty, satisfying meals. (Sample the Poached Salmon and Cucumbers in Chapter 3 and see for yourself.)

Caviar (fish eggs) is exceptionally high in omega-3s, but the following fish also deliver ample amounts — see Figure 8-1.

Farm-raised fish

Twenty percent of seafood for sale is farm-raised, and more and more kinds of seafood are being cultivated. Four species make up about 80 percent of the crop — catfish, crayfish, trout, and salmon — but hybrid striped bass, tilapia, abalone, sturgeon, shrimp, oysters, and clams are also farmed. In fact, the only trout available on the market is farmed. If you want to savor the remarkable flavor of fresh-caught rainbow trout, you have to get out your fishing pole.

Farm-raised fish is harvested when there's a buyer, so it's likely to be very fresh. Such fish is brought to market when it's younger, which is good for profits. This practice also limits the fish's exposure to any toxins that may be in the water.

However, fish farms are sometimes sited on old agricultural land. Pesticides once used on crops and still present in the surrounding soil can make their way into the fishponds via runoff waters. In addition, the water they inhabit may be treated with herbicides and disinfectants, and the fish may be given drugs to prevent or treat disease. Farm-raised fish, which are fed a special diet, may also be lower in omega-3 fatty acids than their wild counterparts.

Eating farm-raised fish is far better than eating no fish at all, but most fish that live in the wild are usually a healthier choice.

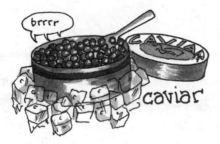

Figure 8-1:
Caviar is high in omega-3s.

✔ Anchovies

✔ Herring

✔ Kippers (little smoked herrings)

✔ Mackerel

✔ Salmon (see Figure 8-2)

✔ Sardines (see Figure 8-3)

✔ Tuna

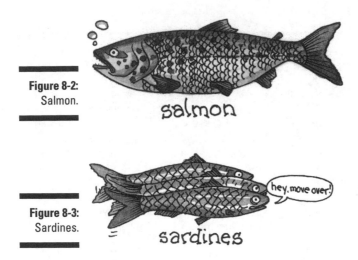

Figure 8-2:
Salmon.

salmon

Figure 8-3:
Sardines.

hey, move over!

sardines

Sardines are a common fish in Europe, where they are eaten in many forms. Sardines are mixed with olives and capers and made into a spread or *tapenade,* a classic provencal mixture of wonderfully salty foods. If this mixture seems odd to you, please give the following recipe a try. Tapenade is just what a slice of French bread is waiting for!

Sardine Tapenade

You can increase your intake of mineral-rich seafood and the healthy oils it contains with this tapenade. This dish originates from the Provence region of southern France, where the Mediterranean sun shines nearly everyday. It is a thick paste that's usually made with the ripe olives of the region, flavored with anchovies, capers, and lemons, and sometimes it includes tuna. This tapenade reverses the ratio and starts with sardines, adding the other ingredients for flavor.

Preparation time: 10 minutes

Cooking time: 5 minutes

Yield: 2 cups

3 4.5-ounce cans water-packed sardines, drained*

½ cup black olives, pitted, preferably marinated

½ cup grated red onion

1½ heaping teaspoon capers

2 anchovies, cut into pieces

1 tablespoon lemon juice

¼ teaspoon herbes de Provence (optional)

1 Drain the sardines and put them in a food processor fitted with a steel blade. Add the black olives, onion, capers, anchovies, lemon juice, and herbs. Process until smooth and light.

2 Serve in a ramekin and accompany with crackers or country-style bread.

*Using fresh sardines is even more nutritious, but one advantage of canned sardines is that the calcium-rich fish bones are quite edible.

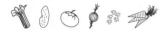

Giving a thumbs-up to shellfish

Yes, shrimp contains more cholesterol than beef. However, shrimp contains very little fat, and the little fat it does contain is predominantly unsaturated, including the heart-healthy omega-3 fatty acids. Because evidence now shows that saturated fat and oxidized cholesterol, rather than simply cholesterol, are prime factors in heart disease, shrimp no longer deserves to be black-listed. Shrimp can be part of a healthy diet if you add it to fish stews or sauté it in its shell and eat it in moderation. (Deep-fried shrimp, of course, is the exception.) Why not enjoy Garlic Shrimp (Chapter 16) tonight for dinner?

Other kinds of shellfish, such as crab and scallops, contain close to the lower levels of cholesterol found in chicken as compared with beef. Enjoy these foods for their unique flavors and high mineral content. Shellfish, in particular, contains *selenium,* a trace mineral that is considered an antioxidant and slows aging.

If you're timid about preparing shellfish at home, shellfish is a good choice when you're eating out, as long as it's not served deep-fried.

Protecting Yourself against Seafood Poisoning

Seafood spoils easily, supporting the growth of common bacteria that can induce symptoms such as queasiness, nausea, vomiting, and diarrhea. Buying fish from a reputable source and knowing how to care for fish after it's in your hands usually protects you from these bacteria.

When you go shopping, always buy your fish last and then go right home and immediately place it in the refrigerator. If you can, have the fish the same night for dinner. Or, if you're going to eat it in the next day or two, store it at 39°F. Keep the fish in a container with a lid so that its odor does not affect the flavor of other foods with which it is stored. You can also keep fish directly on ice if drainage is sufficient to prevent the fish from soaking up water (see Figure 8-4). However, use fish as soon as possible. Fish dries out quickly, destroying the flavor and texture.

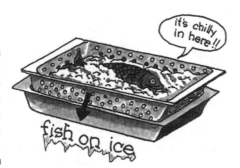

Figure 8-4: Store your fish on ice and use it as soon as possible.

Avoiding Fish from Polluted Waters

Although seafood incorporates the healthful minerals of the sea, it also absorbs pollutants in the water. Industrial waste can work its way into streams, lakes, and coastal waters. These wastes may contain such toxins as the pesticides dioxin and DDT, PCBs (polychlorinated biphenols), and such toxic metals as arsenic, cadmium, lead, and mercury. Exposure to toxic metals can cause medical problems ranging from kidney damage to problems of the nervous system, impaired mental development, and cancer.

Striped bass and bluefish frequently carry PCBs, and catfish and carp often contain contaminants. Swordfish and shark frequently contain mercury above allowable levels. Pregnant women in particular need to avoid these fish, as fetuses are especially vulnerable to this toxic mineral. These fish do have a most satisfying, meaty texture. If you do enjoy eating swordfish and shark, do this just every few months and no more.

So what's left? Many kinds of fish, if you follow these guidelines:

✔ **Eat a variety of fish and shellfish.** You're likely to eat some that are more free of toxins than others.

✔ **Eat smaller fish, which are lower on the food chain or younger than their big brothers and have not had the opportunity to absorb as many pollutants.** (The tuna in cans comes from smaller tunas.)

✔ **Select fish that have habitats offshore, which are the safest.** Next are fish that live nearshore, and last are freshwater fish, caught in lakes and streams. Table 8-1 tells you which common fish come from which habitats.

Table 8-1	Fish That Belong on Your Dinner Plate	
Offshore	*Nearshore*	*Freshwater*
Albacore tuna	Chum salmon	Freshwater bass
Cod	Herring	Lake whitefish
Flounder	Pink salmon	White perch
Haddock	Sardines	Yellow perch
Ocean perch	Sockeye salmon	
Pacific halibut		
Pollack		
Sole		
Yellowfin tuna		

Stay up to date on which fish are health risks. The FDA has initiated a useful Seafood Hotline (800-FDA-4010) that gives information about seafood nutrition and safety. You can also obtain information from the FDA Web site: www.fda.gov. Click Foods and then click Seafood.

Buying Quality Fish

The best place to buy fresh seafood is a dedicated fish store. If you're accustomed to picking up a package of fish from the refrigerated case at your supermarket, treat yourself to a visit to a shop specializing in fish — often a visual treat with all the silver and coral-toned creatures laid out on ice for your review. You can probably find a wider range of fish for sale, and your salesperson can be of help in selecting seafood and guiding you on how to prepare it safely.

In ethnic neighborhoods, you may find shops that sell seafood from displays on the sidewalk, or even from the back of a truck. Don't be tempted. It's not worth the risk to your health.

Here are some general guidelines for buying fish:

- A fish store should not smell like the beach when the tide is out. You should notice a cool, moist freshness to the air, like after a rain, but no smell of fish.

- The fish itself may smell faintly of the sea, but you should not detect a sour or ammonialike odor, which would indicate the growth of bacteria.

- The flesh should bounce back when you gently press the body of the fish with your finger. You don't want the impression of your finger to remain.

- Avoid fish that is displayed directly under very bright display lights, which generate heat.

The plentiful omega-3 fatty acids in fish are very fragile and can easily deteriorate over time and when fish is mishandled. The best quality fish is seafood that is fresh-caught. The next best is fish that is cleaned, processed, and quick-frozen aboard ship within hours of catching. (Avoid "fresh" fish that was previously frozen, and frozen fish that was once fresh but didn't sell — retailers' tricks.) If you do buy frozen fish, look for solidly frozen, tightly wrapped packages free of ice buildup.

Selecting whole fish

You can be smart about shopping for whole fish. Just keep these guidelines in mind.

- Whole fish should be lying on a bed of ice chips as well as covered with chips of ice.

- The skin of the fish you intend to purchase should reflect light. The slightly slimy surface should have a brightness to it.

- The gills of the fish should be a healthy bright pink or red — not green, brown, or gray.

- The scales of the fish should not be sticky or slimy.

- The old rule of a fresh fish having clear eyes is not necessarily true. Some fish remain clear-eyed for weeks, well after they are no longer fit to be eaten. This is true of trout, which loses its flavor long before its eyes cloud.

Selecting fish steaks and filets

Here's what to look for when you're selecting a piece of fish. Be savvy and avoid buying fish that's less than fresh.

- ✔ Select fish steaks and filets, especially tuna steaks, that have been precut and prewrapped. Filets on display may be more attractive, but prepackaging keeps the fish very fresh.

- ✔ Filets of fish on display should be laid directly on ice, but not covered with ice. As the ice on top of the fish melts, the water seeps into the filets and leaches out the flavor.

- ✔ The flesh of a filet should be luminous and translucent so that you can almost see below the surface.

- ✔ If a fish is naturally white, the filet should be white. Any pink is usually a sign of bruising.

Filets of fish need not be boring. You can dress them up with tantalizing seasonings, such as those in this recipe.

Flounder with Flavor

If you want to eat more fish, treat an everyday filet such as flounder to this exotic Yucatan-style sauce.

Preparation time: *15 minutes*

Cooking time: *10 minutes, plus 30 minutes for marinating*

Yield: *4 servings*

1½ pounds flounder filets

6 cloves garlic, crushed

¼ teaspoon ground cumin

½ teaspoon oregano

1 teaspoon achiote (in English, annatto), ground*

3 tablespoons orange juice

2 tablespoons lime juice

Sea salt and freshly ground black pepper to taste

3 tablespoons extra-virgin olive oil

1 medium yellow onion, sliced thin

1 medium red bell pepper, seeded and sliced

1 small fresh hot pepper, seeded and chopped

1 tomato, sliced

2 tablespoons chopped parsley

(continued)

1 Place the filets on a platter in a single layer.

2 In a bowl, put 4 of the garlic cloves and the cumin, oregano, achiote, orange juice, lime juice, and sea salt and pepper. Mix the ingredients into a thin paste.

3 Using a pastry brush, coat the filets on both sides with the spice mixture. Let stand for 30 minutes to marinate.

4 In the meantime, in a medium skillet, heat 2 tablespoons olive oil over medium-high heat. Sauté the onion, bell pepper, and hot pepper to begin to soften the vegetables, about 5 minutes. Add the tomato and cook for another 2 to 3 minutes. Set aside.

5 Coat the bottom of a shallow baking dish with the remaining tablespoon of olive oil. Arrange the marinated fish fillets evenly in the dish, adding any remaining marinade. Top the flounder with the sautéed vegetables and drizzle the remaining oil over the vegetables.

6 Bake at 400°, covered with foil, until the fish flesh is opaque, about 10 minutes. Transfer to warmed, individual serving plates. Garnish each serving with a sprinkled stripe of chopped parsley. Suggested accompaniments include guacamole, stewed pinto beans with garlic, and corn tortillas.

* Achiote, the seeds of a small tropical tree, have a light and flowery flavor.

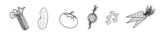

Chic but risky: Raw seafood

The FDA estimates that 85 percent of all illnesses caused by eating seafood involve raw oysters, clams, and mussels. Such shellfish can accumulate bacteria and viruses. *Vibrio Vulnificus* is a bacterium commonly found in Gulf of Mexico oysters that, although not threatening to most people, can be fatal if you have liver disease or a compromised immune system.

If you do hunger for raw shellfish, be very careful of the source — or better yet, eat it cooked. You're engaging in wishful thinking if you think that eating raw oysters with hot sauce or downing them with a margarita will kill the bacteria they carry.

You also need to be very careful if you have a taste for such gourmet foods as sushi, seviche, and raw tuna or swordfish carpaccio, a trendy takeoff on the Italian appetizer usually made with raw meat. Raw fish can contain the larvae of parasites, such as tapeworms and flukes. And marinating fish doesn't kill the parasites or bacteria. Signs that you may have taken in parasites range from mild and temporary digestive problems to severe abdominal pain.

Freezing raw fish at 4°F for a minimum of 60 hours kills the larvae. Find a restaurant that makes sushi with previously frozen fish or prepare sushi this way at home.

Chapter 9

Taking a Fresh Look
at Eggs and Dairy

Staples of the refrigerator section of your supermarket, eggs and dairy products have long been considered a mainstay of the American diet. As science has discovered more about diet and its relation to health, these foods have been targeted for promotion or censure. This chapter talks about how they stack up as components of a healthy, whole-foods diet.

Eggs: Naturally Perfect

Eggs are one of nature's finest products. What a shame that they've gotten such bad press recently! The worry is that cholesterol in the yolk promotes heart disease. But, in fact, the American Heart Association now okays eating up to four eggs a week as a general rule, even if you're watching your cholesterol. If you consume a predominantly vegetarian diet, you can eat even a few more.

The news about eggs is pretty sensational:

▶ **Eggs contain the highest quality protein of any known food.** Eating egg protein in the morning can give you energy that lasts for hours.

Protein quality is judged by how efficiently your body can use it for growth and repair. In eggs, the mix of *amino acids,* which are the building blocks of protein, is ideal; all the essential amino acids — those that the body can't synthesize — are present in the right proportions. Other amino acids can easily by manufactured from these. The Food and Agriculture Organization of the United Nations rates the biological value of the protein in various foods and ranks eggs at the top.

✔ **Eggs provide small to significant amounts of all needed vitamins, with the exception of vitamin C, and several minerals including iron, selenium, and zinc.** They supply B vitamins, including *choline,* which is capable of dissolving cholesterol and fat. Choline is used in the treatment of *atherosclerosis,* a condition in which cholesterol accumulates in the arteries. Eggs are also one of the few food sources of vitamin D, which facilitates the absorption of calcium for bone health. Egg yolks are a source of two special carotenoids, lutein and zeaxanthin, powerful antioxidants, which also filter out blue light, which can damage the eye and cause age-related macular degeneration. (The macula, the yellowish area on the retina, makes possible sharp, detailed vision.)

✔ **One egg provides only 75 calories, and most of the fat in eggs is the healthier, unsaturated kind.** In addition, the cholesterol that you consume when you eat an egg does not automatically increase the amount of cholesterol circulating in your blood. Your liver manufactures cholesterol, a waxy, fatlike substance found in all animal foods, which your body uses to maintain the walls of your cells, insulate your nerves, and manufacture hormones, to name just a few of its functions. If you're like most people, when you consume cholesterol, your body compensates by reducing the amount of cholesterol it's currently producing. Only about 25 percent of the population lacks the ability to regulate cholesterol in this way.

In a 1997 study, researchers at the University of Arizona analyzed the results of more than 224 cholesterol studies conducted over the past 25 years, which included a total of more than 8,000 participants. These studies examined the relation of dietary fat and cholesterol to blood levels of fat and cholesterol. An analysis of the data revealed that, in healthy persons, blood levels of cholesterol are affected more by the amount of saturated fat in the diet than by the amount of cholesterol consumed.

The exception is if you're less than healthy and have elevated cholesterol, you need to restrict the number of eggs you eat. For lunch, a tuna sandwich is a better choice than an egg salad sandwich.

✔ **Eggs are easily digested — an ideal food to cook when you're stressed or convalescing.** When you're feeling under the weather, fix yourself a nice poached egg or have someone else bring you a poached egg served in a pretty English china egg cup and scoop it out with a teaspoon. What a comforting little meal.

Don't judge an egg by its cover

You may prefer to buy brown eggs, thinking that they look more natural — or more "country" if you happen to be a photo stylist — but be assured that there is no nutritional difference between brown and white eggs. Breeds of chickens with reddish brown feathers and ear-lobes — Rhode Island Red, New Hampshire, and Plymouth Rock — lay brown-shelled eggs.

The healthiest ways to cook eggs are poaching and soft-boiling. These methods minimize the effect that cooking has on an egg's cholesterol. When cholesterol is exposed to heat, oxygen, or light, it oxidizes, a natural chemical process quite a bit like rusting. Some studies indicate that oxidized cholesterol may be the culprit in the development of heart disease. Poaching and soft-boiling cook the yolk at relatively low temperatures and keep it safely encased in its surrounding whites and shell.

Frying or scrambling eggs is much more likely to alter the cholesterol. The yolk is in direct contact with the hot cooking surface of the skillet and is exposed to both light and oxygen in the air. When you cook eggs this way or order them in a coffee shop, you're putting harmful oxidized cholesterol on your plate. If you must have a fried egg, keep the yolk a little runny.

In the past few years, the possibility of eggs being tainted with salmonella has become a worry. To knock out this bug, which can cause intestinal problems and even food poisoning, the government recommends you thoroughly cook eggs and not leave the yolk or whites runny. This is good advice for people with weakened immune systems such as AIDS patients. However, another way to lower your risk of salmonella is to be careful of your source of eggs, buying free-range chickens from smaller production facilities rather than eggs produced in massive factorylike conditions where animals are raised in over-crowded and possibly unsanitary settings. Also, look for eggs with thicker shells, which may better protect the eggs from invading bacteria.

If you find you've bought an egg with a cracked shell, throw it out.

Eggs are a versatile food, used in baked goods and sauces. You can also turn them into a main course dish such as this one for lunch or a light supper. And as long as you're eating hen's eggs, why not try a more exotic variety, such as duck eggs, a Chinese specialty, goose eggs, or quail eggs, shown on the cover of this book? Each one has just 14 calories.

Tender Poached Eggs

This recipe is a version of huevos rancheros. The eggs nestle in a salsa sauce, but you can substitute creamed spinach if you prefer.

Preparation time: *10 minutes*

Cooking time: *35 to 40 minutes*

Yield: *4 servings*

1 tablespoon extra-virgin olive oil	*1 teaspoon chili powder*
1 medium onion, chopped	*1 teaspoon oregano*
1 medium organic green bell pepper, chopped*	*½ teaspoon cumin*
2 cloves garlic, crushed	*Sea salt and freshly ground black pepper to taste*
28-ounce can (3½ cups) Glen-Muir organic tomatoes	*8 eggs at room temperature*
2 or 3 green chilies, seeded, deveined, and chopped	

1 In a heavy skillet, over medium heat, heat the oil. Add the onion, pepper, and garlic. Cook until the onion becomes translucent, about 5 to 7 minutes. Add the tomatoes, chilies, chili powder, oregano, and cumin. Add sea salt and pepper to taste. Simmer the tomato mixture, covered, for 20 minutes.

2 With the back of a spoon, make a small depression in the sauce for each egg. To poach the eggs, crack 1 at a time into a cup and gently slide into the simmering sauce. Cover and cook on medium-low heat until the egg whites set, about 6 minutes.

3 Serve in low, individual soup bowls to contain the sauce, accompanied by warm, steamed corn tortillas.

*Commercial bell peppers, which are not organic, are given a coating of wax. If you cook with these peppers, first remove the skin using a potato peeler.

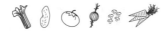

Two halves make a whole

To benefit from the remarkably wide range of nutrients that eggs contain, you need to eat both the white and the yolk. The B-complex vitamins, which are most effective when your diet includes all of them, are distributed in both the yolk and the white. The yolk contains the highest amounts of the B vitamins — biotin, choline, folic acid, inositol, thiamin, vitamin B5, vitamin B6, and vitamin B12 — while the white has more of the riboflavin and niacin. In addition, the yolk contains the fat-soluble vitamins — A, D, and E.

Minerals, too, are distributed in both parts of the egg, with calcium, copper, iodine, iron, manganese, phosphorus, and zinc predominating in the yolk and magnesium and potassium in the white. Each portion also contributes its own array of amino acids that complement each other to build protein.

So what about cholesterol-conscious egg substitutes that are made of only egg whites since only the yolk contains cholesterol? And how about blends of eggs that contain a higher proportion of whites to yolk? I say don't mess with Mother Nature. Egg substitutes don't give you the nutritional benefits of whole eggs, and eggs with lopsided proportions disturb the ideal balance of nutrients in this highly nourishing food.

Dairy Products: A Mixed Blessing

The other food that animals make is milk. Food manufacturers then turn milk into such dairy products as butter, cheese, and yogurt. These foods are high in protein and fats, so they're well-suited for body building.

Dairy products meet the needs of growing children and women during pregnancy. Dieters nibble slivers of cheese, hungry for the protein and satisfying fat. Cheese also makes pizza the most satisfying of fast-food meals (at least in my opinion). Mozzarella, the pizza cheese, now comes in second to cheddar as the American favorite.

Many adults also make a habit of drinking at least one glass of milk a day for the calcium it contains, about 300 mg. Calcium is essential for normal functioning of the heart, nerves, and muscles, and for developing and maintaining strong bones and teeth. (Turn to Chapter 20 for more about bone health.)

Milk: Is it for you?

Mothers' milk, whether produced by cows, cats, or humans, is an ideal food for the infant of that species. Cow's milk has the right mix of proteins, fats, carbohydrates, and nutrients to nourish calves. Human milk is perfectly designed to grow human babies into thriving children. Yet milk in general has long been considered so nutritious that animal milk and milk products have been part of the human diet in countries such as India for thousands of years.

However, many people today find that they are not able to drink milk comfortably. Do you experience any of these signs?

- ✔ If you experience symptoms such as diarrhea, abdominal pain, and bloating, you may be sensitive to lactose, the principal sugar found in milk. About 70 percent of adults throughout the world have difficulty digesting lactose, especially Hispanics, African Americans, and Asians.

- ✔ If you're prone to sneezing, coughing, runny nose, asthma, bronchitis, constipation, diarrhea, skin rashes, general irritability, hyperactivity, or listlessness, you may have a milk allergy. Milk contains at least 25 different proteins that can trigger a reaction.

- ✔ Milk drinkers typically have an accumulation of phlegm and are troubled by nasal congestion. If you often get colds or have a chronically runny nose, try eliminating all milk and cheese from your meals for at least two weeks and see whether your symptoms clear up.

While some individuals avoid milk because they develop one or another of these symptoms, many people shy away from milk because they don't want to drink the fat, or drink milk from which some of the fat has been removed. Again, such manipulated food is no longer the real thing and provides an unbalanced mix of nutrients. You may begin to crave the missing fat and eat more cookies and cakes instead.

The protein in milk is also an issue. While the amount of protein in the various forms of milk is the same, when you remove some fat, you now have a food that is a relatively concentrated source of protein. The amount of protein you are taking in may be a problem. Many adult women these days are drinking lots of milk for the calcium it contains. You may find you can easily drink several glasses of lowfat milk a day because it is less filling than whole milk. But you should be aware that a high-protein diet can be a risk factor for osteoporosis. If you are also eating good amounts of meat, poultry, and fish, you may want to cut back on your milk intake and eat vegetables instead for your source of calcium. (There's more on milk and osteoporosis in Chapter 20.)

If you are thinking, "No way! I love milk," but don't want the fat, you still need to be aware of the way fat content in milk is expressed on labels. The percent of calories from fat sounds teeny, but the actual percentage of calories contributed by fat can be considerable. Take a look at Table 9-1.

Table 9-1	Milk's Fat Content Depends on How You Measure It	
Type of Milk	*% Fat by Weight*	*% of Calories from Fat*
Whole milk	3.5	49
2% milk	2	30
Skim milk	1	2

TECHNICAL STUFF

Modern milk

While traveling in Switzerland, I once ordered the traditional Swiss dish *raclette,* which is made with the cheese of the same name. The cheese is exposed to heat, traditionally from an open fire. Succulent bits are scrapped off as it melts, and you eat these with bread and wine. This particular cheese was so delicious that I asked the waitress where I could buy some. She said that it came from some cows that lived just a few miles down the road; I wouldn't find it even in the local shops. I still can picture those cows living on the grass of Alpine meadows and leading healthy, natural Swiss lives.

Isn't this the sort of cow you vaguely imagine producing the cheese you eat and the milk you drink? Think again. Today's dairy herds live in a much more controlled environment. Antibiotics are routinely given to *prevent* disease, not just to treat it. Cows receive hormones such as estrogen that are meant to fatten them up. Unfortunately, the milk that these cows produce may contain residues of these substances. They are no longer producing old-fashioned milk, but a *milk product.*

About 30 percent of the dairy cows in the U.S. are treated with the genetically engineered hormone called *bovine growth hormone (BGH),* also known as *bovine somatotropin (BST).* If given BGH, a cow will produce 10 to 15 percent more milk. The Food and Drug Administration approved the use of this substance in 1993. However, that same year, Europe banned the use of BGH, and in 1999 Canada also gave it a thumbs-down.

Veterinarians report that cows on BGH are more prone to poor health — udder infection, infertility, lameness, and a generally weakened condition. Scientists and opponents of BGH also question the effect of BGH on humans and are calling for more research. Thankfully, you don't have to resolve this international debate, but if you want to be on the safe side, buy a brand of milk whose label states that the milk is free of this hormone. (If the milk does contain BGH, the producers are not required to say so on the label.) And while you're at it, also buy a brand of milk that is organic, meaning that the cow was fed organic grains. Natural-food stores, innovative new chains of grocery stores such as Trader Joe's, and health-food stores carry such brands. (Flip over to Chapter 4 on shopping to get to know certain brand names.)

Cheese: Treating yourself to the best

Like milk, cheese is a high-calcium food and a good source of vitamin A (important for immunity as well as eyesight). Cheese has a place in a generally healthful diet, enjoyed in small amounts as a condiment or to accent a meal. If you are sensitive to milk, you may also have problems with cheese. However, cheese that is higher in fat is less likely to trigger an allergic response. Fat slows the emptying time of the stomach, which is well-known clinically to reduce the allergic effect.

In addition, because the fat slows the absorption of food into your system, fatty cheese curtails how much insulin you produce and helps to keep blood sugar levels steady. Keeping control over insulin and blood sugar benefits the heart and helps you not gain weight. When you eat low and nonfat cheese, your insulin output is more likely to increase and lead to medical problems. Better to eat regular cheese with all its fat, but only small amounts at a time.

To savor the unique flavors of various cheeses and to make the most of the calories you're eating, buy the best quality you can find. Goat cheese is the darling of caterers and gourmets, as is feta, made from sheep's and goat's milk. Try a mildly flavored version of goat cheese sold in the shape of a log or cone, dusted with herbs or black pepper. Goat's milk is as rich in calcium as cow's milk, and feta is lower in fat than most other cheeses. In addition, such specialty cheeses are likely to be minimally processed because they are often produced on a small scale. Also look for organic cheeses made with organic milk.

The following is a tasty recipe for turning goat cheese into a gourmet offering good enough for company.

Marinated Goat Cheese

If you're hungry for dairy, enjoy this marinated goat cheese. Goat's milk is comparable to cow's milk in nutrition, but goats are usually raised in small herds and more natural conditions.

Preparation time: *10 minutes*

Cooking time: *At least 5 hours for marinating*

Yield: *6 servings*

1 teaspoon cumin seeds	*3 cloves garlic, crushed*
1 teaspoon black peppercorns	*¼ teaspoon sea salt*
¼ teaspoon crushed hot red pepper flakes	*1 log goat cheese, sliced into rounds (about 10 ounces)*
½ cup extra-virgin olive oil	

1 Put the cumin seeds, peppercorns, and red pepper in a small sauté pan. Over high heat, toast, shaking the pan until the spices are fragrant, about 30 seconds.

2 In a small bowl, combine the toasted spices, olive oil, crushed garlic, and salt.

3 Pour the olive oil-spice mixture over the cheese. Marinate, covered, at room temperature for a minimum of 5 hours.

4 Serve the marinated cheese on whole-grain bread or on crackers.

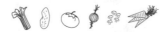

Processed cheeses such as the classic "American" sliced cheese and cheese spreads usually are higher in sodium (1 ounce may contain 400 to 500 mg of sodium), and their vitamin and mineral content is fairly low. They may also contain hydrogenated oils. Cream cheese is also a highly processed cheese and it's relatively low in calcium. Some cheese products, such as Velveeta and Cheez Whiz, must by law be called "cheese food" rather than just "cheese" because they are so processed. Cheese foods contain less calcium and more sodium than regular cheeses and are likely to contain flavorings and chemical stabilizers.

A delicious way to enjoy a little cheese is to use it as a flavoring for other foods. When you make mashed potatoes, add some parmesan.

Yogurt: Introducing friendly bacteria

Yogurt — not the sugary-flavored, fruit-mixed-in, or fruit-on-the-bottom kind, but plain yogurt — belongs in your refrigerator as a staple. Yogurt is high in calcium, and if you're lactose intolerant, you may have less difficulty digesting this milk product.

Shop for brands of yogurt that state on the label "live cultures" or "active cultures." These "friendly" bacteria have several health benefits. Two bacteria that are standard residents of all yogurt are *Lactobacillus bulgaricus* and *Streptococcus thermaphilus*. Research indicates that these bacteria are capable of boosting immunity, reducing the frequency and symptoms of hay fever, and helping to prevent colds.

Some brands of yogurt also have added *Lactobacillus acidophilus* and *Bifidobacteria*, both normally found in the large intestine. Taking antibiotics can kill off the good bacteria in the gut, causing digestive problems, but eating yogurt containing these bacteria can counteract this problem. *Acidophilus* yogurt also appears to help yeast infections, such as *Candida albicans*, and some strains of *Acidophilus* lower cholesterol. *Acidophilus* may also suppress harmful bacteria that create carcinogenic compounds.

The facts about frozen yogurt

Don't kid yourself. Frozen yogurt is not a health food. Like fresh, plain yogurt, frozen yogurt is a source of protein and may contain B vitamins and calcium, but it also contains sugar or sugar substitutes. Furthermore, frozen yogurt does not provide the live bacteria supplied by fresh yogurt, which become part of the beneficial bacteria that inhabit healthy intestines.

The fruit mixture in flavored yogurt kills the friendly bacteria. If you want fruit in your yogurt, add fresh fruit to plain yogurt. You can even increase the bacteria by adding a teaspoonful of supplemental freeze-dried *Acidophilus*.

Yogurt can be a private little meal, a cupful savored in solitude. In Middle Eastern cooking, yogurt also shows up in sauces, desserts, and as a condiment. It's even made into a sort of cream cheese, called *labneh,* which you can taste by making the following recipe.

Yogurt Cream

In the Middle East, this yogurt cream, or labneh, is sometimes eaten for breakfast with olives, but the same combination is good for lunch or a light afternoon snack.

Preparation time: 15 minutes

Cooking time: 8 hours to drain the yogurt

Yield: 2 cups

2 cups plain live or active culture yogurt	*Sea salt to taste*
1 stem fresh mint, leaves removed and finely chopped (about 1 tablespoon)	

1 Fold a large piece of damp cheesecloth in half to form a square and place this over a deep bowl. Pour the yogurt in the center of the cloth, tie the cloth's corners to make a little sack, and then use the loose ends of the sack to tie it onto a wooden spoon long enough to reach over the edges of the bowl. Place the spoon across the bowl so the sack hangs into it. Let sit overnight. (Note)

2 Remove the drained yogurt from the cloth and discard the liquid. Tip the yogurt into a small mixing bowl. Stir in the mint and sea salt. Chill the yogurt cream and serve it in a colorful ceramic bowl.

Note: Yogurt "cheese" funnels are sold at many kitchen stores, giving you an easier way of draining the yogurt.

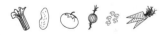

Chapter 10

Quality Fats and Healing Seeds and Nuts

In This Chapter

▶ Choosing healthful fats and oils

▶ Turning seeds and nuts into oils

▶ Avoiding the toxic byproducts of processing

▶ Applauding nutrient-packed seeds and nuts

▶ Cracking down on processed nuts

▶ Storing seeds and nuts for a another day

Fats are one of the primary nutrients, along with protein and carbohydrates. Fats have a place in every meal you eat because you need them for health. Even though fatty foods are a worry to the vast majority of people trying to slim down and diet, they perform many essential functions. High in calories, they supply energy and warmth. Fat tissue cushions and protects vital organs. Molecules of fat act as carriers for the fat-soluble vitamins A, D, E, and K. Fats are the raw materials from which hormones are formed. Fats also function as flavor carriers in food, delivering tantalizing tastes to your palate. In this chapter, we explore the healthiest fats to cook with and the array of seeds and nuts that supply healing oils.

Fat and Oils

Of all food categories, fats are undoubtedly the most talked about, written about, worried about, measured, manipulated, and misunderstood. Here's what you need to keep in mind: High-quality fats and oils are healthy, and your body needs them to function properly. Poor-quality fats and oils are unhealthy, and you should go out of your way to avoid them. You may need to cut back on the quantity of fatty foods you're eating, but quality is all-important.

Fats (such as butter, which is solid at room temperature, and cooking oils, which are liquid at room temperature) are fragile substances. Heat, oxygen and especially light can attack and break down their structure. In fact, light can break down oils a thousand times faster than oxygen. Cooking fats at high temperatures, as in frying, converts a perfectly acceptable fat into a poisonous toxin. The way cooking oils are commonly processed and refined (which the following section explains) also produces a product that contains toxic compounds, and such oils are also stripped of nutrients.

Understanding how cooking oil is refined

Seeds, nuts, and other plant foods have been used for thousands of years as a source of cooking oils. In times past, oils were extracted mechanically simply by pressing and were produced in small amounts more or less for immediate use. Then, around 1900, the business of refining cooking fats was launched. Crisco first appeared on the market around this time. The great majority of cooking oils that you now find on supermarket shelves are processed. This section outlines the typical steps taken in refining oil (see Figure 10-1). (Remember that heat, oxygen, and light deteriorate oils.)

Extracting the oil

Seeds are first prepared for processing, and then the oil is extracted using one or the other of a variety of methods.

- **Cleaning and cooking:** Before the seeds are mechanically pressed, they are cooked for up to two hours at an average of 248°F to facilitate pressing. This cracks the seed and opens it to oxygen.

- **Mechanical or expeller pressing:** The seeds are pressed with the pressure of several tons per square inch. This process generates heat, and the seeds can reach temperatures of between 185° and 203°F, during which time heated oils react with oxygen 100 times faster than at room temperature. If, during this process, oxygen and air are not eliminated, essential fatty acids in the oil are damaged.

- **Solvent extraction:** An alternative method of extracting oil from seeds is to grind the seeds into a fine meal and then, at an elevated temperature, dissolve the meal by using a solvent such as hexane, a known carcinogen. The resulting mixture of oil and solvent is then heated to about 302°F to evaporate the solvent, which is then reused. Oils refined in this way may contain traces of these solvents. The protein, fiber, vitamin, and mineral content is reduced during this process.

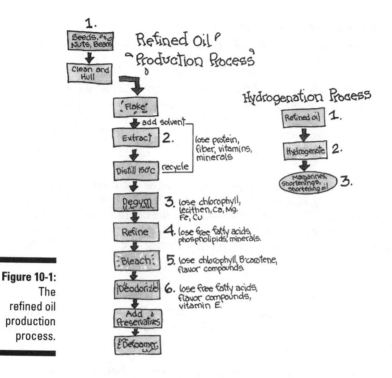

Figure 10-1:
The refined oil production process.

Up to this point, the oil is not *refined.* In fact, an oil extracted with a solvent can be labeled unrefined, as can a mixture of expeller-pressed and solvent-extracted oil. Oils labeled cold-pressed may also be refined. To produce a refined oil, the following further steps are taken. (Are you starting to get the picture of how processed most oils are?)

Refining the oil

The refining process involves several steps, which, one by one, strip the oil of nutrients.

✓ **Degumming:** Degumming occurs at 140°F and uses phosphoric acid and water. This process reduces levels of chlorophyll, calcium, magnesium, iron, and copper in the oil. In addition, lecithin, which is required for brain and nerve function, is extracted and sold separately.

✓ **Refining:** The oil is mixed with sodium hydroxide or with a combination of sodium hydroxide and sodium bicarbonate. Again heated, the mixture is agitated and the oil and chemicals separated. This process depletes *free fatty acids* (essential components of fat molecules, which when removed can form soaps with sodium hydroxide, which dissolve into the watery part of the mixture), *phospholipids* (a class of compounds that contain phosphorus and are important elements in cell membranes), and minerals.

Removing color and odor from the oil

Uniquely colored and flavored oils are turned into oils that all look and taste alike.

- ✔ **Bleaching:** Bleaching the oil by using filters and chemicals removes *chlorophyll* (the green pigment that synthesizes carbohydrates in plants by using carbon dioxide and water) and beta-carotene (an orange pigment and antioxidant). The oil is heated to 230°F for 15 to 30 minutes. Bleaching alters the structure of essential fatty acids, producing toxic compounds.

- ✔ **Deodorizing:** Deodorizing removes substances with strong odors and unappealing tastes, as well as peroxides that develop during processing and some pesticide residues. However, deodorizing also removes aromatic oils, free fatty acids, and vitamin E. The deodorizing process occurs at 464° to 518°F — frying temperatures! — and lasts for 30 to 60 minutes.

Preparing the oil for bottling

To extend the oil's shelf life, manufacturers add synthetic antioxidant chemicals. In addition, they add defoaming agents, and sometimes also treat the oil to keep it from clouding if you store it in your refrigerator.

You can tell whether a manufacturer is selling a line of refined oils because the oils in all the bottles will be virtually the same color. A truly unrefined and minimally processed oil has the color and flavor of the nut or seed from which it was produced. Extra-virgin olive oil has a greenish tint and the distinct flavor of olives.

What you don't want for dinner: Chemical byproducts of the refining process

The refining process generates *free radicals* — molecular fragments with a single unpaired electron, which darts about and readily reacts with whatever it comes in contact with. When this occurs, the free radical steals an electron from another molecule, triggering a chain reaction that is damaging to biological processes. Free radicals can damage cell walls and even the nucleus of the cell, which controls cell reproduction, a function that runs wild in cancer. Free radicals play a key role in the aging process.

When oils are refined, many other unnatural fat molecules form. As oils are deodorized at exceptionally high temperatures for a length of time, chemical bonds between atoms shift, and molecules develop a twist in their structure. This type of molecule is called a *transfatty acid.*

Margarine: Not better than butter

At one time, margarine was preferred over butter because it's made with polyunsaturated fats rather than saturated fats. But now we know that there are problems with margarine because of the way it's made.

Margarine is composed of vegetable oils, which have gone through the steps in refining oil that I describe earlier in the chapter. Because margarine is used as a substitute for butter, these liquid vegetable oils are put through a process that makes them semi-solid at room temperature, just like the butter it's trying to imitate. This process is called *hydrogenation*. (When an oil is hydrogenated, hydrogen atoms are added to a polyunsaturated fat in order to saturate it and make it solid.) Hydrogenation puts an unnatural twist in the structure of many of the fat molecules, producing transfatty acids. Margarine can contain as much as 50 percent transfatty acids.

Always choose butter over margarine.

You don't want to run into some of the problems that transfatty acids cause:

- ✔ Transfatty acids are sticky, and like saturated fat, remain solid at body temperature. They can increase your risk of blood clots and, consequently, heart disease and stroke.

- ✔ These misshapen molecules take the place of normal fat molecules in cell walls, but they cannot perform the same tasks. The permeability of the cell membrane is altered, possibly promoting allergic reactions and lowering immunity.

- ✔ Twisted transfatty acids have altered electrical properties and interfere with the flow of energy within the body.

- ✔ Transfatty acids raise cholesterol levels.

Unfortunately, the types of oils that are particularly susceptible to such alterations are monounsaturated and polyunsaturated vegetable oils, which physicians and nutritionists routinely recommend for lowering your risk of heart disease. Monounsaturated and polyunsaturated oils do indeed lower blood levels of cholesterol, but when you consume these oils in their refined form, they can no longer be considered health foods or quality fats.

To find out more about the fats and oils that you regularly eat, I highly recommend *Fats that Heal, Fats that Kill,* the bestselling, authoritative, and thoroughly entertaining book by Udo Erasmus, published by Alive Books in a new edition in 1999.

Finding the finest fats and the best oils

High-quality fats are a source of fat-soluble vitamins, minerals, lecithin, essential fatty acids, phytohormones, and natural antioxidants. The quality fats and oils described in the following sections deserve a place on your table.

Unsalted butter

The virtue of organic butter, besides its delectable flavor, is that it's relatively unprocessed and stable at high temperatures and does not form toxic compounds such as transfatty acids. Butter is also a source of vitamin A and some vitamin E, a natural antioxidant that helps prevent it from going rancid.

The finest quality butter is the unsalted kind, which is made from cream that is very fresh. I also highly recommend organic butter, made from milk produced by cows that have grazed on organic feed, free of pesticides. These accumulate in fatty tissue and can concentrate in fatty butter.

Coconut oil and lard also contain saturated fats. Coconut oil is commonly used in cooking in other countries, and lard is a staple of old-fashioned Southern cooking in the United States. Of course, a diet high in saturated fats such as these increases your risk of *arteriosclerosis,* or hardening of the arteries. But again, these fats are relatively stable at high temperatures and have their uses.

A few years ago, movie theatres stopped cooking popcorn in coconut oil and began using polyunsaturated vegetable oils instead. However, when that oil is allowed to stay hot for the length of a double feature or longer, it becomes junk food. It's best to enjoy your popcorn at home, drizzled with a little butter (unless you want to sneak your own into the theatre).

Another source of saturated fat is coconut oil, which in small amounts can be part of a healthy diet. Coconut tastes great in cakes and cookies.

Orange-Scented Coconut Macaroons

A deficiency of saturated fat can leave you with dry skin and hair. These orange-scented coconut macaroons are a delicious way to replenish these important fats.

Preparation time: *5 minutes*

Cooking time: *20 minutes*

Yield: *24 cookies*

2½ cups unsweetened shredded coconut

1 cup whole-wheat pastry flour

Zest of 1 organic orange

1 cup maple syrup

1 teaspoon vanilla

1 Preheat oven to 350°. Put the coconut and flour in a medium bowl and combine.

2 Put the zest in a small bowl and add the maple syrup and vanilla. Stir to combine.

3 Add the maple syrup mixture to the dry ingredients and combine.

4 Drop the cookie dough by teaspoonful on a buttered baking sheet. Bake until edges are nicely brown, about 20 minutes. With a spatula, transfer the macaroons to a cooling rack. Immediately store the ones you don't eat in an airtight container.

Extra-virgin olive oil

Extra-virgin olive oil is the first pressing of the olives, made without heat or chemicals. Nutrients are retained, and the oil is not likely to contain trans-fatty acids. Olives are high in monounsaturated fats, which are associated with a lower incidence of heart disease, and they are the star ingredient of what has been identified by researchers as the healthful Mediterranean diet. Compared to polyunsaturated fats, such as those found in safflower oil, corn oil, and soybean oil, monounsaturated fats are less likely to oxidize — a process that may contribute to narrowing of the arteries.

You can find extra-virgin olive oil in most stores, produced by such national brands as Bertolli and Colavita. ("Pure" on a label just means that the bottle contains only that kind of oil. If you find the words "light" or "extra light" on the label, these words refer to flavor, not calories, which remain the same for all fats: 9 calories per gram.)

You can use whole olives to add healing oils to pasta dishes and salads. A mix of minced olives, herbs, and garlic is irresistible. Try this recipe and see if you agree.

Become an olive oil connoisseur

Olive oils are as varied as wines. While Italy is a major source, many delicious varieties are produced in Spain, from subtly flavored oils in the north to lusty versions in the south. An oil that offers a nice balance is L'Estornell extra-virgin olive oil produced in Catalonia from organically grown Arbequina olives.

Mediterranean Olives

Let yourself nibble on this olive paste, spread on hearty country bread, and give your body the fat it needs. Then you won't be so hungry for far less healthy French fries.

Preparation time: 10 minutes

Cooking time: None

Yield: About 4 to 6 servings

1 pound jumbo green and black unpitted olives	*3 crushed bay leaves*
	1 tablespoon whole anise seeds
1 teaspoon dried rosemary, or 1 tablespoon fresh rosemary	*4 garlic cloves, crushed*
1 teaspoon dried thyme, or 1 tablespoon fresh thyme	*½ cup vinegar (white wine, rice, or sherry)*
	2 tablespoons anchovy paste
1 teaspoon ground cumin	*Filtered water to cover*

1 Put the olives in a large strainer to drain. Discard the liquid.

2 With the side of a broad knife, crush the olives lightly.

3 Put the rosemary, thyme, cumin, bay leaves, anise seeds, garlic, vinegar, and anchovy paste in a bowl and stir to combine. Add the olives and mix well.

4 Transfer the olives to a jar with a tightly fitting lid. Add the filtered water until jar is filled. Close jar securely and refrigerate to marinate olives, at least 3 or 4 days. Garnish salads, sandwiches, and grilled meats and use as an appetizer.

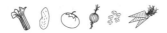

Flaxseed oil

Flaxseed oil, which may be unfamiliar to you, belongs in your kitchen as a staple. Flaxseed is a superb source of omega-3 essential fatty acids, the essential fatty acids also found in fish and walnuts.

Omega-3 fatty acids help thin the blood and widen the arteries. In contrast, the omega-6 fatty acids promote the thickening of the blood and the narrowing of arteries. Together, these two essential fatty acids, when kept in balance, help sustain the health of the circulatory system and help prevent high blood pressure. Essential fatty acids are also a critical parts of all cell walls and brain tissue. As recently as 100 years ago, our diet provided 2 parts omega-6 fatty acids to 1 part omega-3 fatty acids, considered to be a healthy ratio. Unfortunately, the typical diet today provides 20 to 25 parts omega-6 fatty acids to 1 part omega-3 fatty acids.

An estimated optimal dose of omega-6 fatty acids is 9 grams a day, and 6 grams of omega-3 fatty acids (1 tablespoon).

Flaxseed oil is very fragile and breaks down easily when exposed to light, heat, and oxygen. *Never* heat it. Instead, use it cold as a component of salad dressings, made fresh for each meal, or add it to a hot food once it's ready to serve. Flaxseed oil is also available as a supplement.

Flaxseed has a nice, buttery flavor. If you find that you don't like the taste, the oil is probably rancid, and you should throw it out.

You can find flaxseed oil in the refrigerated section of natural-food stores. It's sold packaged in small, opaque bottles to ensure freshness. Some labels state that the oil is high in *lignans,* which are a type of insoluble fiber that helps reduce the risk of cancer.

As you increase your intake of flaxseed oil, as well as other sources of essential fatty acids, also be sure to increase your consumption of fruits and vegetables rich in antioxidants. Essential fatty acids break down easily, forming free radicals that the antioxidants do away with.

Another very important source of omega-3 fatty acids is seafood. The omega-3s are in the plant material fish eat, and the omega-3s make their way up the food chain.

Shanghai Steamed Fish

This fish dish supplies omega-3 essential fatty acids and is prepared with sesame oil, which adds a delicious, nutty flavor.

Preparation time: *10 minutes*

Cooking time: *35 minutes*

Yield: *4 servings*

1 2-pound whole sea bass, red snapper, flounder, or pompano, scaled and cleaned

Sea salt and pepper to taste

1 tablespoon butter

2 tablespoons soy sauce

2-inch length of ginger root, peeled and slivered

2 scallions, trimmed and chopped

2 tablespoons toasted sesame oil

Scallion tassels for garnish (optional)

(continued)

1 Adjust height of oven shelf so that it is a little higher than the oven center. Preheat oven to 325°. Fit a baking dish with an oiled rack high enough to allow juices to accumulate in the dish without touching the fish.

2 Place the whole fish on the oiled rack. Season insides with salt and pepper. Drizzle the butter and soy sauce over the fish skin so that it is evenly coated. Top the fish with a scattering of the ginger and scallions.

3 Bake until done, about 30 to 35 minutes. The fish is done when the flesh is opaque and pulls away from the bone.

4 Use 2 spatulas to lift the fish from the baking dish and transfer to a warmed serving platter. Over the top of the fish, drizzle the sesame oil. Garnish with the scallion tassels. Serve immediately.

Note: To make a scallion tassel, cut a scallion into 2-inch strips. Gently flatten the scallion with 1 hand while, with the point of a sharp paring knife, you make several lengthwise cuts into each end. (Take care not to cut all the way through the length of the scallion.) Drop the cut scallion into a bowl of ice water for an hour or longer. Chilling curls the ends of the scallion, making a fancy tassel!

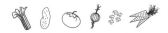

Unrefined sesame oil and other unrefined vegetable oils

Unrefined sesame oil makes a flavorful addition to many dishes. It's absolutely delicious lightly toasted. (Simply heat it for a minute or two in a sauté pan.)

You can also buy unrefined safflower oil, but it feels very heavy on the tongue. Try making a salad dressing with it and see what you think. I personally think it is better suited to baked goods. You may also want to experiment with walnut, hazelnut, and grapeseed oils to add flavor to salad dressings and cooked dishes.

Vegetable oils that are widely available and sold in supermarkets, corner groceries, and all-night delis are fully refined. The oils that fall into this category include canola, sunflower, safflower, corn, soybean, and peanut oil. Thousands of food products, such as baked goods, are made with these oils. Look for unrefined versions of these oils in natural-food stores.

Labeling oil as "pure" or "100%" means that only oil is in the product. It does not mean that the oil is unrefined. You may also find labels that say "enriched with vitamin E." Vitamin E, a natural preservative, is lost in processing; added vitamin E replaces what was removed.

Shopping for healthful oils

To make sure that the oil you cook with is the freshest, healthiest possible, buy the smallest quantities you expect to need, use them up, and then buy more. Notice the color and savor the aroma of these natural products. Search out oils with color and flavor. Ideally, oil should have opaque packaging.

Also search out brands with labels stating that the oil is cold-pressed and unrefined or unprocessed. I recommend these brands:

- **Omega Nutrition** packages its oils in opaque black bottles. The nuts and seeds are mechanically pressed in small batches at low temperatures, between 82 and 92°F. Common oils such as canola, soy, and safflower oils are in this line of unrefined oil products.

- **Loriva Culinary Oils** produces a range of unrefined oils, including extra-virgin sesame oil, California walnut oil, toasted sesame oil, garlic-flavored oil, and basil-flavored oil.

- **Montana Amber** offers a line of unrefined, organic oils extracted at low temperatures. These oils are produced on demand at low volume. The company sells first-pressing, high-oleic, organic safflower oil. Oleic acid is a heart-friendly monosaturated fatty acid.

- **Spectrum Naturals** sells a range of oils. Its cold-pressed, unrefined oils include peanut oil and the organic oils, such as canola, flaxseed, and extra-virgin olive oil. Spectrum also sells expeller-pressed/unrefined and expeller-pressed/refined oils. In the refining process, no chemicals are used in pressing, and no chemical preservatives or defoaming agents are added.

- **Barleans** produces a high-quality flaxseed oil sold in an opaque plastic bottle. This oil is high in lignans, compounds thought to help prevent cancer.

- **House brands** are another option, such as Wild Oats' extra-virgin organic olive oil.

Storing butter and oils

As fats and oils can easily go rancid, you need to take special care in how you store them once you bring them into your kitchen. Keep oils away from heat, oxygen, and light. Store them in a cool place in tightly closed opaque containers. Here are some guidelines on how long butter and oils will last.

- **You can store sticks of unsalted butter frozen in the freezer for up to six months.** In the refrigerator you can store one stick for daily use, which will keep for about two weeks.

✔ **Store cooking oils in opaque containers such as ceramic bottles and under refrigeration.** Keep only small amounts unrefrigerated for daily use. This oil, too, should be in an opaque container.

✔ **Store flaxseed oil in the refrigerator even before you have first opened the bottle.** Once opened, flaxseed oil lasts three to six weeks. It keeps frozen in the freezer for six months.

To increase the shelf life of your oils, you can add a capsule or two of vitamin E, a powerful antioxidant that helps keep the oil from going rancid. Just break open the capsule and pour the vitamin E into the oil.

Cooking with unrefined oils

You can use many unrefined vegetable oils in recipes that involve boiling and steaming, cooking methods in which the food reaches only 212°F. You can also use these oils for light sautéing, as well as in baking. The maximum temperature of the interior of baked goods reaches only about 240°F. (Just remember to grease your baking pans with butter, not oil.) Frying is never a good idea, but if you must, use butter or refined oils. Choose those low in essential fatty acids and high in saturated and monounsaturated fatty acides, such as high-oleic safflower and sunflower oil, peanut oil, and canola oil. Add garlic and onions to the oil you are using and fry these, too. Sulfite compounds in these foods can help minimize the effects of the free radicals in the oil. Table 10-1 gives you guidelines on heating unrefined oils.

Table 10-1	Maximum Cooking Temperatures for Certain Types of Unrefined Oils
Oils	*Maximum Cooking Temperature*
Unrefined flaxseed	No heat
Unrefined sesame	250°F
Unrefined walnut	250°F
Unrefined peanut	275°F
Unrefined safflower	300°F
Unrefined soy	300°F
Unrefined high-oleic safflower	325°F
Unrefined high-oleic sunflower	325°F
Extra-virgin olive oil	325°F

Seeds and Nuts: Concentrated Nourishment

Birds and squirrels search about for seeds and nuts to sustain themselves and to store away for future meals. These creatures are after the array of nutrients that seeds and nuts contain. What a contrast with our own eating habits, with nuts demoted to cocktail snacks and seeds having the connotation of hippie health food. If the only nuts you eat are the peanuts handed out in little packets on airplanes, you have a whole category of food to discover!

Potent little packages

Every type of seed and nut provides a wide range of minerals. Seeds and nuts are first-rate plant sources of protein. They also provide fiber, which helps maintain the health of the digestive tract. Nuts and seeds supply nearly all the B vitamins, with the exception of B12. The B-complex vitamins support normal functioning of the nervous system, including the brain, and the production of energy within the cells.

Some have exceptionally high amounts of certain nutrients. For example:

- Pistachios are high in folic acid, which is essential during pregnancy.

- Almonds, hazelnuts, and Brazil nuts are especially high in vitamin E, a fat-soluble vitamin that helps ease a woman's passage through menopause.

- Almonds, pistachios, hazelnuts, and pumpkin seeds provide calcium and magnesium, both of which are needed to maintain the structure of bones and prevent osteoporosis.

- Sunflower seeds and pistachios are high in iron, which makes the transport of oxygen in the blood possible.

- Chestnuts and sunflower seeds provide potassium, a mineral that helps regulate blood pressure.

- Pumpkin seeds and sesame seeds supply zinc, used by the prostate gland to produce fertile sperm.

- Brazil nuts are unique in that they are a superb source of selenium, a trace mineral that functions as an antioxidant and protects against heart disease.

Seeds and nuts also contain special compounds that ward off disease. Flax seeds have anti-tumor properties and are linked to a low incidence of colon and breast cancer. In addition, flax seeds contain phytoestrogens, which help balance hormone levels. The ellagic acid in walnuts has anticancer properties, as does oleic acid, found in almonds. Studies have linked a low intake of nuts and seeds, which provide vitamin E, with a greater risk of Parkinson's disease. Nuts also contain magnesium, an essential mineral for bone health.

Magnesium Munchies

The nuts, seeds, and fruit in this recipe contain especially high levels of magnesium, which is as important as calcium for keeping bones strong.

Preparation time: *5 minutes*

Cooking time: *5 minutes*

Yield: *4 cups*

1 cup almonds

1 cup cashews

1 cup pumpkin seeds

½ cup chopped dried figs

½ cup raisins

2 tablespoons organic unsalted butter

1 teaspoon ground ginger

1 teaspoon ground cinnamon

Sea salt to taste

1 Combine the almonds, cashews, pumpkin seeds, figs, and raisins in a small bowl.

2 Over low heat, melt the butter in a sauté pan. Add the ginger and cinnamon and toast spices, keeping heat low, about 1 minute.

3 Add the nut-fruit mixture. Toss with the spice-butter mixture to coat. Lightly toast the nuts over medium heat, stirring continuously, about 3 minutes. Add sea salt to taste.

4 Transfer mixture to a bowl and cool, occasionally stirring to allow moisture to escape. When cool, store the mix in an airtight glass jar.

Note: *These ingredients are often sold in bulk at natural-food stores. I find that buying just the amount of nuts, seeds, and dried fruit I need for the recipe is the most economical. If you buy these already packaged, you risk having leftovers go stale.*

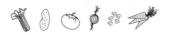

Protected oils

There's no better container for oils than the nuts and seeds that contain them. They're locked within the meat and protected from light, oxygen, and heat. These elements degrade fats and turn them rancid. It's far, far better to eat a handful of pecans, pistachios, or cashews than french fries soaked in hot cooking oils. Seeds and nuts contain a high percentage of polyunsaturated and monounsaturated oils, which are associated with a lower risk of heart disease. Almonds are especially high in monounsaturates. Seeds and nuts also contain essential fatty acids, fats that are fundamental components of all cell walls and are necessary for the formation of hormones and the health of the nervous system. The American diet is very deficient in these quality fats. Pumpkin seeds and sunflower seeds deserve to be regulars on your food shopping list.

Chestnuts contain only 1 percent to 3 percent fat, making them much lower in calories than other nuts. They provide vitamin B6, vitamin E, and potassium.

Walnut Pesto Pasta

There's more to nuts than cocktail peanuts. In many classic cuisines, nuts form the base of delicious sauces. From Italy comes pesto, traditionally made with pine nuts. Put a healthful twist on this standard and use walnuts instead. You'll increase your intake of essential fatty acids, which help restore vitality, and their flavor needs no apology!

Preparation time: *15 minutes*

Cooking time: *12 minutes*

Yield: *4 servings (2 cups pesto; freeze ⅔ cup in a small container for another use)*

1 bunch fresh sweet basil leaves, washed, patted dry (2 cups well packed)	*¾ cup extra-virgin olive oil*
4 cloves garlic, crushed	*Sea salt and freshly ground black pepper to taste*
1 cup walnuts	*2 to 3 quarts filtered salted water*
¼ cup grated Parmesan cheese*	*1 pound pasta***
¼ cup grated Romano cheese	

1 Put the basil and garlic in a blender or food processor. Pulse to produce a very coarse paste. Add the walnuts and cheese and pulse to a coarse consistency. With the motor running, slowly pour the oil through the feed tube of the food processor or top center opening of the blender; process until mixture is a coarse ground sauce, adding more oil if a thinner sauce is desired.

2 Transfer to a small bowl. Season with salt and pepper to taste.

3 In the meantime, boil salted water in a large saucepan. Add 1 package pasta. Cook according to package instructions.

(continued)

4 Toss the pasta with 1⅓ cups pesto sauce. Refrigerate or freeze the remaining sauce for another use, such as salad dressing. Arrange slices of tomato and fresh mozzarella on a serving platter and drizzle these with the pesto sauce.

Using 2 cheeses enhances flavor, but you can use either one alone.

**The heavier texture and taste of whole-wheat pasta versus common refined semolina pasta requires the commanding flavors of a sauce such as this pesto. If whole-wheat pasta doesn't appeal to you, try some of the new pasta products, such as 50 percent whole-wheat pasta and whole-grain brown rice pasta.

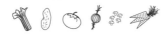

Buying seeds and nuts: Freshness first

The precious oils in seeds and nuts are fragile by nature and break down into toxic compounds when exposed to light, oxygen, and heat. Especially with high-fat nuts, such as pecans and walnuts, buy whole nuts rather than nuts broken into bits or ground up — a process that exposes their oils to the air. (If you must have almonds cut into perfect little white slivers, it's probably better to buy them sliced, because a food processor won't do the job attractively, and you risk losing a thumb if you cut almonds with a knife.)

Roasted nuts and nut butters have a wonderful, rich flavor. However, roasted nuts are nutritionally inferior to raw nuts. Roasted nuts are actually *fried* nuts; coconut oil, which is high in saturated fats, is usually used as the cooking oil. With exposure to heat, the fats in nuts can break down into substances that are toxic to the body. Roasting also forces oils to the surface of the nut, where they turn rancid faster. To add insult to injury, roasted nuts are heavily salted and may have added sugar, flavorings, and preservatives. ("Dry-roasted" nuts are not cooked in oil, but they may contain added flavorings and preservatives.) You can be sure of the quality of roasted nuts if you start with fresh raw nuts and toast them yourself.

Oh, those omega-3s

Omega-3 fatty acids, a type of polyunsaturated fat, are essential for good health. They lower cholesterol and help treat asthma, arthritis, allergies, inflammation, skin conditions, stress reactions, and symptoms of PMS, such as water retention.

Of the oils in flax seeds, as much as 57 percent are the omega-3 fatty acids. English walnuts are the only common nut that contains these. Both of these foods should be staples in your healing foods kitchen.

Peanut butter and beyond

Peanuts, which are actually legumes and not nuts, *fresh out of the shell* are a very healthful food. Unfortunately, common brands of peanut butter usually contain hydrogenated oils, salt, or sugar. Natural-food stores often sell peanut butter ground fresh at the store. (Buying your peanuts from a reputable source is important because peanuts are susceptible to a mold that is carcinogenic.)

If you've never tried almond butter, rush to your nearest natural-food store and buy a jar. Almond butter is delicious smeared on toast, added to desserts, and licked off a spoon. You may also find butters made from cashews, filberts, macadamia nuts, pecans, and pistachios.

And try butter made from sesame seeds, called *tahini,* a traditional Middle Eastern preparation. Tahini is a nondairy source of calcium. To avoid eating sesame seeds that have been hulled using chemical solvents, buy organic tahini made from sesame seeds that are mechanically hulled.

Storing seeds and nuts

Consuming rancid oils in seeds and nuts that have been improperly stored can undermine your long-term health. Here are some guidelines for squirreling these foods away safely:

- Store seeds and nuts out of the shell in tightly closed containers, such as jars. Keep these in the refrigerator. Seeds and nuts stored this way can stay fresh for up to several months.

- To extend their shelf life, put seeds and nuts in tightly closed containers and freeze them.

- Chop or grind nuts immediately before you want to eat them or use them in cooking. Even refrigerated, they spoil quickly.

- If you discover that the seeds or nuts you've stored smell rancid or taste bitter, *don't* be thrifty and eat them anyway. Throw them out.

Remember, nuts and seeds are not just for snacks. You can incorporate them into all sorts of dishes. Traditional recipes offer many ways to include nuts and seeds into everyday dishes. Experiment with this one!

Ali Baba's Toasted Sesame/Nut Rub

Use this recipe to dress up lamb or pork chops. In the final stage of pan-broiling chops, sprinkle the rub on the meat and, using a fork, press the mixture down so that it will adhere. Turn the chops over and repeat this procedure. Then cook for about 30 seconds on each side. Serve immediately, with lemon wedges.

Preparation time: *5 minutes*

Cooking time: *10 minutes*

Yield: *A generous ½ cup*

2 tablespoons raw sesame seeds

¼ cup raw pistachios

¼ cup raw almonds

1 teaspoon dried thyme

1 teaspoon allspice

Salt and freshly ground black pepper to taste

1 In a small sauté pan, warm sesame seeds over medium heat until fragrant, about 3 minutes. Shake pan frequently to prevent burning. Set aside. Next heat the pistachios and almonds and roast over medium heat until they are just browned, about 4 to 5 minutes.

2 Transfer the pistachios and almonds to a food processor or spice grinder. Process until coarsely ground. Add the sesame seeds, thyme, allspice, and salt and pepper. Continue to process until the nut mixture has the consistency of coarse meal and is finely ground. Use to season lamb or pork chops.

Chapter 11

Healing Herbs, Spices, and Flavorings

. . . .

. . . .

Many herbs, spices, and assorted flavorings have healing properties. These substances offer abundant proof of the medicinal treasures that nature provides. Herbalists and healers in ancient times relied on these foods for treating the ill. The Greek physician Hippocrates wrote of the healing powers of watercress. In the Middle Ages, innkeepers maintained herb gardens for treating ailing travelers. And in Victorian times, ladies carried sachets of lavender, in easy reach in case they needed to calm their nerves.

More recently, physicians have begun to prescribe traditional herbal medicines along with modern medications. In Germany, herbs are on par with commercial pharmaceuticals. And chemists are now identifying active compounds in these flavors that may account for their therapeutic effects.

This chapter tells you about the health benefits of many common herbs and spices and how they can ease symptoms when you're ill. You also find out about the healing qualities of certain flavorings and have a look at different sweeteners. You can add delicious flavorings to your cooking and give your health a boost as well.

Culinary Herbs That Gently Heal

Herbs are the fragrant leaves of various plants that commonly grow in temperate zones and do not have woody stems. (*Spices,* in contrast, are not obtained from the leaves, but the bark, buds, fruit, roots, seeds, and stems of various plants and trees.) Many of today's culinary herbs were used medicinally in the monasteries of Europe long ago. The knowledge of their healing properties was recorded in manuscripts and, during the Dark Ages, was preserved by women who passed on the knowledge of them by word of mouth. But then, with the Renaissance and the age of exploration by sea, herbalism took a giant leap forward, as exotic plants were brought home for study. Soon universities had "physic" gardens full of herbs, which physicians studied and apothecaries ground with mortar and pestle.

Now's your chance to work with these same herbs, in your own kitchen, adding them to the foods you cook. Over time, their subtle health-promoting properties can do their part in bringing you good health. And should you be sick, you can use these herbs to help you recover.

If you explore the world's cuisines, you'll find that fresh herbs are much more widely used than in American cooking. Many traditional cuisines incorporate fresh herbs into everyday dishes, such as Thai salads, in which lettuce is mixed with generous amounts of basil and cilantro; or Persian omelets, which you make with 2 parts egg and 1 part dill. Then there's the chamomile tea you find everywhere in Mexico, and rosemary used to flavor all sorts of roasts and savory dishes in European cooking. So don't limit your use of fresh herbs to garnishing with a sprig. Cook with a variety of herbs on a regular basis. In the following list, I cover some common herbs (see Figure 11-1) and their traditional medicinal uses.

If you want to use herbs to treat a chronic ailment, make a tea by using the leaves and start with one cup a day, building up to three cups per day. Beneficial results should be evident within two weeks. Side effects to watch for include headaches, nausea, and vomiting. To find out about how to prepare medicinal teas and tonics, refer to *Herbal Remedies For Dummies,* by Christopher Hobbs (IDG Books Worldwide, Inc.).

- ✔ **Basil:** Soothes nerves, clears bronchial congestion, fights infection, clears the mind, lifts depression, and aids digestion. Add basil to salads, pasta dishes, soups, sandwiches, and use to flavor homebaked bread.

- ✔ **Fennel seeds:** Traditionally used to stimulate lactation, menstrual flow, and libido; contains phytohormones, compounds that help balance your own hormones (find out more about these in Chapter 17); use to treat PMS and symptoms of menopause; also a digestive aid. Add fennel to fish stews, and munch on them after a heavy meal.

✔ **Lemon balm:** Soothes nerves, relaxes muscles, relieves depression, lessens menstrual cramps, eases digestion, fights bacterial and viral infections (including herpes), and relieves pain. Enjoy lemon balm in salad, in fish dishes, desserts, and especially as a tea.

✔ **Marjoram:** Helps regulate the menstrual cycle, reduces menstrual cramping, relieves stomach upset and babies' colic, and relieves headaches. Add fresh marjoram leaves to bath water to relieve pain and soothe nerves. Include in stuffings for game, soups, and salad dressings.

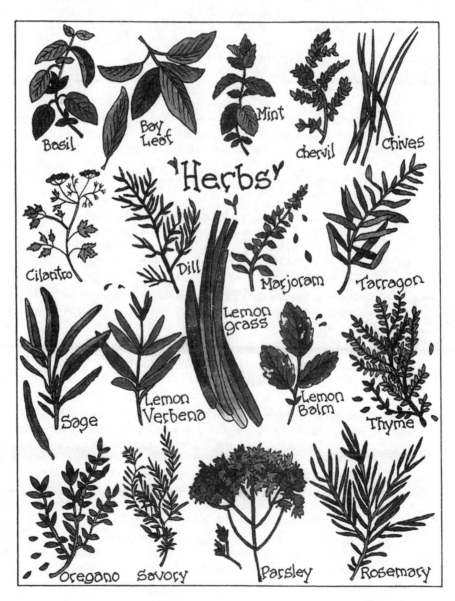

Figure 11-1:
Some common herbs.

After-dinner mints and other herbal digestive aids

There is herbal wisdom in the after-dinner mint! These sweets aid digestion after a fatty meal, clearing the palate and easing the stomach. Many other herbs and spices are credited with reducing after-meal bloating and gas. Caraway seeds, cayenne pepper, coriander, fennel seeds, ginger, and the Mexican herb epazote are considered digestive aids. Some people find that as they switch to whole grains and beans, and more raw foods, that their digestion goes through a period of adjustment and needs a little help. (Also take a look at Chapter 20 in the section on digestion.)

- **Mint:** Aids digestion, relieves fatigue, reduces menstrual cramping, treats nausea and motion sickness, acts as a remedy for colds by stimulating the flow of mucous, and aids coughs, sore throats, headaches, and fever. Add to Middle Eastern dishes, fruit salads, and desserts. Use as a condiment and especially as a soothing tea to benefit from its volatile oil, menthol, which you can inhale.

- **Parsley:** Sweetens the breath, helps heal gum disease (gingivitis), relieves indigestion, and enhances the immune system; especially high in vitamin C, beta-carotene, iron, and magnesium. Enjoy parsley in a cream sauce for fish filet, add to soups and salads — and yes, add as garnish and then be sure that you eat it!

To brighten the flavor of a recipe that calls for dried herbs, first mix the herbs with chopped fresh parsley and then use this mixture to season the dish.

- **Rosemary:** Increases the flow of bile to promote digestion, invigorates circulation, helps relieve headaches, serves as a tonic for stress, supports normal communication between nerves, and improves memory. Use to flavor lamb roast, potatoes, salads, soups, and breads.

- **Sage:** Inhibits the growth of bacteria to ease colds and sore throats, helps heal mouth sores and receding gums when used as a mouthwash, helps balance hormones, thereby lessening menstrual cramping and menopausal hot flashes, and contains plentiful minerals and antioxidants. The medicinal use of sage is not recommended for pregnant women and nursing mothers, but if you use small amounts of sage in cooking, it's typically considered safe. Add to poultry stuffings, roasted vegetables, and meat sauces and use as a tea.

- **Tarragon:** Stimulates appetite, aids digestion, relieves colic, helps regulate the menstrual cycle, and lessens the pain associated with joint disease. Use tarragon to flavor lamb and fish, carrots, and deviled eggs.

Cooking with French lavender

French lavender, a decorative flowering plant that is at home in sunny, dry terrain (including Provence and my backyard), has a flavor reminiscent of rosemary and can be used as a culinary herb. It's delicious added to Yogurt Cream (recipe in Chapter 9) and spooned over fruit. Lavender promotes relaxation, but rather than dulling the spirits, it has an uplifting effect.

Lavender also induces sleep. Researchers working with elderly patients in a nursing home in England compared the effects of a standard tranquilizer with lavender for the ability to induce sleep. When lavender oil was diffused into the air, the patients slept as well as when they had taken the medication, according to results published in the British medical journal *The Lancet*. Furthermore, these individuals slept more quietly and showed no side effects the following day.

✔ **Thyme:** Fights bacterial and fungal infections, helps bring up phlegm, relaxes the respiratory tract, is useful as a mouthwash, promotes digestion, alleviates nausea, and counteracts altitude sickness. Use thyme when you cook poultry and roasts and add it to salads and soup.

✔ **Watercress:** Clears bronchial congestion, lessens cough, promotes digestion, strengthens gums, lowers high blood sugar, reduces fluid retention, and contains many vitamins and minerals, including vitamin A and calcium. (Also turn to Chapter 20, in the section on water retention, for more about watercress.)

You can bring fresh herbs to your table in many ways — in salads, chopped fine and mixed with olive oil, parmesan cheese, and garlic to make a pasta sauce, or served as part of the little Italian open-faced sandwiches known as *bruschetta*.

Warm Bruschetta with Fresh Basil

In this recipe, basil leaves are eaten in quantity like lettuce and made into a little salad that sits atop garlic toast.

Preparation time: 10 minutes

Cooking time: 10 minutes

Yield: 4 servings

(continued)

2 large ripe tomatoes, diced

¼ pound fresh mozzarella cheese, diced

½ cup basil leaves, chopped, plus 8 leaves for garnish

½ cup homemade basil-scented olive oil or plain extra-virgin olive oil

2 tablespoons balsamic vinegar

1 clove garlic, minced

4 1½- to 2-inch slices of round, flat loaf of freshly baked bread with a substantial texture*

1 tablespoon capers

Freshly ground black pepper to taste

1 Preheat the broiler.

2 Combine the tomatoes, cheese, and basil in a small bowl and set aside.

3 In a bowl, whisk together the olive oil, vinegar, and garlic and set aside.

4 Cut each piece of bread lengthwise into 4 slices of equal width.

5 Arrange the bread slices on a baking sheet and place 6 inches under the broiler. Allow the slices to lightly toast for about 4 to 6 minutes and then remove from heat.

6 Brush the bruschetta lightly with some of the salad dressing. Fan 4 bread slices on each of 4 individual salad plates.**

7 Top the bruschetta with the tomato mixture. Drizzle the remaining dressing over the garnished bruschetta. Place 2 basil leaves where the pieces of bruschetta come together. Strew with capers and add a grind or 2 of pepper. Serve immediately.

*You need bread that absorbs the juices of the food you place on top, but one that's strong enough not to fall apart after it absorbs the liquids.

**Serve on heavy, white kitchen porcelain for an Italian chef look or on colorful glazed ceramics for a country look.

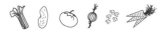

Fresh is better

Fresh herbs have medicinal benefits that can be lost when the green herb is dried. You may think of fresh herbs as a gourmet luxury (they can be expensive), but eating fresh herbs regularly is one more way to promote your good health. If you do cook with dried herbs, use those that have retained the color and scent of the original plant, which is a sign that healing compounds, such as essential oils, are still present. Discard all dried herbs that have turned gray and feel like sawdust in your mouth.

Herbs used in the small quantities needed to add flavor to a dish are not considered a health risk. However, taken in volume, their active compounds may be potentially toxic. Consult an herbalist before taking high doses.

Treating Ailments with Exotic Spices

Feeling a bit under the weather? Need a pick-me-up? Have some curry or even a baked apple spiked with cinnamon and cloves. The active compounds in the colorful and pungent spices that flavor such foods have remarkable health-promoting properties. Today, people appreciate the classic dishes of traditional cuisines around the world for their rich and complex flavorings, but there is more to these dishes than meets the tongue.

Following are some common spices (see Figure 11-2) and their healing properties:

- **Cardamom:** Promotes normal digestion and reduces gas and spasms of the colon. This Asian spice is said to have grown in the Hanging Gardens of Babylon and is praised in *The Arabian Nights* as an aphrodisiac. Its exotic scent may well free the imagination!

- **Cinnamon:** Promotes good digestion, helps to control diarrhea, fights bacterial infection, helps reduce menstrual cramping, restores energy after overeating, and enhances liver function, allowing the release of toxins from the body. This aromatic spice is actually dried bark. The bark oil is antibacterial, inhibiting the growth of several common bacteria, including strains of bacteria that cause traveler's diarrhea, food poisoning, and yeast infection.

- **Clove:** Sweetens the breath and functions as an antiseptic. Oil of clove, which you can purchase in most pharmacies, temporarily stops the pain of toothache when a drop or two is dabbed on the problem area.

- **Ginger:** Warms the body, increases circulation, promotes sweating and the release of toxins from the body for the treatment of colds and flu, aids digestion, eases arthritis pain, and helps lessen the risk of clogged arteries. Studies show that taking powdered ginger before boarding a boat prevents *mal-de-mer,* or seasickness, quite effectively — it's used as a standard remedy on cruise ships. As little as half a teaspoon of powdered ginger has been found to relieve postoperative nausea, a side effect of anesthesia. Even the amount of ginger in gingersnaps or ginger ale may be adequate to relieve mild queasiness.

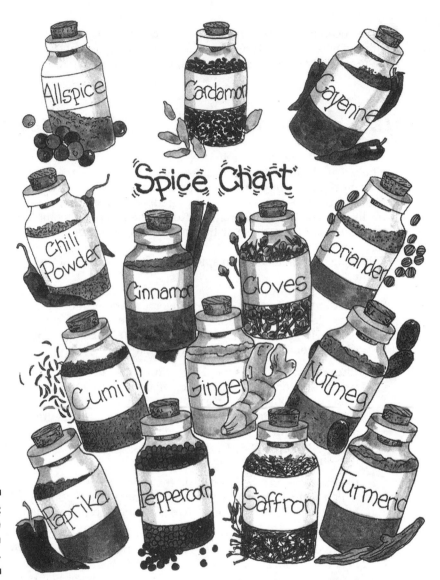

Figure 11-2:
Some common spices.

✔ **Mustard seed:** Stimulates appetite, aids digestion, relieves chronic constipation, and helps arrest the onset of a cold. Mustard is a relative of broccoli and cabbage, and its active constituents are mustard oils, which contain allyl-isothiocyanate. To benefit from mustard's healing properties, add one of the many varieties now available — French Dijon, whole-grain German mustard, English mustard powder, and American ballpark mustard — to salad dressings, roasted meats, vegetables, and sandwiches.

Mustard greens are considered a traditional tonic for the liver. Many groceries now carry this vegetable, a standard ingredient in Southern cooking.

✔ **Turmeric:** Reduces inflammation, making it useful in the treatment of such conditions as hay fever, muscle injury, and arthritis. Also treats itchiness and skin disease when applied externally, according to Ayurvedic medical treatises dating back 3,000 years (for more on Ayurveda, turn to Chapter 2). The active component of brightly colored, yellow-orange turmeric is *curcumin,* which in studies has been shown to be as effective at reducing inflammation as common anti-inflammatory drugs, but without the side effects.

Spice can turn a ho-hum, ordinary ingredient like chicken into a culinary masterpiece! Give this one a try.

North African Roast Chicken with Almonds and Dried Fruits

The array of spices and dried fruit in this recipe turns ordinary chicken into an exotic dish, a great choice for a buffet dinner party. The sweet potatoes, very high in beta-carotene, add a unique flavor to this "chicken stew."

Preparation time: *20 minutes*

Cooking time: *1 hour*

Yield: *4 servings*

1 chicken, preferably naturally raised, quartered

Freshly ground black pepper to taste

2 tablespoons extra-virgin olive oil

1 onion, thinly sliced

1 tablespoon minced garlic

2 medium sweet potatoes, with skins, cut into 2-inch chunks

1 tablespoon ground cumin

1 tablespoon ground cinnamon

1 tablespoon ground coriander

4 cups chicken stock

½ lemon, in segments and cut into ½-inch chunks, plus the central pith*

¼ cup currants

¼ cup dried figs

¼ cup dried unsulphured apricots**

¼ cup blanched almonds, coarsely chopped

(continued)

1 Preheat oven to 350°. Sprinkle the chicken with pepper. In a large sauté pan, heat the olive oil over medium heat until hot but not smoking. Add the chicken parts and cook, turning every couple minutes, until well browned on all sides, 5 to 7 minutes. Remove and set aside on a large plate.

2 Add the onion slices to the sauté pan and sauté over medium heat, stirring frequently, until they begin to brown, 5 to 7 minutes. Add the garlic and cook, stirring frequently, for 1 additional minute. Add the potatoes and spices and cook, still stirring frequently, for 1 more minute. Add the stock, reserved chicken, and all the remaining ingredients and bring to a boil.

3 Cover the sauté pan, put it in the preheated oven, and cook until the chicken is tender and cooked through, 25 to 30 minutes. Let sit 5 minutes. Season with pepper and serve.

Suggested accompaniments: Steamed spinach, whole-grain couscous

*To segment the lemon, peel it to the flesh and then separate the segments. Keep intact the membrane. The white pith in the center of the lemon is where the healthful flavonoids are.

**If you're sensitive to sulphur, you can buy unsulphured apricots in natural-food stores.

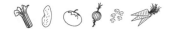

Condiments That Deliver More Than Flavor

Certain foods used as flavorings also have medicinal value. For example, onion and garlic (see Chapter 6) have long been revered for their many healing properties. Condiments such as chili peppers, horseradish, licorice, and certain sweeteners also provide unique health benefits. Ancient peoples recognized the value of these foods, paying them ceremonial honor. King Tut was entombed with piles of licorice.

The following condiments have medicinal value that you want to be aware of:

✔ **Chili peppers:** Warm the body, promote good digestion, act as a mild diuretic to help remove toxins, and used to treat respiratory ailments (see Figure 11-3). Capsaicin, one of the compounds that give hot peppers their bite, has powerful medicinal properties. The hotter the pepper, the more capsaicin it delivers. Cayenne pepper is made from special cayenne chilies. Adding a pinch of cayenne to hot water and sipping this eases a congested chest. Cayenne also makes a good substitute for black pepper, which can be irritating to the stomach.

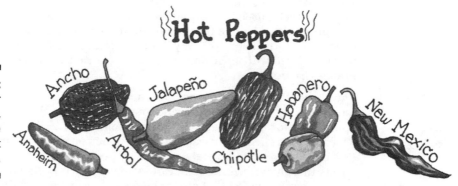

Figure 11-3:
The hotter
the pepper,
the more
capsaicin it
delivers.

Capsaicin dampens pain by triggering the release of *endorphins*, the body's natural opiates, produced in the brain, which raise the pain threshold. (Chocolate also causes the release of endorphins.) It's administered as a cream to reduce the pain of shingles and arthritis. The mild irritation that this substance produces confuses nerve cells and interferes with the relaying of pain signals to the brain. Capsaicin also stimulates the flow of digestive juices, thereby protecting the lining of the stomach from damage by acids and alcohol. (Yes, margaritas and hot salsa do go together.) Research also suggests that capsaicin lowers blood pressure and can even play a role in blocking the development of cancer.

You may have been told that the hot bits in chilies are in the seeds and membranes, but actually, capsaicin and other fiery compounds are in the soft, seed-bearing core of these vegetables. That's why you also need to remove this, too, if you want to cut down the heat.

✔ **Horseradish root:** Promotes urination and removal of toxins, stimulates circulation, strengthens immunity, fights bacterial infection in the lungs and urinary tract, and treats gout and rheumatism. The healing properties of hot-tasting horseradish root are due to the mustard oil it contains. To benefit from horseradish, you need to use the fresh root.

Horseradish root is not recommended for persons who have low thyroid function or who are taking thyroxine.

✔ **Licorice root:** Lessens bronchial congestion, helps balance estrogen to curtail symptoms of PMS and menopause, and treats inflammation associated with asthma and allergies. It also helps heal ulcers, supports liver and kidney function, promotes cardiovascular health, acts as an antidote to toxins such as diphtheria and tetanus, and fights bacterial and viral infection, including hepatitis B. Licorice root is an excellent source of vitamin C and beta-carotene.

The major active compound is *glycyrrhizin,* which gives the root its taste (a bittersweet aniseed flavor) and its decongestant and anti-inflammatory properties. Licorice tea is made from the root, but check the label of licorice candy before you buy it for its therapeutic properties. Much of it is flavored with anise and contains no licorice. Look for imported brands that do.

The glycyrrhizin in licorice root can cause side effects such as fluid retention, high blood pressure, and low potassium levels and is not appropriate for persons at risk for these conditions. Even licorice candy, which contains licorice extract, should not be consumed in large quantities and should be completely avoided by people sensitive to the side effects that glycyrrhizin causes. However, you can now find licorice extracts on the market that are for medicinal purposes and that have had the glycyrrhizin removed.

Sweeteners

Young and old have a taste for sweet foods. It's a natural survival instinct. The sweetest fruit, at the peak of the season, contain more health-giving nutrients than fruit that is not as ripe, or already going bad. Our ancestors learned to eat the sweetest fruit, and we're still on the hunt for sweet foods. Of course, these days we overdo it. Americans eat on average 155 pounds of sugar a year. This overconsumption of sugar plays a role in the development of many health conditions, including tooth decay, obesity, diabetes, heart disease, and various psychological and emotional problems, including those related to PMS and syndromes involving stress and burnout.

Take a look at the kinds of sugar you have to choose from. Some sweets are more nutritious than others.

Refined sugar: Pure white and empty

Refined white sugar has no nutritional value except for providing calories. When sugar is processed, its vitamins, minerals, amino acids, and trace elements are stripped away. Sugar is easily assimilated and converted into blood sugar, which the cells use for energy. However, in order for your body to turn sugar into energy, the chemical reactions involved require several B vitamins (vitamin B5, thiamin, niacin, and riboflavin) plus magnesium. Eating sugar uses up these nutrients so that they are not available to perform other functions in your body such as maintaining your nervous system or building bones. You can use refined white sugar as a source of energy, but you deplete your reserves of these nutrients when you do.

Food products contain main forms of sugar with various names. Look for corn syrup, corn sweeteners, high fructose corn syrup, dextrose, dextrin, malt, fructose, fruit juice concentrate, invert sugar, and evaporated cane juice. Often several of these sugars are listed and, if added together, may be one of the most plentiful ingredients in the food that you're buying.

Sugar can also be addicting. Withdrawal symptoms include weakness, poor concentration, depression, and a strong craving for sugary foods.

Replacing white sugar with natural and nutritious sweeteners

You do have options if you have a sweet tooth. The following sweeteners also provide some vitamins and minerals, and some, like honey, even have a medicinal effect.

However, don't kid yourself. All these foods are sugars, and eating these sweeteners in quantity will have the same effect on your system. Sugars of all sorts cause insulin levels to rise. (Insulin is the hormone that manages blood sugar and allows you to store sugar in your cells for later use). And abnormally high levels of insulin can lead to medical problems, including diabetes, hypertension, atherosclerosis, and coronary artery disease. If you do use sweeteners, use them in moderation.

- **Maple syrup:** Rich in potassium and calcium. Check to make sure that it's labeled "pure" maple syrup, or it may be mixed with corn syrup. A product that calls itself "pancake syrup" may contain no more than 2 to 3 percent maple syrup, with the remainder consisting of corn syrup or sugar syrup, plus artificial flavoring and color.

  Grade C maple syrup, which is dark brown and strongly flavored, is preferred because it is higher in mineral content than the more delicately flavored, amber-colored Grade A maple syrup.

- **Date sugar:** Made from ground, dehydrated dates. A good source of folic acid and potassium, plus other nutrients and complex carbohydrates found in dried dates. Nearly as sweet as sugar. Can be used as you would brown sugar.

- **Blackstrap molasses:** The syrup left over when cane sugar is made into white table sugar. Rich in iron, calcium, and potassium, with a strong bitter flavor. The milder-tasting light and medium molasses deliver only half to a third of the nutrients.

  Molasses contains sulphur. Therefore, if you have a sensitivity to sulphur, which can cause symptoms ranging from nausea to difficulty in breathing, use unsulphured or Barbados molasses.

✔ **Honey:** Supplies an exceptionally wide range of vitamins, minerals, and amino acids, as well as several phytonutrients that function as antioxidants. Darker colored honeys, such as buckwheat, have greater antioxidant activity. Honey kills bacteria and can be used to treat infection. Look for New Zealand raw Manuka honey sold in specialty stores. In studies, Manuka honey has been proven to prevent the growth of common kitchen bacteria such as *Staphylococcus aureas*.

The potency of honey varies, with tree honey such as orange more effective than honey produced from low-growing flowers like clover. And raw honey has more antibacterial activity than honey that is heat-treated during pasteurization, true of most honey on the market. Honeycomb is the least treated form of all.

To preserve raw honey's antibacterial properties, use it at room temperature or add it to foods after they are cooked.

✔ **Stevia:** Stevia is an herb that grows primarily in South America, where it has been used as a sweetener for more than 600 years. Although stevia is noncaloric, it is 250 to 300 times sweeter than sugar. You can find stevia in natural-food stores. For more about stevia, check out the stevia Web site `www.fastlane.net/~kirkland/stevia/stevia.htm`.

A little stevia goes a long way. A squirt or two in your tea sweetens the brew, but a lot of stevia can produce a bitter taste.

Sugar substitutes

Aspartame, a chemical sweetener, is about 200 times sweeter than sugar. It is sold under the names NutraSweet and Equal. One of aspartame's components, *methanol,* can convert to formaldehyde and formic acid, substances that have a toxic effect on the thymus gland. People who are sensitive to aspartame report such symptoms as recurrent headaches, dizziness, nausea, malaise, and visual disturbances. Aspartame is used as a sweetener in dozens of categories of diet foods.

Another component of aspartame is *phenylalanine,* an amino acid. In an individual who has the inherited disease phenylketonuria, phenylalanine can accumulate and cause seizures and mental retardation.

Saccharin is another controversial artificial sweetener. The use of saccharin has been implicated in the development of cancer.

The advent of sugar substitutes has not dampened the appetite for sugar. As consumption of these substances has risen, so has the consumption of sugar. And dieters beware: According to several studies, individuals who consume sugar substitutes tend to eat more food, perhaps to compensate for the missing calories.

Chapter 12

Selecting the Healthiest Beverages

· ·

In This Chapter

▶ Giving yourself ample, pure water

▶ Quenching thirst with nourishing juices

▶ Assessing the pros and cons of coffee

▶ Treating ailments with a cup of tea

▶ Nixing colas and alcohol

· ·

> **Recipes in This Chapter**
>
> ↻ California Sunrise
> ↻ Icy Pear Cooler
> ↻ Uncoffee Cappuccino
> ↻ Fizzy Fruit Cocktail
>
>

*W*hat kinds of drinks do you use to quench your thirst and wash down a meal? Start keeping track. Do you rely on liquids that are sweet or on beverages that contain caffeine?

Although you may think that what you drink is an inconsequential part of a meal, don't discount the nutritional impact of what you sip. A glass full of super-sweet fruit juice, or a cup of coffee or tea buzzing with caffeine, affects your system as much as any gooey dessert does. You may go out of your way to eat healthy salads and avoid greasy foods; beverages require the same careful selection. But don't worry — you have many healthful drinks to choose from.

Water: The Ultimate Thirst Quencher

Water is the ideal beverage. It replenishes fluids in the system, but because it doesn't need to be digested or metabolized by the body, it provides benefits with a minimum expenditure of energy. Water is a primary and fundamental nutrient, just like protein, fat, and carbohydrates. The reason for this is that water does much more than quench thirst. Water's crucial functions within the body include the following:

> ## You may be thirstier than you think
>
> The first sign of thirst is not having a dry mouth. A dry mouth is a sign that you've been thirsty for a long while and need some water right now! A sign of dehydration that happens well before is fatigue, both physical and mental.
>
> You probably aren't drinking as much water as you need. This is the norm, because colas, tea, coffee, and juices are the beverages of choice for most people. In addition, you may have to rediscover the sensation of thirst. In many adults, this survival mechanism has oddly faded, which perhaps is a sign of chronic dehydration. The body no longer recognizes the signals that fluids are needed and no longer asks for water.

- Transports vitamins and minerals
- Takes part in water-dependent chemical reactions
- Plays a role in energy production
- Acts as an adhesive to bond cell structures
- Provides lubrication around joints
- Serves as a shock absorber inside the spinal cord and eyes
- Acts as a solvent for substances, such as mineral salts, that maintain the vital balance between acidity and alkalinity in body tissues
- Provides a vehicle for waste removal from the body
- Plumps up cells so that wrinkles are less apparent

Without water, these functions begin to fail. However, as crucial as water is to human existence, the body does not have a large reserve of water to draw on. You need to drink water throughout the day, every day.

If you hit a mid-afternoon low, instead of grabbing a cup of coffee, which is a diuretic and increases urination, quickly drink one or more glasses of cool water. This remedy for fatigue brings true refreshment.

Increasing your intake of water

To make sure that your body is well hydrated, try to drink eight glasses of water a day. If you're not accustomed to drinking this much water, you may at first feel like you're drowning, but try to sip water throughout the day.

What you sip can add up. Keep containers of water in the rooms where you spend most of your time so that you're reminded to drink some, and you have no excuses. Fill pitchers, carafes, jars, and bottles with water and keep them within easy reach.

Making sure that you're drinking water of the highest quality

The U.S. water supply contains approximately 1,000 chemicals and other impurities, including chlorine, lead, mercury, benzene, bacteria, industrial wastes, mining wastes, pesticide runoff from farms, toxins from leaking municipal landfills, feces, and radon, a radioactive byproduct of uranium decay. These compounds can burden the immune system and overwork the liver, which is designed to inactivate toxins.

Filtering water

You have a great deal more control over the quality of your water when you use a water filter. A good water-filtering system incorporates several methods of filtering water. Activated carbon filters cleanse water by using either granular or solid block carbon. Reverse-osmosis systems depend on water pressure and a range of selective membranes that remove specific contaminants. Copper-zinc alloy (KDF) systems use an electrochemical process. You can also buy a distillation system that boils the water and condenses the steam. You need to buy a system that filters out the particular contaminants that your water contains — a good reason for having your water tested.

When shopping for a filter, look for those that are able to remove organisms that are less than 1 micron in size, such as the common human parasite *Giardia lamblia*.

A bonus of filtering is that filtered water tastes better because the chlorine is removed. Chlorine in water may be a health risk. Chlorine can react with other substances and produce carcinogenic compounds called *trihalomethanes*.

Figuring out which water-filtering system to buy and understanding what each type has to offer can be complicated. A good resource to help you through the process is the National Sanitation Foundation (NSF), at 3475 Plymouth Road, Ann Arbor, MI 48105; 800-673-8010. Call for a booklet on filtering or visit the NSF Web site at www.nsf.org.

One highly recommended source for water filters, as well as air filters, is Environmental Protection Products, 100 Carney St., Glen Cove, NY 11542; 800-444-3563; www.cwrenviro@worldnet.att.net.

The first time you turn on the faucet each day, make sure that you let it run a minute or two before you take water for drinking or cooking. This will help flush out bacteria and contaminating minerals, such as lead, a component of all water pipes, which can accumulate in dormant water. Also use cold water from the tap because minerals tend to leach out into hot water, not cold. However, hot water does have one advantage — a lower level of potentially toxic chlorine, which becomes volatile in hot water and escapes into the air. (Water filters remove both lead and chlorine.)

The Environmental Protection Agency is responsible for monitoring the quality of water, but it currently tests for only 80 contaminants. However, you can find out more about the quality of your water supply. Begin by asking your municipal water company for its analysis of the quality of the water it supplies. If that approach doesn't supply the information you need, try these suggestions:

✔ **Have an independent lab test your water.** The lab sends you a water collection kit, which you return with a sample that it can assess for purity. Here are four avenues to pursue:

- National Testing Laboratories, Inc., 6555 Wilson Mills Rd., Cleveland, OH 44143; 800-458-3330

- Spectrum Labs, Inc., 301 W. County Rd. E2, New Brighton, MN 55112; 800-447-5221

- Water Quality Association, 4151 Naperville Road, Lisle, IL 60532-1088; 630-505-0160; www.wqa.org.

- The EPA Safe Drinking Water Hotline at 800-426-4791 can give you the name and phone number of the drinking water laboratory certification officer in your state, who has a list of approved labs in your area. Also ask for the federal limits of contaminants, a document titled *National Primary Drinking Water Standards.* You can compare these figures with your test results. (You can access the water area of the EPA Web site at www.epa.gov/safewater.)

✔ **If you drink bottled water, write to the bottlers and ask for the results of their water quality tests.** Just because water is bottled does not guarantee safety. Some of the bottled water is just tap water, and even bottled spring water may contain contaminants.

You may also want to select a filter that removes fluoride, a trace element that is routinely added to water. After decades of debate over the benefits and risks of this process, there is evidence that fluoride reduces tooth decay, but some studies link fluoride with an increased risk of bone cancer and a crippling skeletal disease characterized by dense, hard, but very fragile bones. In addition, children under the age of nine who have received higher levels of fluoride than recommended can develop dark brown mottling and spotting of teeth.

In some cases, the teeth can become chalky white in appearance. Watch for these signs of overexposure. Higher levels of fluoride in water are found in the northern Plains states and the Southwest states. The best way to avoid tooth decay is not by drinking fluoridated water, but by avoiding sugar and eating a whole-foods diet.

Nourishing Juices from Fruits and Vegetables

A glass of fruit or vegetable juice is a nourishing mini-meal. Freshly extracted juice is full of vitamins, minerals, and natural sugars. Carrot juice, for example, supplies extraordinarily high levels of vitamin A in the form of beta-carotene. Pineapple juice supplies several B vitamins that support hair and skin health, as well as copper and a small amount of magnesium and potassium.

Freshly prepared juice also contains living enzymes, which are proteins that catalyze chemical reactions. They are present in raw foods, including fruit and vegetable juices. Enzymes can trigger the breakdown of cell walls, eventually causing a food to spoil. Eating foods that contain enzymes aids in their digestion.

The only part of the fruit that is missing in juice is the fiber, which is separated from the juice in the juicing process. Fruit, not fruit juice, supplies fiber, which helps keep the digestive tract healthy and helps steady blood sugar. However, fruit juice still has a place in a healing foods diet, giving you an easy way to increase your intake of nutrients.

Inventing juice drinks is great fun. Here, I've mixed a fruit with a juice to come up with this one.

California Sunrise

You can make fruity beverages with a combination of fruit juices and freshly pureed fruit. By starting with whole fruit to make this drink, you increase your intake of fruit as well as the vitamins, minerals, and fiber it contains. Eating melon with other foods that contain protein and fat may result in digestive upset. For this reason, it's best to enjoy this melon-based frappe as a between-meal treat.

Preparation time: *10 minutes*

Cooking time: *None*

Yield: *4 servings*

(continued)

3 cups seedless chilled watermelon   *1 teaspoon fresh-squeezed lemon juice*

1⅓ cup fresh-squeezed, chilled orange juice

1 Put the watermelon chunks in a food processor and blend until most of the fruit is pureed, leaving small bits of fruit for texture.

2 Pour the pureed watermelon into a pitcher. Add the orange juice and lemon juice. Stir to blend.

Note: By using chilled fruit, you can avoid adding ice, which would dilute this drink.

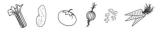

After having juice, drink a little water to rinse off your teeth and remove sugars in the juice that can cause tooth decay. Also, have only one glass of sweet fruit or vegetable juice at a time because, like candy, fruit juice is a highly concentrated sweet that can trigger swings in blood sugar levels. Fruit juice is not recommended for individuals with diseases that involve sugar sensitivity such as hypoglycemia and diabetes.

To be a savvy shopper and make sure that you're buying quality juices, keep the following points in mind:

✔ A juice bottle may be labeled strawberry, kiwi, or tangerine, but it may actually contain more pear, apple, or grape juice than anything else. Check to see whether the first ingredients listed are these juices, with the more exotic and expensive fruit juices coming toward the end of the list. Best to search out the real thing or make your own.

✔ If a label doesn't state "100% juice," the juice probably has been diluted with water, plus some form of refined sugar, such as high-fructose corn syrup. Juice blends often have water as their first ingredient.

✔ Many vegetable juices are high in sodium. However, you can find low sodium versions of standard juices, such as V-8 juice.

✔ Look for fresh-made juices in the refrigerated section of your market. These juices are likely to have higher levels of the more perishable vitamins, as well as enzymes. The bottle should carry a date that lets you know how long the juice will stay fresh and safe to drink.

Icy Pear Cooler

By diluting the pear juice with ginger tea, you get a sweet beverage that's less likely to give you a sugar rush.

Preparation time: 30 minutes

Cooking time: 3 minutes

Yield: 6 servings

2 cups filtered water

1 bag Stash Ginger Lemon tea

1 quart 100% pear juice

A couple of squeezes of lemon juice

1 Bring the filtered water to a boil. Pour into a teapot, add the tea bag, and let steep for 5 minutes. Discard tea bag. Set tea aside until cooled to room temperature.

2 In a pitcher, mix together the tea and pear juice.

3 To the juice mixture, add lemon juice to taste.

4 Pour into tall, ice-filled glasses and enjoy.

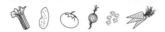

Coffee: Friend and Foe

I've loved coffee ever since my mother put a teaspoonful in my glass of milk, but I also know that I feel much better when I'm not using coffee as a stimulant.

The caffeine in coffee can indeed boost your physical energy, improve muscle function, increase mental alertness, and impart a sense of well-being. Caffeine produces these benefits due to its effect on the adrenal glands, which help sustain your energy level by triggering the release of stored sugars to use as fuel. Normally, as energy reserves are used up, a protective mechanism in the adrenals stops this process and allows your body to rest. However, caffeine disables this shutoff mechanism and allows you to keep going. The problem with caffeine is that it enables you to keep working and using up your energy until you drop.

Caffeine, which is also in tea, colas, and chocolate, has other marks against it. It is a diuretic, increasing urination and thereby promoting the loss of minerals and water-soluble vitamins. Caffeine can also trigger anxiety, sleeplessness, irregular heart beat, and low blood sugar.

In women, caffeine may increase the risk of infertility and miscarriages. In addition, some studies (but not all) have found an association with caffeine consumption and fibrocystic disease of the breast characterized by breast tenderness and benign lumps in the breast. Some women report a significant lessening of breast tenderness after going off caffeinated coffee and tea. And newborns of mothers who used caffeine during pregnancy show signs of caffeine withdrawal. Caffeine is transmitted through mother's milk.

Are you addicted to caffeine?

One day, I was eating at a Los Angeles restaurant and happened to chat with a woman who was seated at the next table. She told me that she hadn't thought that she was addicted to caffeine until the day of the Northridge earthquake. Due to the quake, all her utilities were turned off, including her electricity, and she wasn't able to make coffee that morning. At about 10 a.m., she began to have an enormous craving and, despite the strong after-tremors, was willing to drive to a local coffee shop to have a cup.

Here are some signs that *you* may be dependent on caffeine:

✔ You have some caffeinated beverage every day, even if it is only a small amount.

✔ You are plagued by brain fog in the morning before your first cup of coffee or caffeinated tea.

✔ You use coffee to control your daily cycle of energy.

✔ You rely on caffeinated coffee or tea to help you move your bowels.

✔ You experience withdrawal symptoms, such as headache, irritability, and even depression, after abstaining from caffeine for 24 to 36 hours.

You are less likely to experience withdrawal headaches as you stop using caffeine if you gradually reduce the dose you take each day. You can begin drinking a mix of regular and decaffeinated coffee or tea, or you can follow Table 12-1 and trade down to a beverage, which naturally contains a smaller amount.

Table 12-1   Switching Hot Beverages to Lower the Caffeine Dose

Beverage	Amount of Caffeine Per 6 Fluid Ounce Cup
Drip-brewed coffee	140 mg
Instant coffee	70 mg
Tea	50 mg
Japanese green tea	25 mg
Cocoa	5 mg
Decaf coffee (brewed and instant)	4 mg, 2 to 8 mg

Uncoffee Cappuccino

I am forever experimenting with coffee substitutes. Many grain and herb substitute coffees are on the market, but the brand used in this recipe is exceptionally coffeelike.

Preparation time: *10 minutes*

Cooking time: *5 minutes*

Yield: *1 large cup*

1 rounded tablespoon Teeccino coffee substitute, or 1 rounded tablespoon café d'orzo*

2 cups filtered water

Stevia (an herbal, nonsugar sweetener)**

¼ cup whole milk

Dash of powdered cinnamon

1 In a drip coffee maker, put the coffee substitute in a filter and brew normally. (You can also prepare the coffee substitute by using a filter cone or a French press pot, following the usual procedures.)

2 In a small saucepan over low heat, warm the milk.

3 Whip the milk with a small whisk or a small electric beater to generate foam.

4 Pour the brewed coffee into a coffee cup. Sweeten to taste with stevia.

5 Pour the warm milk and froth into the coffee.

6 Sprinkle the cappuccino froth with cinnamon, take a sip, and pretend that you're in Venice.

*You can find this brand in natural-food stores.

**Stevia is available at natural-food stores and through mail-order and private distributors. Take a look at Chapter 11 for lots more about this remarkable sweetener.

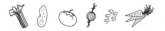

Tea: Social and Medicinal

If you're switching from coffee to tea or are a confirmed tea drinker, you'll be glad to know that recent research has revealed many healing properties of tea. Scientists have identified active compounds in black, green, and oolong teas that provide a variety of health benefits. (All three teas come from the same plant, but each is processed differently and has a unique taste.) Teas contain flavonoids, which act as antioxidants, slow the aging process, and protect against heart disease. Polyphenols, specifically tannins in tea, exhibit antiviral activity and may even prove one day to be of use against cancer.

Green tea contains estrogenic compounds that have a structure similar to our own hormones and play a roll in balancing hormones. Because of this, the habit of drinking green tea, common in Asia, has been linked to the ability of Japanese women to pass through menopause with few symptoms.

Enjoying a nice cup of tea (but not the whole pot)

Sipping a cup of tea can be both restorative and soothing, but drinking cup after cup throughout the day is not recommended. The amount of caffeine in this quantity of tea adds up, just as if you were drinking several strong cups of coffee. Even decaffeinated tea has its drawbacks.

Compounds in tea also interact with important nutrients. Tea contains enzymes that split thiamin (vitamin B1), making it unavailable. Even the beneficial tannins have a downside and can block the absorption of calcium, iron, thiamin, and vitamin B12. Tea also contains *oxalates,* mineral salts formed from oxalic acid, that bind with calcium, potentially leading to the formation of kidney stones. And just like coffee, tea is a diuretic, containing not just caffeine but also *theophylline,* which can make you want "to go."

To make a proper cup of tea, you need to steep the teabag or leaves for five minutes to develop the full flavor. However, if you're concerned about your caffeine intake, you can reduce your tea's caffeine content by nearly half by steeping the tea for only one minute.

Herbal teas that belong in your collection

Tea companies are making the most of the rapidly expanding interest in herbal medicine. Blends of tea that provide a wide range of health benefits are now available in supermarkets as well as natural-food stores. Look for these ingredients:

- **Ginger:** Energizes, warms the system, and eases digestion
- **Chamomile:** Calms, relaxes, and promotes sleep
- **Peppermint:** Aids digestion and lessens menstrual cramps
- **Ginseng:** Counteracts fatigue and acts as a general tonic
- **Senna:** Prevents constipation

> ✔ **Red raspberry leaf:** Benefits women by strengthening the pelvic area
>
> ✔ **St. John's Wort:** Alleviates depression and relieves pain and inflammation
>
> ✔ **Echinacea:** Wards off colds and flu and strengthens the immune system

Drinking any sort of beverage — whether coffee, tea, or chicken soup — when it's very hot can damage the tissues in your upper intestinal tract and esophagus and increase your risk of developing esophageal cancer. Let it cool for a minute or two!

Colas: Just Say No

Colas and soft drinks have no place in a healing foods diet. These beverages are caffeine-sugar-phosphorus cocktails that stress your system and deplete your mineral reserves. The caffeine in cola can give you the jitters just like the caffeine in coffee, the sugar can ultimately cause you to feel tired, and the phosphorus has the ability to draw calcium from your bones. You also need to be wary of aspartame, a common sugar substitute used in diet colas, which is considered safe by the Food and Drug Administration. Some scientists believe that high doses of this substance can adversely affect neurotransmitters in the brain that control thinking, behavior, and mood. (Aspartame can also cause seizures in persons with the genetic disorder phenylketonuria.) Use colas as treats if you must, but please experiment with the following Fizzy Fruit Cocktail, to give yourself a healthier option when you want a sweet, fizzy drink.

Fizzy Fruit Cocktail

A great duo is fruit juice and club soda spiked with a squeeze of lemon or lime. This mixture drinks like a bubbly cola but does not contain the refined sugar and caffeine. When you are out, order cranberry juice, club soda, and a squeeze of lime. Here's a version that I made at home.

Preparation time: *3 minutes*

Cooking time: *None*

Yield: *1 serving*

1 cup Knudsen's 100% pomegranate juice   *1 squeeze lime*

1 generous splash club soda

(continued)

1 Pour the pomegranate juice and club soda into a tall glass. Stir once to combine.

2 Add the lime juice to the juice mixture.

3 Add an ice cube or two. Enjoy!

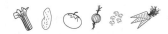

Alcoholic Beverages: Risks and Recommendations

Alcohol and its breakdown products are toxic to the liver and can eventually poison the system if you consume them in great enough quantities for a long enough time. Alcoholism can cause destruction of liver tissue, problems with blood sugar, hypertension, and oral cancer. Individuals consuming much of their calories as alcohol also tend not to eat enough food and risk vitamin and mineral deficiencies and low protein intake that can weaken immunity.

That said, the recent interest in phytonutrients (see Chapter 6) has brought to light certain compounds in wine and beer that have notable health benefits. The French drink wine with their meals and enjoy a relatively low rate of heart disease. Researchers think that compounds called *polyphenols,* found in red grapes and red wine, do the trick. (Polyphenols are not present in white wine.) Flavonoids are present in dark brews of beer, such as stout. Lighter beers contain smaller amounts. Flavonoids remove free radicals, molecules that can damage your arteries, and also help prevent blood platelets from sticking together and forming clots.

Your liver has the task of breaking down alcohol so that the alcohol does no harm. If you're eating healthy foods that do not burden the liver, you should be able to tolerate a shot of tequila or a glass of beaujolais nouveau on special occasions. Indulge in quality, not quantity, and enjoy the best you can afford.

Part IV
Treating Medical Problems with Healing Foods

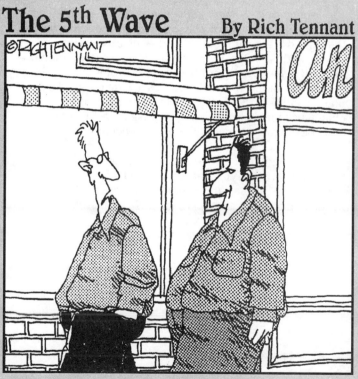

The 5th Wave   By Rich Tennant

"The doctor said my wife suffered from an iron deficiency, so I went home and had all her clothes pressed."

In this part . . .

You can use food as your first line of defense in preventing common ailments and disease. After all, four of the ten leading causes of death and disease in the United States are diet-related — heart disease, cancer, stroke, and diabetes. Even respiratory diseases, pneumonia, and influenza, other major health problems, can be affected by diet. This part includes a wide range of complaints and takes you step by step through ways of changing your diet to lessen your risk of these conditions and speed your recovery should they occur.

So, bon appetit! Get out your pots and pans, reach for a fork, and start enjoying the many special foods that can help prevent disease and support your body when it needs to mend.

Chapter 13

Wakeup Foods for Fatigue

● ●

In This Chapter

▶ Refreshing your body and mind with water

▶ Choosing foods with energizing nutrients

▶ Starting the day with a power breakfast

● ●

> **Recipes in This Chapter**
>
> ▶ Busy-Day Bouillabaisse
>
> ↻ Breakfast Wakeup Muffins
>
> 🥄 🌰 🍶 ⚘ 🌿

*F*atigue is the complaint that doctors most frequently hear from their patients. Are you one of the millions of people who push through tiredness to get through the day? In this achievement-oriented world, you certainly have "permission" to go beyond your limits, both physically and mentally, and to ignore the normal signals from your body that it's time to stop and rest.

Life can be very demanding, even if you're not a super-achiever. You may not be able to take a break from rearing children, caring for aging parents, or trying to launch a business. So what can you do? Plenty, from learning relaxation techniques to going for massages to making sure that what you eat and drink restores your energy rather than depleting it. This chapter helps you take care of the eating and drinking part.

A little exercise can revive your energy, but at the end of an exhausting day, taking it easy and getting a good night's rest is a better strategy for the long term. Save the exercising for the morning. Exercising when you're tired from hours of activity only depletes you more. Besides, exercising late in the day or at night can be overstimulating and keep you from falling asleep.

Refreshing Yourself with Water

Fatigue, both physical and mental, can be a sign that your body is dehydrated. If you're working late at night and feeling tired, try having a glass or two of fresh water instead of reaching for yet another cup of coffee, and you should perk up within a few minutes. You may be surprised to find how thirsty you really are! Water plays an essential role in metabolism, as a component of the many chemical reactions that are *hydrolytic* (meaning that water is an essential part of the reaction and splits molecules in two) and in the production of energy, which occurs within cells.

Water is especially energizing if you drink several glassfuls *quickly.*

Coffee and caffeinated teas give you a quick energy boost, but this high is soon followed by a low, especially if you're overly tired. If you consume more caffeine to restore your energy, you perpetuate an ever-declining energy cycle. In addition, both coffee and tea function as diuretics, increasing urination. To combat this effect, make sure that for every cup of coffee you drink, you drink twice that quantity of water.

Sugar also depletes the body of energy. Gulping down a sugary cola can give you an energy surge, but your body rapidly absorbs the sugar and stores it in the cells. Then your blood sugar drops and your tiredness returns. (The same thing can happen when you eat a piece of pie or cake.)

Eating Foods That Contain Energizing Nutrients

Eating a diet of whole foods gives you more long-lasting energy than foods that are refined and highly processed. Whole foods supply the many vitamins, minerals, and healthy fats that help in the production of energy and bring life-giving oxygen to the cells — in particular, the B vitamins, vitamin C, vitamin E, iron, magnesium, potassium, zinc, and essential fatty acids. If you are deficient in any one of these nutrients, you may feel tired; and having even marginal deficiencies of several of these nutrients can slow you down.

Table 13-1 gives you the lowdown on these essential nutrients — where they come from and how they work in your body.

Table 13-1	Energizing Nutrients	
Nutrient	*Sources*	*How It Works*
B vitamins	Whole wheat, pinto beans, potatoes, avocado, almonds, sunflower seeds, tuna, chicken, liver, yogurt	The cells convert glucose, or blood sugar, into energy with the help of four B vitamins: thiamin, niacin, riboflavin, and pantothenic acid. The adrenal glands, which enable you to withstand stress, also require B vitamins. And according to studies, fatigue is a common symptom of deficiencies of folic acid, pantothenic acid, and vitamin B12.

Nutrient	Sources	How It Works
Vitamin C	Sweet red peppers, broccoli, brussels sprouts, papayas, citrus, strawberries, oysters, liver, rose hips, sauerkraut	Vitamin C supports adrenal gland function and your ability to physically manage stress. When the adrenals are over-worked without proper nourishment, fatigue and even exhaustion can result.
Vitamin E	Millet, whole oats, navy beans, sweet potatoes, asparagus, mangoes, Brazil nuts, sunflower seeds, shrimp, eggs, lamb	As an antioxidant, vitamin E protects the B vitamins and vitamin C, as well as oxygen, from being damaged and destroyed by free radicals. (Find out more about this in Chapter 6.) In this way, vitamin E increases the amount of oxygen traveling in the blood and reaching cells to enliven body functions.
Iron	Brown rice, wild rice, chickpeas, parsley, raisins, pistachios, pumpkin seeds, clams, eggs, liver, beef, pork, lamb, blackstrap molasses	Oxygen in the blood is transported by red blood cells, in part, made up of iron. When the blood lacks sufficient iron (a condition known as *anemia*), fatigue is the primary symptom. Studies show that iron deficiency causes a reduction in both physical and mental activity.
Magnesium	Buckwheat, soybeans, lima beans, spinach, beets, figs, plantains, cashews, pumpkin seeds, shrimp, egg yolk, blackstrap molasses	The conversion of glucose into energy, which makes use of the B vitamins, depends on sufficient supplies of this mineral.
Potassium	Whole rye, millet, beans, potatoes, beet greens, raisins, papayas, pistachios, sunflower seeds, cod, flounder, beef	This mineral, which is far more abundant in whole foods than processed foods, plays a vital role in energy production within the cells. A clinical sign of potassium deficiency is chronic muscular weakness.

(continued)

Table 13-1 *(continued)*

Nutrient	Sources	How It Works
Zinc	Brown rice, cornmeal, Great Northern beans, mushrooms, seaweed, Brazil nuts, cashews, pumpkin seeds, oysters, chicken, duck, beef, lamb	Enzymes catalyze and accelerate the pace of chemical reactions. Zinc is a constituent of many enzymes involved in the digestion and metabolizing of food, functions required for energy production. In addition, several studies have found that when a zinc deficiency is corrected, muscle strength and endurance improve, and your need for sleep diminishes.
Essential fatty acids	Seed oils, organic eggs, organ meats, wild game, whole grains, mackerel, herring, sardines, salmon, tuna, flax seeds, walnuts	These fats, which must be supplied through the diet, transport energizing oxygen.

A delicious way to enjoy walnuts, which have high amounts of omega-3 essential fatty acids, the kind you are most likely to be low on, is to make a salad of fresh sliced pears, mixed salad greens, and walnuts, dressed with a Dijon mustard vinaigrette, and garnished with crumbled goat cheese (chèvre). Or enjoy a fish stew, also high in omega-3. This recipe requires little time or effort.

Busy-Day Bouillabaisse

Eating more fish is a good anti-aging strategy. Minerals in fish help keep bones strong to prevent osteoporosis. The oils in fish are especially abundant in brain cells and in the retina of the eye, supporting mental function and eyesight.

Preparation time: *15 minutes*

Cooking time: *1 hour, 10 minutes*

Yield: *4 generous servings*

1 small bulb fennel, tops removed and chopped

1 small onion, peeled and chopped

1 tablespoon extra-virgin olive oil

2 cloves garlic, minced

1 28-ounce can diced tomatoes

4 sprigs parsley, leaves only, minced

½ teaspoon dried basil

1 fresh, small chilie, minced (1 tablespoon)

1½ cups water or fish stock

1½ pounds of several kinds of seafood (red snapper, bass, cod, and shrimp)

1 In a large stew pot, sauté the fennel and onion in olive oil for 5 to 7 minutes. Add the garlic for another minute and then add the tomatoes, parsley, basil, and chilie. Stir together and cook the tomato sauce over medium heat for 1 hour, adding the water or fish stock as needed.

2 Add the fish to the tomato sauce, lower heat, and cook until fish is opaque, about 10 minutes. If using shrimp, add these in the last few minutes.

3 Ladle bouillabaisse into warmed individual soup bowls and serve immediately with garlic whole-grain French bread and salad.

A Menu for Lasting Energy

Foods that are high in fat can burden your system and make you feel tired. To keep your energy level high, fill your refrigerator and your dinner plate with an array of fresh fruits and vegetables. Go out of your way to eat whole grains. Buy whole-wheat bagels rather than ones made of white flour. (Whole-wheat bagels are good toasted.) Order brown rice rather than white rice when you're at your local Chinese restaurant, and if they don't serve it, suggest that they do. Select leaner cuts of meat, cut back on red meats, and eat more fish. Beans are an excellent lowfat, protein alternative. Nuts and seeds supply vitamins, minerals, and essential fatty acids and provide protein, too.

While the majority of people have more energy when they stoke up on plant foods, some people can eat lots of meat and still feel full of vim and vigor. Notice what kinds of food you eat leave you feeling most energized.

Breakfast is a particularly important meal in terms of how much energy you have throughout the day, so don't shortchange yourself. Eat a real meal. If you eat only something starchy, like toast or an English muffin, and wash it down with coffee, you'll have energy for a couple of hours at most. Instead, give yourself some protein and fat as well. Foods that supply protein and fat burn more slowly than carbohydrates and can keep your body, and your brain, going until lunch. If you're a slow starter in the morning, you particularly need to make the effort to feed yourself.

Brain fog

If you usually greet the day fuzzy-headed, your liver may be underperforming. The liver performs many functions, including metabolizing fats and breaking down toxic substances such as alcohol, drugs, and chemicals. When the liver is overworked, toxins accumulate in the system, and brain fog results.

To improve your liver function, cut back on dietary fats and increase your intake of greens, grains, and legumes. Make sure to get enough choline, folic acid, and vitamin B12 in your diet. These nutrients support liver function and are found in, respectively, eggs, romaine lettuce, and meats. Eat most foods lightly cooked rather than raw and steam foods rather than cooking with fat. In addition, drink plenty of filtered water. You may also want to supplement your diet with the liver-cleansing herb milk thistle, the active ingredient of which is silymarin.

Try one of the following breakfasts for extra pep:

- ✔ Whole-grain toast with almond butter and all-fruit preserves
- ✔ Poached eggs and home fries with rye toast
- ✔ Sautéed polenta and turkey sausage
- ✔ A toasted whole-wheat bagel with smoked salmon
- ✔ Whole-grain pancakes and nitratefree bacon
- ✔ A homemade Breakfast Wakeup Muffin (see the following recipe)

Breakfast Wakeup Muffins

I was going to call these muffins "power muffins," but they're so light and delicate that they're more like a gentle wakeup call. They supply many energizing nutrients: B vitamins, magnesium, potassium, zinc, and essential fatty acids, as well as some protein. In addition, they contain lots of fresh ginger, which is a natural stimulant.

Preparation time: *15 minutes*

Cooking time: *20 minutes*

Yield: *12 muffins*

2 cups whole-wheat pastry flour

2 teaspoons baking powder

½ teaspoon baking soda

¼ teaspoon salt

2 eggs

1 ½ cups fresh-squeezed orange juice (2 oranges)

¼ cup unrefined safflower oil

½ cup grated fresh ginger root

½ cup pitted and chopped dates

½ cup chopped walnuts

12 muffin cups, buttered or lined with paper muffin cups

1 Preheat oven to 350°. In a large bowl, mix together the whole-wheat pastry flour, baking powder, baking soda, and salt.

2 In a medium bowl, beat the eggs. Add the orange juice, oil, and ginger root and whisk together with the eggs.

3 Add the orange juice mixture to the flour mixture, stirring just to moisten the flour. Mix in the dates and walnuts.

4 Distribute the batter evenly among the 12 muffin cups. Bake the muffins until the tops begin to brown, about 20 minutes. Serve warm.

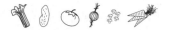

When Fatigue Is a Symptom

Feeling tired can be a symptom of various common ailments and health conditions, as well as a generally weakened immune system. For more information, see Appendix A.

The most common complaint of women passing through menopause is fatigue. Feeling depleted is also associated with more serious conditions, such as mononucleosis, candida, diabetes, and cancer. If your fatigue persists, even after you make the necessary dietary changes and get reasonable amounts of exercise and rest, consult with an informed health professional to rule out any underlying medical problems.

Chronic fatigue syndrome (CFS), which can last for months or years, is characterized by incapacitating fatigue that can come and go. The precise cause is not known, but several factors may be involved. (The Epstein-Barr family of viruses, once thought to cause CFS, has been ruled out.) In some patients, the cause of the disease may be viral. Other factors may include stress, lowered immunity, hormone problems, depression, environmental toxins, and mineral deficiencies. Some patients benefit from injections of magnesium sulfate. Thiamin, vitamin B6, folate, vitamin B12, manganese, iron, molybdenum, and essential fatty acids are also given as supplements.

Arriving bright-eyed and bushy-tailed

If you have to take a night flight from New York to attend a power breakfast in Geneva in the morning, you can minimize your jetlag by choosing your food and drinks carefully. Here are a couple of tips:

✔ A day or two before you fly, avoid caffeine and alcohol and make sure not to drink wine or liquor en route. Instead, have a glass of water every hour you are onboard the plane. (You'll probably need to cart along your own supply of mineral water to supplement what the flight attendants will bring you.)

✔ In your carry-on luggage, pack your own snacks. Mineral-rich fruits and nuts are your best bets — bananas that come in their own tidy packaging, almonds, cashews, pistachios,

and walnuts (shelled, of course, to spare your neighbors). Another good snack food is dried fruit such as dried figs, papaya, mango, and pitted dates (as long as you keep drinking your water!), which is manageable to eat in cramped quarters.

✔ The first few days of your trip, dine *al fresco*. Eat lunch at a sidewalk café and sit outdoors in the sun so that your eyes receive sunlight. This bright light will help you stay awake and adjust to a new time zone. Bright light suppresses your production of *melatonin*, a hormone that helps you fall asleep. Afternoon and early evening light is best. You can expect your internal clock to adjust to the local time by up to three hours per day.

Recovering from chronic conditions takes time. Eating properly and taking supplements can both contribute to your recovery, but if an ailment has developed over a period of time, it usually takes considerable time to correct.

General recommendations for CFS include a diet of whole foods that supply antioxidants, such as the antioxidant vitamins beta-carotene, C, and E, the minerals magnesium and selenium, and B complex vitamins, as well as essential fatty acids. Avoiding foods high in poor-quality fat, refined sugar, caffeine, and alcohol is also very important.

Chapter 14

Improving Your Mood with Food

• •

• •

*I*f you feel moody, anxious, or down in the dumps, you can use food to change how you feel. Food affects your body chemistry, including the aspect of that chemistry that influences mood. Depending on their levels, neurotransmitters in the brain, hormones, and blood sugar can raise your spirits or bring them down. In fact, every meal you eat affects your emotions to some degree. The trick is to have this effect of food work in your favor. This chapter shows you how to ensure that it does.

Calming Down

Eating carbohydrates such as potatoes, cereals, and sweets can help you feel relaxed and give you a sense of general well-being. Such foods trigger your body to produce more *serotonin,* an important neurotransmitter that has a calming effect. When you're all worked up, have a couple of handfuls of popcorn or one or two slices of whole-grain bread with all-fruit preserves. You can feel a difference in 20 to 30 minutes, and the effect should last two to three hours.

In a nutshell, here's how the process works in your body: The body synthesizes serotonin from the amino acid tryptophan. When you eat carbohydrates, your body produces insulin, which increases tryptophan's uptake by the central nervous system. More tryptophan reaches the brain and more serotonin is produced, resulting in a calming effect.

Be forewarned: Carbohydrates are not soothing if you eat them with protein at the same meal. The many other amino acids in protein compete with tryptophan and crowd it out, so no boost in serotonin occurs. Toast is fine. Toast with a slice of ham on it is not. Combining fat with carbohydrate also cuts down on serotonin. A plain baked potato works fine. A baked potato with butter and sour cream is not as effective. Having a small amount of fat along with a starch can enhance the effect of the carbohydrate, however. Eating fatty foods increases your level of *endorphins,* chemicals in the brain that produce a positive mood.

Choosing quality carbohydrates

If you're going to use carbohydrates to calm yourself, choose those that are the most nutritious. Sure, the sugar in candy can quickly calm you. But if you're always relying on sweets to reduce anxiety, you'll be depleting your system of the very nutrients you need for managing stress, the B vitamins, which sugar uses up as it is metabolized. In addition, the conversion of tryptophan to serotonin requires the two B vitamins niacin and vitamin B6, plus the mineral magnesium, also depleted by sugar. Whole grains provide good amounts of all these nutrients.

You probably already have on your kitchen shelf some of the foods you can use as a calming snack. Experiment with these nutritious whole foods. Many people find that even a small portion of any of these foods is calming.

- Whole-grain cereals such as millet, cream of brown rice, and cream of whole wheat, cooked in water, not milk, topped with maple syrup
- Puffed rice cakes
- Whole-grain bread with honey
- Plain baked potato
- Dried fruit

Eating any of these singly or combining them, as I do in this recipe for a soothing cereal, increases their potency.

Peaceful Porridge

Oats, cooked in water along with some dried fruit, are a reliable remedy for stress. The complex carbohydrates in the grain and especially the concentrated sugars in the dried fruit quickly go to work to calm you down.

Preparation time: *3 minutes*

Cooking time: *5 minutes*

Yield: *1 serving*

1 cup filtered water	*½ cup whole oats*
1 heaping tablespoon diced dried fruit, such as apricots, raisins, prunes, or apples	*Salt to taste*

1 Put the water and fruit into a small pot. Cover the pot and bring water to boil.

2 Add the oatmeal and salt (if using) and cook, uncovered, over medium heat for 5 minutes, stirring occasionally.

3 Spoon the porridge into a bowl, settle into a cozy armchair, and be gentle with yourself as you munch.

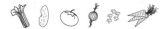

Getting a quick tryptophan fix

Some foods contain tryptophan, so you can boost your own levels directly by eating them. Bananas, almonds, cashews, eggs, beef, and pork are good sources. Turkey has the reputation of being high in tryptophan because everyone falls asleep after eating a huge Thanksgiving dinner, but people do not doze off because of the turkey. The many sweet and starchy carbohydrate-rich side dishes are the reason. The proof is that you probably feel the same way after Christmas dinner, even when turkey is not served!

Coffee at the end of a meal can pull you out of the lethargy that follows. But be careful with coffee. It can bring on jitters. Some people have cured their chronic anxiety simply by going off all caffeine.

Perking Up

If you're feeling lackluster and not up to speed, you may need protein foods. When you eat protein, as the theory goes, the amino acid tyrosine in the protein crosses into the brain, where it's converted to dopamine and in turn norepinephrine. These two stimulating neurotramitters, dopamine and norepinephrine, produce alertness, a faster reaction time, and an increased ability to concentrate. The effects of eating protein last about two to three hours.

When you compose a protein meal to increase your alertness, limit your intake of fat and carbohydrates for maximum effect. For example, have some tuna or snack on a cup of plain yogurt. Or try this thoroughly satisfying chicken salad that is full of crunch and flavor.

Chicken Salad Pick-Me-Up

This main-course salad is high in protein, which quickens body and mind, and low in carbohydrates, which slow you down. Crunching on all the lettuce can also be very stimulating! This recipe includes cashews and a delicious dressing, both sources of fat. If you're eating this salad for medicinal purposes, skip the cashews and go light on the dressing to maximize its energizing effect.

Preparation time: *10 minutes (excluding dressing)*

Cooking time: *15 minutes*

Yield: *4 servings*

4 cups chicken broth*

4 halves chicken breast (about 1½ pounds), skin and bone removed

½ head iceberg lettuce

2 to 3 scallions

Five-Spice Sesame Dressing (see next recipe)

2 heaping tablespoons cashews

1 In a medium pot, bring the chicken broth to a boil over medium-high heat. Lower the heat to medium-low and add the chicken breasts. Cook until the chicken breasts are cooked through, about 10 to 15 minutes.

2 When the chicken is cooked, remove from the broth and place on a plate to cool. You can freeze the chicken broth and use it at another time.

3 On a cutting board with a sharp knife, cut the lettuce into narrow strips about ⅜-inch wide. Trim and chop the scallions into ¼-inch lengths. Combine the lettuce and scallions in a large bowl.

4 Using your hands, shred the chicken breast into bite-sized pieces. Add to the lettuce mixture. Add Five-Spice Sesame Dressing to taste and toss. Serve on individual plates and top each salad with some of the cashews.

*To make a quick chicken stock, take the bones that you removed from the chicken breasts and put them in a medium pot filled with 2 quarts filtered water. Add a carrot, an onion, and a small stalk of celery. Simmer, uncovered, for 30 minutes.

Five-Spice Sesame Dressing

Using quality oils in a dressing makes it worth the added calories. The grape seed oil functions as a powerful antioxidant, and unrefined sesame oil supplies vitamin E.

Preparation time: *5 minutes*

Cooking time: *None*

Yield: *¼ cup*

¼ cup grape seed oil	2 tablespoons rice vinegar
¼ cup unrefined sesame oil	2 teaspoons honey
2 tablespoons soy sauce	1 teaspoon five-spice powder*

1 In a small bowl, whisk together all ingredients.

2 Use the dressing with Chicken Salad Pick-Me-Up or use as a dressing for peeled and sliced cucumbers.

*Five-spice powder is a mixture of dried anise, anise pepper, fennel seeds, cloves, and cinnamon, sold in Asian and gourmet markets.

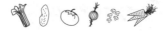

Cheering Up

Feeling a little depressed can be linked to poor nutrition. Both sugar and caffeine give you an energy lift, but the up is always followed by a down. These foods have a depressant effect, as does alcohol.

Chocolate chemistry

There's no denying that chocolate is a remarkable substance. Chocolate contains phenylethylamine, a mood enhancer, and theobromine, which has a stimulating, caffeine-like effect and triggers the release of endorphins. These chemicals produce the euphoric sensation of being in love. But make sure that you're not using chocolate as a crutch for coping with day-to-day stresses. Have it only once in a while, and when you crave some chocolate, have the best so that you really feel satisfied.

Having a deficiency of virtually any nutrient can also result in depression. In particular, you may lack vitamin C, zinc, or the B vitamins, including thiamin, niacin, vitamin B6, and in particular folic acid. If you eat a predominantly refined and processed foods diet and don't take vitamin supplements, you're likely to be low in these nutrients. To boost your levels, enjoy some of these foods:

- ✔ **Thiamin:** Pork, beef, liver, pistachios, and whole grains
- ✔ **Niacin:** Liver, salmon, chicken, lamb, trout, and whole grains
- ✔ **Vitamin B6:** Meats, egg yolks, beans, kale, and blackstrap molasses
- ✔ **Folic acid:** Salmon, asparagus, boysenberries, whole grains, and lentils
- ✔ **Vitamin C:** Citrus, sweet peppers, broccoli, papayas, and rose hips
- ✔ **Zinc:** Seafood, liver, mushrooms, pumpkin seeds, brown rice, and Brazil nuts

Studies show that St. John's Wort is effective for mild to moderate depression. For more information about these and other herbs, see *Herbal Remedies For Dummies* by Christopher Hobbs, L.Ac. (IDG Books Worldwide, Inc.)

Staying Even-Tempered

You can use food to keep you from emotional extremes caused by swings in blood sugar levels and hormone imbalances. There may be days when you have just cause for feeling the way you do, but I'm referring to those times when emotions overtake you for no apparent reason or when you overreact to a situation. A change in diet can help you stay on an even keel.

Steadying blood sugar levels

Low blood sugar, or *hypoglycemia,* can leave you low on energy, and it can also trigger emotions. If glucose levels drop gradually, you may experience some emotional instability, but a sudden drop can trigger anxiety. The primary fuel of your brain is blood sugar, or glucose. When the brain does not receive sufficient glucose, this triggers the release of hormones, which increase blood sugar levels, such as adrenaline, the hormone your body produces when you are under stress. Such episodes can be very disruptive of both work and social life and can be physically depleting. Observing the following dietary guidelines (and taking a look at the section on blood glucose in Chapter 20) to manage glucose levels is well worth the effort.

✔ Eat three meals a day and, if necessary, a mid-morning and mid-afternoon snack.

✔ At each meal, include protein, complex carbohydrates, and fats.

✔ Avoid all concentrated sweets, including refined white table sugar, honey, maple syrup, and fruit juice. Have whole fruit instead.

Balancing female hormones

Abrupt changes in levels of estrogen and progesterone trigger the emotional symptoms associated with PMS and menopause. When estrogen levels peak, a woman is likely to feel irritable and anxious or suffer mood swings. Excessive levels of progesterone, in relation to estrogen, can trigger weepiness and depression.

Phytohormones, which are hormonelike compounds found in foods, can help minimize the swings in hormone levels. Eating more plant-food-based meals adds phytohormones to your diet. Specific foods that are high in phytohormones include soybeans, currants, and buckwheat. (See Chapter 17 for more information about diet and mood.)

Toxic emotions

Alcohol can overburden the liver, which must break down this toxic substance before the body can eliminate it. Researchers at UCLA have identified certain toxins that the liver releases when it is damaged by alcohol. These toxins travel to the brain and may be the reason a drinker feels "liverish," or angry.

Taking certain food additives into your system and being exposed to environmental toxins can also trigger extremes of emotion, anxiety, and depression. The heavy metal cadmium in cigarettes can accumulate in the brain and affect mood and behavior. Hair analysis is a cost-effective and accurate diagnostic tool to discover whether you have an accumulation of toxic metals in your body tissues. Search out a holistically oriented physician or a nutritionist who regularly orders these tests, or tell your current physician about this lab that performs hair analysis: Analytical Research Labs, 2225 W. Alice Ave., Phoenix, AZ 85021; phone 602-995-1581, fax 602-371-8873. If the tests show your body has an accumulation of heavy metal, the company will also test your drinking water to determine whether it's the source.

Chapter 15

Eating for a Healthy Heart

• •

• •

*A*s you age, the walls of the arteries throughout your body normally begin to thicken and lose elasticity, a condition known as *arteriosclerosis*. Although this process is essentially determined by genetics, the accumulation of fats on artery walls, called *atherosclerosis,* is the result of poor diet and lifestyle. Together, these conditions raise your risk of heart attack and stroke.

Fortunately, you can prevent atherosclerosis, especially through diet. You probably know the standard advice about watching your intake of fat, cholesterol, and sodium. General recommendations are painted in broad strokes. But the details about what to eat are also important to know. For example, some fats are associated with a lower risk of heart disease; eating a lot of sugar is another risk factor; certain forms of cholesterol are more harmful than others; antioxidant vitamins are especially healthful; and high blood pressure is associated with several minerals, not just sodium.

Every time you sit down to eat or plan a meal, you have the chance to give yourself foods that heal the heart. Use this chapter to guide your choices and sample the recipes to find out how tasty heart healthy foods can be.

Making Sure That Your Diet Is Heart-Healthy

Heart disease is the No.1 cause of death in the United States. It reached this position as the American diet shifted from one of predominately fresh, natural foods to one including many processed and ready-made foods that are typically high in unhealthy refined fats, salt, and sugar. Yet an abundant variety of heart-healthy foods, such as fruits and vegetables, are available in markets. Whole grains, too, lower the risk of coronary heart disease, and fortunately, whole-grain baked goods are available in a greater variety than ever before. You just need to know how to pick and choose foods to purchase and prepare.

First, you need to be aware of what ingredients, such as sugar and certain fats, you should stay away from. Eating such foods, even though you are also eating some foods that are good for you, can still increase your risk of heart disease. Read on to find out about what ingredients to avoid.

Fats and oils

The American Heart Association's general dietary guideline is to consume no more than 30 percent of your calories as fat. But many health experts believe that a truly heart-healthy diet should contain no more than 20 to 25 percent of calories from fat. The percentage of fat in the average American's diet is about 40 percent.

If you are overweight and eat many fast foods or cook with a lot of fat, your fat intake is probably too high. Cutting back on desserts and rich sauces, ordering salad dressing on the side in restaurants, and practicing similar habits are a good way to start reducing your fat intake.

One study conducted by the Monell Chemical Senses Center in Philadelphia and reported in the *American Journal of Clinical Nutrition* in 1993 shows that as you reduce your fat intake, your desire for fatty foods diminishes — not overnight, but after a few months. Certainly, your tastes can change. But rather than drastically cutting back your fat consumption, you'll probably have more success if you find a reduced amount that you can stick with. In my experience of working with patients who are put on a diet that restricts fat to only 10 to 15 percent of total calories, most people find such a diet very difficult to comply with over the long term. (And yes, there are exceptions. Some individuals recovering from life-threatening heart disease gladly accept very lowfat diets rather than risk another heart attack.)

To keep your heart healthy, eat foods that are naturally low in fats, such as grains, beans, vegetables, and fruit. In accordance with a whole-foods diet, I also recommend full-fat yogurt and cheeses (foods such as skim milk and nonfat yogurt no longer have their natural ratio of nutrients and are now concentrated sources of protein) as well as almonds, walnuts, pumpkin seeds, and the like. If you eat these foods in modest quantities, your fat intake need not be excessive. In addition, if you satisfy your body's legitimate need for fat with wholesome foods, you'll be less likely to eat cheeseburgers and french fries.

Legumes, including beans and lentils, are a natural source of lowfat protein. An easy way to start eating more beans, if you aren't in the habit, is to spoon them on toast and have them for breakfast or add them to soup. And lentils, such as those in the following recipe, make a great side dish with meats.

Lentils and Leftovers

Lentils supply lowfat protein and soluble fiber, which lowers your cholesterol and *triglyceride* levels (dietary fats in the blood, which can raise cholesterol). And adding spinach, either fresh or from last night's dinner, makes this dish even more nutritious. Serve it as a side dish with lamb or increase the amount of liquid and serve it as a soup.

Preparation time: *15 minutes*

Cooking time: *1 hour, 5 minutes*

Yield: *6 servings as a side dish*

1 tablespoon unsalted, organic butter

1 medium onion, thinly sliced

1 small stalk celery, thinly sliced (½ cup)

1 carrot, thinly sliced (½ cup)

1 cup dried lentils, washed and drained

½ teaspoon dried thyme, or several sprigs of fresh thyme

3 cups chicken stock

Salt and hot pepper flakes to taste

1 bunch fresh spinach, washed and drained (½ cup or more)

Leftovers (cooked spinach or other vegetables such as cooked cabbage, broccoli, broccoli rabe, dandelion greens, kale, or potatoes may be substituted)

2 tablespoons richly flavored extra-virgin olive oil

1 In a medium soup pot, melt the butter over low heat. Add the onion, celery, and carrot and sauté over medium heat for 15 minutes, or until the onions become translucent.

2 To the vegetable mixture, add the lentils, thyme, and chicken stock. Cover and cook for about 45 minutes. Add the salt and hot pepper flakes and spinach or leftover vegetables and cook for an additional 3 to 4 minutes. Stir in the olive oil and serve.

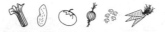

Transfatty acids

Hydrogenated oils (refined oils that are further processed to make them solid at room temperature) and oils and fats heated to high temperatures contain *transfatty acids* — unnatural, manmade molecules. Studies have linked their consumption to a higher risk of heart disease.

You find hydrogenated and partially hydrogenated oils in the ingredient lists of many food products, including cakes, crackers, cookies, and shortening. Hydrogenated soybean oil is used extensively. Margarine also contains trans-fatty acids (this is the reason people have switched back to butter). Fried foods are also a source.

In the past few years, the national campaign to consume smaller amounts of saturated fat has resulted in these fats being replaced, usually by monounsaturated and polyunsaturated oils that are less likely to clog your arteries. However, most oils on the market are refined, and the refining processes generate transfatty acids. Although saturated fat intake may have declined, the intake of transfatty acids has increased.

You may think that you can't win, but you do have a choice of healthy fats. You can cook with butter in modest amounts. Heating it to high temperatures does not create transfatty acids. And unrefined cooking oils, such as extra-virgin olive oil, are never processed at high temperatures or hydrogenated. You can safely use these oils as salad dressings or when cooking at lower temperatures. (See Chapter 10 for details.)

When sugar is fat

Your body can convert sugars and starches into fat. When you eat sugary and starchy foods, your body breaks down these substances into glucose. Some of the glucose is converted into energy to meet immediate needs. The remaining is either stored in cells for future use or turned into fat.

In the process of being turned into energy, a molecule of glucose passes through many stages. At one point, the 6-carbon glucose molecule becomes 2-carbon acetates. Vinegar is a familiar form of acetate. Now, wouldn't you know, the body prefers fat to vinegar, which is less healthful to have in your tissues. The body quickly converts these acetates to fat, specifically saturated fats and cholesterol, and this is what you get more of when you have too much glucose. And when your body can't use all the extra fat and cholesterol, it deposits it in your arteries and organs, including the heart.

In this way, white table sugar, the sugars in fruit, beer, and even milk, and such healthy sweeteners as maple syrup can generate fat and cholesterol when you eat more than you need. They are digested quickly and can flood your system with glucose, especially when you eat these foods quickly and in large amounts. Refined flour (the kind in white bread) has a similar effect. Foods that are high in both sugar and unhealthy fats, such as jelly donuts, deliver a double whammy!

Lowfat can mean high sugar!

Many lowfat and fatfree diet food products are loaded with sugar. Such items can have two to four times the amount of sugar of a nonlowfat product. Check the labels.

A heart-healthy diet needs to rely on complex carbohydrates, like whole grains, corn, and starchy vegetables such as cauliflower and broccoli, which are digested and break down more slowly. These foods provide a gradual supply of glucose, which is less likely to become fat. Such foods also supply the vitamins and minerals your body requires to turn sugars and starches into energy. High intake of sugar threatens heart health also in another way. Eating a piece of pie à la mode can send insulin levels soaring. (*Insulin* is the hormone in charge of storing sugar for later use.) Elevated levels of insulin can lead to hardening and thickening of heart valves, arteries, and veins.

Cholesterol

High levels of cholesterol in your blood increase the likelihood that cholesterol will deposit on the walls of your arteries, initiating the development of atherosclerosis. Cholesterol comes in two forms:

- **Low-density lipoproteins (LDL)** are a major contributor to atherosclerosis and carry most of the cholesterol.

- **High-density lipoproteins (HDL)** protect your arteries by removing cholesterol from the artery walls and returning it to the liver for disposal.

While you should know your overall cholesterol level, it is also important to know your levels of these two forms of cholesterol and their ratio to each other. Table 15-1 lists the recommended levels.

Table 15-1	Recommended Levels of Cholesterol		
Type of Cholesterol	*Desirable (mg per deciliter)*	*Borderline High*	*High*
Total cholesterol	Under 200	200 to 239	Over 240
Total cholesterol compared to HDL	A ratio of about 4.5:1		
HDL	Over 45		
LDL	Under 120		

The cholesterol in your body comes from two sources. Your liver manufactures the majority, which becomes part of the walls of your cells and performs many other vital functions. But only about 15 percent of your body's cholesterol comes from the cholesterol-containing foods that you eat. Cholesterol is present in animal foods — meats, poultry, dairy products, and seafood. (Because plants do not have livers, plant foods do not contain cholesterol.)

Normally, the body is able to compensate for the amount of cholesterol in the diet, with your liver producing less if your intake of cholesterol increases and producing more if there is a lack. If you have normal levels of cholesterol, you can include such nutritious foods as eggs and shrimp, which do contain cholesterol. However, in about 25 percent of the population, the liver is not able to adequately manage cholesterol levels, and the cholesterol level rises. These people need to limit their intake of cholesterol as well as their intake of saturated fat. (Unfortunately, there is no test to find out if you are one of the 25 percent. If you have exceptionally elevated levels of cholesterol, even though you follow the dietary recommendations to lower cholesterol, this may be a sign that your liver is overproducing and not adequately breaking down the excess cholesterol in your system.)

The type of fat you eat is as important as how much you eat, because the body can use fats as the raw material from which to manufacture cholesterol. For example, the saturated fats found in red meats increase LDL cholesterol. At one time, replacing saturated fats with polyunsaturated fats such as safflower and corn oil was strongly advised, but eating quantities of these polyunsaturated fats appears to lower HDL, the more desirable form of cholesterol. Now the focus is more on monounsaturated fats, such as olive oil, to lower LDL.

 Oils that contain essential fatty acids are very beneficial to the heart and circulatory system. The omega-3 fatty acids lower blood pressure and help prevent blood clots, and some studies show they increase HDL, the beneficial form of cholesterol in certain individuals. Flaxseed oil and walnuts are excellent sources of these essential fatty acids, as are the fattier fish, such as salmon and tuna.

Foods that contain *soluble* fiber can lower cholesterol to some extent as well. These foods include oat bran, dried beans, the skin of baked potatoes, and oranges. *Insoluble* fiber, which is found in wheat bran, has no effect on cholesterol.

Something good about cholesterol

If you're laboring to remove as much cholesterol as you can from your diet, consider this. Sex hormones are made from cholesterol. Some of the cholesterol you eat is converted through a series of chemical reactions to hormones such as estrogen and testosterone.

Oxidized cholesterol

Researchers now believe that before LDL can deposit itself in arterial walls, it must be *oxidized* (chemically changed) by *free radicals,* which are highly reactive molecules. The oxidized LDL damages the cell walls, setting the stage for the buildup of fats and other materials that eventually narrow arteries. In other words, your cholesterol reading does not tell the whole story. This may be the reason some people with high cholesterol do not develop heart disease.

Lifestyle and heart disease

Everyday habits of smoking and drinking coffee and alcohol can threaten the health of your heart and circulatory system to some degree. If you indulge, be aware of the risks.

- ✔ **Smoking:** The most serious risk factor for coronary heart disease (CHD) is smoking. However, the heart is forgiving. Even after a person has smoked for many years, his or her risk of CHD returns to that of a non-smoker just two or three years after he or she stops smoking.

- ✔ **Coffee:** Research attempting to link coffee to increases in cholesterol has had mixed results. However, there is evidence that the oils and sediment in espresso, cappuccino, French press, and Turkish coffee can cause harm. To remove much of the oils, brew coffee in a drip pot using a paper filter. (Buy the brown, unbleached filters.)

- ✔ **Alcohol:** There's some evidence that light consumption of alcohol may reduce the risk of a blood vessel being blocked by a blood clot *(embolism),* but excessive drinking can impair heart function. With continued use of alcohol, heart muscle action and electrical conductivity within the heart can decrease. In women in particular, alcohol can damage the heart.

Antioxidants

Given that oxidized cholesterol appears to be the culprit in cardiovascular disease, researchers have turned their attention to the antioxidant vitamins beta-carotene, vitamin C, vitamin E, and selenium. Although the findings of this research have not been totally consistent, the results generally demonstrate that a diet high in antioxidants is associated with a significantly lower risk of heart disease, as well as a lower incidence of signs of heart disease such as chest pains, or *angina pectoris.*

You may decide to take an antioxidant supplement, but eating a variety of foods that supply antioxidant nutrients is still necessary. Take a quick look at Chapter 6 on fruits and vegetables to find out more about antioxidants. I list all sorts of antioxidant-rich foods and also describe the different types of antioxidants more fully.

Even people who don't like vegetables will enjoy this recipe for carrots, a great source of the antioxidant beta-carotene. They're sweet and always brighten up a dinner plate. I guarantee that the carrots in this recipe will not be refused.

Beta-Carotene Carrots — Three Ways

Beta-carotene is better absorbed when the food that contains it is lightly cooked, as in this recipe. These three ways of dressing steamed carrots are equally delicious and easy to prepare.

Preparation time: *5 minutes*

Cooking time: *15 minutes*

Yield: *4 servings*

> *4 medium carrots*
>
> *½ cup filtered water*
>
> *One of the following combinations: 1 tablespoon all-fruit, sugarfree*

> *marmalade and 1 tablespoon organic, unsalted butter; or 1 tablespoon chopped fresh tarragon and 2 table-spoons cream; or 1 tablespoon flaxseed oil and ½ teaspoon ground cinnamon*

1 Cut the carrots into quarters and then into 3-inch lengths.

2 Put 1 cup water in a saucepan fitted with a steamer. Place the carrots on the steamer and cook, covered, over medium heat until tender, about 10 to 15 minutes.

3 To the cooked carrots, add your choice of combination.

4 With a wooden spoon, gently toss the carrots in the seasonings. Serve as part of a meal that includes hummus and grilled chicken breast.

> ***Note:*** *You can also toss the carrots with a vinaigrette dressing made with extra-virgin olive oil and mustard and enjoy these vegetables cold as a side dish.*

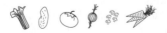

Homocysteine and your heart

At one time, the level of *homocysteine*, an amino acid, in your blood was thought to be a sure indicator of your risk of heart disease, including blood clots, clogged arteries, heart attacks, and strokes. But now this notion has become very controversial. Homocysteine levels may rise only after heart disease has developed and a patient has had a coronary.

Protein is made from this amino acid, but this requires vitamin B6, vitamin B12, and folic acid, in order to keep homocysteine levels low. Individuals with elevated homocysteine levels commonly have deficiencies of these nutrients.

To be on the safe side, make sure that you don't run out of these vitamins. Meats, whole grains, legumes, and green leafy vegetables are good sources of vitamin B6. B12 is found in organ meats, pork, fish, eggs, milk, and cheese. And food sources of folic acid include beets, cantaloupe, turkey, whole barley, and cranberries. A general recommendation is 400 mcg of folic acid a day in food or supplemented. A beet, a large serving of asparagus, and a cup of corn contains a total of about 350 mcg of folic acid. You can make a delicious salad using avocados, an excellent source of folic acid, mixed with pink grapefruit and slivers of radish, served on a few leaves of Boston lettuce, and dressed with vinaigrette.

Combating Hypertension

Hypertension, or high blood pressure, is a risk factor for heart disease. It is either *secondary* hypertension, due to conditions such as kidney damage, or, as in over 90 percent of cases, *essential* hypertension, when the cause is said to be unknown. In fact, a significant amount of research indicates that a variety of genetic, environmental, and nutritional factors, such as those following, can lead to this condition:

- ✔ Excess weight, lack of exercise, alcohol, and smoking can all be factors in chronic hypertension.

- ✔ Consuming caffeine can cause elevated blood pressure that lasts a few days.

- ✔ Exposure to the toxic metals lead and cadmium can be a factor.

- ✔ Stress can trigger high blood pressure. Research consistently shows that individuals with stressful jobs, especially at the lower end of the economic ladder, have higher blood pressure. (Take a look *at Stress Management For Dummies,* by Allen Elkin, Ph.D., IDG Books Worldwide, Inc., for ways to calm down and chill out.)

A diet high in sodium does not cause hypertension. In addition, only about 10 to 20 percent of Americans are salt-sensitive. And only about half of all individuals with hypertension have this sensitivity.

If your blood pressure is normal, don't bother buying high-priced low-salt grocery items. You have no reason to trim your salt intake. However, the recommended moderate amount is only 1 teaspoon, or about 2,400 mg of sodium, a day.

Sodium and potassium

A diet that is low in potassium and high in sodium can bring on hypertension in susceptible persons. When these two minerals are out of balance, fluid volume in tissues can increase and the mechanisms that regulate blood pressure can become impaired. In some cases, when salt-sensitive individuals are given enough potassium, blood pressure levels are dramatically lowered.

Individuals with hypertension also need to make sure to restrict their sodium intake while increasing their intake of potassium-rich foods. If you need to cut back your sodium intake, go out of your way to eat fresh and minimally processed foods and avoid eating such high-salt items as catsup, luncheon meats, canned soups, and frozen dinners. If you want to salt something you've cooked, add the salt at the table, not to the cooking pot. Good food sources of potassium are bananas, broccoli, potatoes, red beans, oranges, nectarines, and melon.

Magnesium and calcium

Research shows that deficiencies of magnesium and calcium can lead to hypertension. To avoid deficiencies, be sure to regularly eat foods such as broccoli and figs, as well as dark leafy greens such as kale, yogurt, seafood, and nuts.

A good reason to cook with onions and garlic

Onions and garlic belong to the same family of foods and promote heart health in similar ways. These flavorings play a role in preventing blood clots, lowering cholesterol levels, reducing blood pressure, and normalizing blood lipids. If you have a hamburger or a steak, you can counteract the effects of the saturated fat in the meat by having on the side, a salad made with raw onion and garlic.

Enjoying the Heart-Healthy Way of Eating

If you combine all the assorted dietary advice for maintaining a healthy heart, you have meals that are predominantly vegetarian, composed of grains, legumes, fruits, vegetables, seeds, and nuts, with moderate amounts of dairy, meat, and fish. This way of eating is typical of traditional diets in other cultures, such as China, where heart disease is low. The ability of the traditional Chinese diet to prevent heart disease was confirmed in the 1991 China Health Study, a massive survey of the diet and health habits of Chinese people, conducted by Cornell University in association with researchers in China.

Especially eat all those fruits and vegetables that contain phytonutrients that protect the heart. (Take a look at Chapter 6 and Appendix B for specifics.) Red grapes and red wine are recommended. The French who drink red wine have a low rate of heart disease. Red wine contains several flavonoids, which benefit circulation and function as antioxidants, protecting arteries from damage. You can use red wine to poach other fruit, as I've done here in this recipe for poached pears, an elegant dessert with medicinal benefits!

Pears Poached in Red Wine

Red wine contains tannins and two flavonoids, quercetin (a powerful antioxidant described in Chapter 6) and *anthocyanin,* a red pigment shown to lower cholesterol levels and reduce blood pressure. Hence *red* wine rather than white wine is recommended. Pears also have a plus. They are an excellent source of soluble fiber, which lowers cholesterol.

Preparation time: *5 minutes*

Cooking time: *10 minutes*

Yield: *4 servings*

2 Bosc pears

1½ cups good-quality red wine

¼ teaspoon freshly grated nutmeg

4 whole cloves

Plain full-fat yogurt for garnish

(continued)

1 Peel and quarter the pears. Remove the core and slice each quarter into 3 or 4 slices lengthwise.

2 Put the pear slices, wine, nutmeg, and cloves into a small saucepan.

3 Cook over medium-low heat, simmering until tender but still firm, about 10 minutes.

4 Spoon into individual serving dishes and top with a dollop of yogurt.

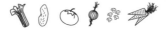

Chapter 16

Reducing Your Risk of Cancer at Every Meal

● ●

In This Chapter

▶ Following dietary guidelines to help prevent some forms of cancer

▶ Increasing your intake of antioxidants

▶ Adding cancer-protective phytonutrients to your cooking

▶ Avoiding foods that may promote cancer

● ●

Recipes in This Chapter

↻ Antioxidant Cocktail

▶ Garlic Shrimp

▶ Simmered Chicken with Citrus

↻ Red Onions with Vinegar and Chilies

You can use food to reduce your risk of cancer. Research shows that the right sort of diet, when coupled with a healthy weight and regular exercise, can help prevent about 30 to 40 percent of cancer cases worldwide. In particular, eating fresh fruits and vegetables appears to protect you from most forms of cancer. General population studies show that people who eat five or more servings a day have half the cancer risk of people who eat just two servings a day.

Conversely, research shows that people with cancer have lower intakes of raw and fresh fruits and vegetables. In particular, they eat less citrus, leafy green vegetables, carrots, lettuce, and cruciferous vegetables such as broccoli and cabbage. Intake of fiber and whole grains may also help prevent some forms of cancer.

The association of meat and saturated fat consumption with cancer risk is not as well established; however, some studies show a link with ovarian cancer and cancers of the breast, as well as endometrium, colon, lung, and prostate. Maintaining normal weight for height is also recommended. The results of the American Cancer Society's 12-year Cancer Prevention Study show a significant increase in the incidence of cancers of the uterus, gallbladder, kidney, stomach, colon, and breast associated with obesity. This was especially true for men and women who were 40 percent or more overweight.

Every time you plan a meal or go shopping for food, you can make choices that can potentially reduce your cancer risk. Active compounds that may help prevent and alter the course of cancer are in dozens and dozens of foods. In this chapter, I tell you about the foods to favor and those to avoid so that you'll be on your way to a healthy future.

Eating in a Cancer-Protective Way

The effect of diet on cancer risk has been a prime focus of scientific research in recent years. One organization, the American Institute for Cancer Research, tackled the enormous job of reviewing the results of the thousands of nutrition and cancer studies that have been conducted worldwide. A panel of experts from seven countries assessed more than 4,500 recent studies. The panel analyzed and distilled the results of these studies to provide dietary advice applicable to people everywhere. Based on this mega-analysis, in 1997, the American Institute for Cancer Research released the following dietary guidelines:

- Eat a varied diet based primarily on foods of plant origin.

- Have a variety of fruits and vegetables — five servings or more a day — and eat this much year-round.

- Consume a variety of minimally processed, starchy staple foods — that is, whole grains, legumes, root vegetables, and tubers. Many of these foods are also sources of protein. They should provide 45 to 60 percent of total calories. Limit the consumption of refined sugar.

- Red meat, if eaten at all, should provide less than 10 percent of total calories, limited to one 3-ounce portion a day. Fish and poultry are preferred. And cook meat and fish at relatively low temperatures to avoid charring and burning. Meat and fish broiled and grilled by direct flame, and cured and smoked meats should be consumed only occasionally, if at all.

- Limit intake of oils and fats, particularly those of animal origin. Total dietary fat should provide from 15 percent to a maximum of 30 percent of total calories.

- Restrict salt intake from all sources to less than 6 g a day. (This is equivalent to about 1 teaspoon of salt, which contains 2,300 mg of sodium.)

- Drinking alcoholic beverages is not recommended. If alcohol is consumed, men should have no more than two drinks a day and women no more than one drink a day.

No smoking!

Lung cancer is the deadliest form of cancer, with only 13 percent of people surviving longer than five years. Yet most cases of lung cancer can be prevented simply by avoiding tobacco products, including cigarettes, cigars, and chewing tobacco. If you smoke, eating the right foods can reduce your risk of cancer by 20 to 30 percent, but you still have a high risk of lung cancer even if you eat a good diet and exercise. Other causes of lung cancer include radiation, radon, asbestos, arsenic, air pollution, and secondary smoke.

When you smoke and drink alcohol at the same time, the carcinogenic compounds in the smoke become more soluble and are more easily carried into the cells. Drinking alcohol in combination with smoking increases your chance of contracting cancers of the mouth, throat, larynx, and esophagus.

Looking at the Cancer-Fighting Compounds in Fruits and Vegetables

Researchers are identifying more and more compounds in produce that help prevent the initiation of cancerous cell growth. Some even may arrest growth after it has begun. These substances include common vitamins and minerals, as well as a collection of phytonutrients with less familiar names. All these nutrients work together to help lower your risk of cancer.

How do you get *all* of these nutrients? By eating a *variety* of fruits and vegetables. No bingeing on broccoli!

Antioxidants, which slow the aging process, may be a factor in the development of some forms of cancer. Folate and iodine, as well as a host of phytonutrients, also hold promise for giving you protection. Here's a quick runthrough of these nutrients.

Antioxidants

Cancer develops when DNA becomes damaged, primarily by *free radicals* — unstable molecules that are chemically incomplete. Free radicals readily react with other molecules, causing a chain reaction that can damage cells. Antioxidants to the rescue! These compounds combine with free radicals before they do their damage. Even when compounds that produce free radicals are present, your DNA will be protected if you have sufficient levels of antioxidants in body tissues.

Scientists are examining specific antioxidants for their effects on cancer, including beta-carotene (a form of vitamin A found in plants), vitamin C, vitamin E, and selenium, and existing research is continuing to be reviewed and updated. For example, new research suggests that carotenoids do not protect against lung cancer as once thought. What is known for sure is that antioxidants work together. Consuming only one type of antioxidant is not as beneficial as eating a variety of foods that supply all of them. If you want to know more about antioxidants, take a quick look at Chapter 6, which is on fruits and vegetables, for more on antioxidants and food sources. And while you're at it, you can sip this drink, which is full of antioxidants, while you read about them!

Antioxidant Cocktail

An easy way to down your antioxidants is to drink them. This cocktail is spiked with chili pepper, which is also cancer-protective.

Preparation time: *5 minutes*

Cooking time: *None*

Yield: *2 servings*

8 medium carrots*

1 bell pepper

1 tomato

1 hot chili pepper, to taste

Sea salt to taste

1 Set up an electric juicer and a low, wide-mouthed container to receive the juice. Then feed in the carrots, bell pepper, tomato, and chili pepper.

2 Stir the cocktail to combine the juices and add a dash of sea salt. Pour into long-stemmed glasses and serve at room temperature for maximum flavor.

*Use organic vegetables or make sure that you peel them.

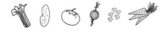

Folate

Folate naturally occurs in more than 150 forms in nature. (One of those forms is folic acid, a B vitamin most commonly found in vitamin supplements.) Folate plays a unique role in slowing cancer. It has the ability to repair DNA after it's been damaged — especially important in the progressive stage of cancer when it has begun to spread.

DNA normally contains a methyl group. Free radicals can knock off the methyl group on DNA. But folate contains methyl groups and can donate them to replace those that were removed, thereby repairing the DNA.

Folate is destroyed by heat, so the best source is raw foods. One easy way to increase your intake of folate is to eat more guacamole made with fresh, mashed avocados, a great source of this nutrient. Other foods that contain good amounts of folate and that you can enjoy raw are boysenberries, cantaloupe, alfalfa sprouts, broccoli, and cauliflower.

Iodine

One theory regarding the increase in the incidence of cancer is that it is due to exposure to radioactive materials in the environment. Sea vegetables, including seaweeds such as nori and kombu, contain iodine, a mineral that protects against radiation.

Phytonutrients

Various compounds in fruits and vegetables appear to play a role in preventing and reversing cancerous processes within the body. A natural arsenal has evolved to fight the seeds of this modern disease. These phytonutrients help explain why a diet high in fruits and vegetables is associated with lower rates of cancer. Here are some of the compounds now being studied and where you can find them in foods.

- **Allium and allyl sulfides** in garlic, onions, leeks, chives, and shallots are associated with a reduced risk of stomach and colon cancer.

- **Anthocyanins,** red pigments found in red grape skins, citrus, berries, and yams, function as antioxidants, protecting DNA from damage.

- **Catechins** protect against stomach cancer and are found in berries and black and green tea.

- **Ellagic acid** inhibits cancerous cells and detoxifies certain carcinogens. It is widely distributed in fruits and vegetables, but particularly high amounts are present in apples, berries, cherries, grapes, and walnuts, as well as other nuts.

- **Indoles** are present in broccoli, cabbage, brussels sprouts, turnips, and dark leafy greens such as kale. Indoles act on enzymes, which are important to the body's cancer-fighting mechanisms. A specific indole, indole-3-carbinol, is thought to protect against breast cancer.

- **Isoflavonoids** (genistein and daidzein) in soybeans appear to deactivate excess estrogen and thereby lower the risk of hormonelike cancers of the breast, cervix, and uterus. Fresh soybeans provide the most genistein, but processing the soybeans lowers the amount. Tempeh and miso come in second place, and highly processed soy products come in last.

- **Lignans** in flax seed and whole grains block estrogen and are thought to reduce the risk of breast cancer.

- **Lycopenes,** powerful carotenoids and a reddish pigment, are associated with a reduced risk of prostate cancer and cancers of the digestive tract. Rosy foods like tomatoes, red grapefruit, watermelon, and apricots contain lycopenes.

- **Monoterpenes** help prevent cancer by increasing the production of liver enzymes that detoxify carcinogenic substances. Citrus contains monoterpenes.

- **P-coumaric acid and chlorogenic acid** occur together in such common fruits and vegetables as pineapple, strawberries, peppers, and tomatoes. They detoxify nitrosamines, such as those in deli meats and bacon, which are known to be carcinogenic.

- **Phthalides** are anticancerous compounds found in celery, carrots, and various herbs, including parsley, dill, fennel, and coriander.

- **Polyphenols** in green tea are associated with a lower risk of stomach cancer.

- **Protease inhibitors** in beans, potatoes, rice, and eggplant may inhibit the development of cancer.

- **Quercetin,** abundant in yellow and red onions, but not white, and also present in shallots, red grapes, Italian yellow squash, and broccoli, protects DNA from damage, inhibits tumor stimulating enzymes, and inactivates several cancer-causing agents.

- **Sulforaphane** is present in cruciferous vegetables such as broccoli and cauliflower. This compound neutralizes carcinogens and speeds their removal from the body.

- **Triterpenoids** in citrus fruits and soybeans block estrogen and its ability to increase the risk of cancer.

As you can see from this long list of active compounds and the many foods that contain them, you have a wide choice of ingredients to cook with if you want to follow a cancer-protective diet. Even flavorings such as hot chili peppers, turmeric, and cumin help prevent carcinogens from attaching to DNA and initiating cancer. To begin adding these ingredients to your meals, the three following recipes, which are full of bright and lively flavors, are a good place to start.

Garlic Shrimp

Shrimp is exceptionally high in selenium, a powerful antioxidant that is thought to help prevent skin cancer. U.S. farmland is depleted of selenium, but the oceans (and seafood living in these waters) are still a rich source. The garlic and red pepper flakes also protect against cancer.

Preparation time: 5 minutes (20 minutes if prepping shrimp)

Cooking time: 10 minutes

Yield: 4 servings

5 garlic cloves, peeled

½ bunch cilantro, stems removed (½ cup)

1 tablespoon extra-virgin olive oil

½ teaspoon red pepper flakes

1 pound large shrimp, peeled and deveined, with tails left on

1 With the side of a broad knife, crush the garlic cloves to release the juices. Let sit for 15 minutes.*

2 In a food processor, put the garlic and cilantro. Blend until smooth.

3 Heat the oil in a large, heavy skillet over medium heat. Add the pepper flakes and toast for a few seconds. Immediately add the shrimp. Cook, stirring, for 2 minutes.

4 Add the garlic-cilantro mixture and continue to cook the shrimp on low heat, stirring, an additional 5 minutes or until opaque.

5 Serve immediately. This shrimp is good with black beans, brown rice, and sautéed plantains.

*To benefit from garlic, you first need to chop or crush garlic to activate certain enzymes. These enzymes trigger the production of compounds that fight cancer.

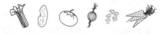

Benefits of starchy foods

Potatoes and other starchy foods, such as grains, also play a role in cancer prevention. When you eat starch, not all of it is digested in your stomach. Some reaches your colon, where bacteria break it down into short-chain fatty acids. These fats may inhibit cancerous growths on the walls of the intestines. Whole-grain complex carbohydrates, which supply fiber, also speed the elimination of waste products, reducing the chance of colon cancer.

Simmered Chicken with Citrus

The cancer-protective ingredients in this chicken dish — garlic, chili peppers, and cumin, plus orange, grapefruit, and lime juices — also contribute animated flavors.

Preparation time: *15 minutes*

Cooking time: *1 hour, 10 minutes, plus 8 hours for marinating*

Yield: *4 servings*

1 orange	*2 bay leaves*
1 pink grapefruit	*1 teaspoon ground allspice*
2 limes	*1 teaspoon dried oregano*
2 chili peppers, stem and seeds removed, minced, or to taste	*½ teaspoon dried cumin*
3 large cloves garlic, chopped	*1 chicken, preferably organic and residue-free, skin removed, quartered*
1 teaspoon salt	*1 tablespoon extra-virgin olive oil*
2 teaspoons freshly ground black pepper	

1 Cut the orange, grapefruit, and limes in half. Using a manual citrus juicer, squeeze the juice from the citrus and collect it in a medium bowl. Set aside. With a paring knife, remove any membranes and remaining pulp from the fruits. Cut this into manageable pieces and add these to the juice.*

2 To the bowl that contains the citrus juice and pulp, add the chili peppers, garlic, salt, pepper, bay leaves, allspice, oregano, and cumin and mix the marinade thoroughly.

3 Arrange the chicken in a baking dish and pour the marinade over the chicken. Marinate, covered, in the refrigerator overnight.

4 Remove the chicken from the marinade, reserving the marinade. Heat the olive oil in a large skillet or casserole over medium-high heat and brown the chicken pieces on all sides.

5 Add the reserved marinade to the browned chicken and bring the marinade to a boil over high heat. Immediately reduce the heat to low and simmer the chicken, covered, for 50 minutes, adding up to 1 cup water if necessary during cooking. Stir the chicken every once in a while during cooking to prevent it from sticking to the pan.

6 Serve the chicken with the cooked citrus marinade on the side. Suggested accompaniments include steamed broccoli and rice (preferably whole-grain brown rice, which contains the antioxidant selenium) and Red Onions with Vinegar and Chilies (see next recipe).

*The membranes and the fluffy white stem in the core of these fruits contain cancer-protective flavonoids.

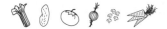

Red Onions with Vinegar and Chilies

Red onions contain quercetin, a compound that fights cancer, as do yellow onions, but not white! These warm, pickled red onions provide just the right flavor accent to the Simmered Chicken with Citrus.

Preparation time: *10 minutes*

Cooking time: *5 minutes*

Yield: *2 cups*

1 medium red onion, peeled and thinly sliced

¼ cup cider vinegar

½ cup water

1 chilie, serrano or jalapeno pepper, chopped

1 bay leaf

1 clove garlic, crushed

¼ teaspoon cumin

¼ teaspoon oregano

1 In a medium saucepan, combine all ingredients.

2 Cover the pot and bring to a boil over high heat. Lower the heat and simmer the onion mixture for 5 minutes.

3 Remove from heat and serve warm.

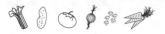

Avoiding Carcinogens in Food

The populations of countries where the diet includes substantial amounts of smoked foods and meats treated with nitrates and nitrites, used as preservatives, have higher rates of cancer of the stomach and esophagus. Foods in the American diet that are prepared in these ways include hot dogs, bacon, and ham. To be safe, look for brands of uncured, nitratefree meat products such as bacon in natural-food stores.

Intake of pesticides may also increase the risk of cancer, although studies have had mixed results. However, in one study, conducted in 1992 at Hartford Hospital in Connecticut and published in the *Archives of Environmental Health,* women with breast cancer had 50 to 60 percent higher concentrations of PCBs, DDT, and DDE in their breast tissue than women who did not have breast cancer. These chemicals can increase estrogenic activity and suppress immune function — another reason to eat organic foods.

For further information about diet and specific forms of cancer, contact these organizations and request a copy of their educational materials:

- ✔ **American Cancer Society:** 800-227-2345, www.cancer.org
- ✔ **National Cancer Institute:** 800-422-6237, www.nci.nih.gov
- ✔ **American Institute for Cancer Research:** 800-843-8114, www.aicr.org

Hot, hot foods and beverages cool some before you consume them.

Cancer of the mouth and pharynx is promoted by drinking very hot beverages, a common practice in such places as Afghanistan and China, where the incidence of this type of cancer is high

HAA HAAs are no laughing matter

Cooking meat, poultry, or fish at high temperatures — 480°F and higher — results in the formation of carcinogenic compounds called heterocyclic aromatic amines (HAAs). Meats cooked over an open flame on a barbecue may reach 700°F. Hot foods and beverages naturally cool some before you consume them.

Chapter 17

Healing Foods for Women

. . . .

In This Chapter

▶ Managing PMS with food

▶ Treating common symptoms

▶ Minimizing painful cramps

▶ Correcting heavy flow with diet

▶ Eating during pregnancy

▶ Munching your way through menopause

▶ Healing foods for symptoms

▶ Discovering special nutrients

. . . .

*A*natomy books a hundred years ago showed the male body in detail but delicately omitted illustration of the female form and its more private parts. The female body was thought of as a sort of lesser version of male physiology. Some physical complaints were assumed imaginary or simply emotional.

Yes, we've come a long way since these Victorian times. Premenstrual syndrome (PMS) is now acknowledged as an identifiable medical condition with various protocols for treatment. The word *menopause* can now be mentioned in polite society, and it isn't the end of the world if people notice you perspiring from a hot flash. There's also a new respect for subtle differences in female anatomy; for example, women's arteries are more delicate than men's, requiring special care during heart surgery.

However, these are recent advances, and we still don't have all the answers. Several research projects are now underway. One, the Women's Health Initiative, was launched in 1994 to help decide how diet, hormone therapy, calcium, and vitamin D may prevent heart disease, cancer, and bone fractures. This is the first such study to examine the health of a very large number of women over a long period of time. We can learn from the results, but we won't have them until the year 2008.

In the meantime, you can do much to ensure your well-being by choosing the right foods to eat. Certain nutrients and changes in diet are known to alleviate specific symptoms of PMS and menopause. This chapter shows you how nourishing foods can support female health.

Treating Premenstrual Syndrome (PMS) with Specific Foods

For most women, the subject of *premenstrual syndrome* (a collection of symptoms that can occur usually beginning sometime during the week before menstruation begins) needs little introduction. An estimated 97 percent of females have PMS at some point in life. For about 40 percent of these women, symptoms are significantly intense, and for about 5 percent, PMS disrupts their usual routines for a day or two each month. Yet simple remedies for various symptoms of PMS abound. You can use food to balance hormones and increase or diminish their production, thereby taming monthly woes.

What's going on in there?

PMS is triggered by an imbalance in sex hormones. These hormones direct a woman's monthly menstrual cycle. In the first half of the month, estrogen output is on the rise, and then it rapidly declines at ovulation. Then progesterone production kicks in and increases in the days leading up to your period. However, output can vary, and too much or too little of a hormone at the wrong time can trigger PMS symptoms.

But your hormone production may be off for many reasons, including taking birth control pills, gynecological problems such as endometriosis or fibroids, multiple childbirths, lack of exercise, stress, and simply being over 30. However, it's also more than likely that what you are eating is affecting your cycle.

Normal hormone production depends upon having a ready supply of certain vitamins, minerals, and, yes, fats, both essential fatty acids and saturated fats. When you consume saturated fats, such as those found in butter and animal foods, your body converts them into reproductive hormones. This is why women who diet or exercise themselves into a state of extremely low body fat stop having their periods, a medical condition known as *amenorrhea*.

Choosing foods to treat common symptoms

As many as 150 symptoms of PMS have been identified, covering a range from cravings for sugar and crying spells to migraines and backache. These symptoms are commonly grouped into various categories, each associated with specific nutritional deficiencies that probably developed over a period of many years. Each group of symptoms can be treated with specific dietary changes. Take a look at some of the most common problems.

Irritability, nervous tension, mood swings, and anxiety

Irritability, nervous tension, mood swings, and anxiety are all symptoms characteristic of *estrogen dominance,* which occurs when your body makes too much of this hormone in relation to progesterone. Your body may be producing excess estrogen itself, but estrogen can accumulate in the system in several other diet-related ways.

If your body is lacking B-complex vitamins, for example, the liver can't perform its normal function of inactivating excess estrogen. If you're lacking fiber, estrogen in the process of being excreted via the intestines can be reabsorbed back into the bloodstream. And estrogen in the food supply — in meats and dairy products from animals raised with supplemental hormones — can add to your own supply of estrogen. If you're suffering from PMS, make sure to eat these foods only if they are organic.

I also highly recommend organic produce. Regular produce may be sprayed with pesticides that mimic estrogen. While the body quickly metabolizes natural estrogens, the synthetic estrogenlike compounds that are byproducts of pesticides tend to accumulate in body tissue. These can be potent at even low levels, especially when several are present. Such compounds can upset your own hormone balance.

The emotional symptoms of PMS can also be triggered by rapid drops in blood sugar (see Chapter 20), as well as low levels of *endorphins,* brain chemicals that make you feel that all is right with the world.

Eat a natural foods diet and give yourself sufficient protein to help stabilize your blood sugar. Such foods also provide B-complex vitamins, minerals, and fiber, and these ingredients are free of added hormones. (For more on this way of eating, flip through Part III.)

Go out of your way to eat foods that contain these nutrients: B complex, vitamin B6, choline, inositol, vitamin C, magnesium, and zinc. (The foods that are high in these are at the end of this chapter.)

Foods that contain phyto-estrogens also help tame emotions. This creamy soup, a combination of whole soybeans and lima beans, is a delicious way to increase your intake. (Turn ahead in this chapter for more on phytohormones in the section on menopause.) Flavonoids, covered in Chapter 6, also help balance hormones.

Puree of Green Soybean Soup

The mild flavor of fresh soybeans combines well with the more familiar taste of lima beans. Soybeans supply phyto-estrogens that help balance hormones, while lima beans, which are exceptionally high in magnesium, help quell PMS emotions. This soup makes a refreshing and slightly tart starter course.

Preparation time: *10 minutes*

Cooking time: *1 hour, 20 minutes*

Yield: *6 servings*

2 cups fresh lima beans, or 1 cup dried lima beans

1 quart filtered water

2 cups green soybeans, removed from pod

2 ½ cups chicken stock

1 teaspoon lemon juice

½ cup buttermilk

Sea salt and freshly ground black pepper to taste

1 In a medium saucepan, put the lima beans and water to cover. Simmer, covered, until tender, 15 to 20 minutes, if using fresh beans, and 45 minutes to 1 hour, if using dried beans.

2 In the meantime, bring 1 quart filtered water to a boil. Add the soybeans, lower heat to simmer, and cook, covered, until tender, about 10 to 15 minutes.

3 Drain both pots of beans. Put the beans in a food processor and puree, adding some of the chicken broth if needed to facilitate the pureeing.

4 Put the pureed beans, remaining chicken broth, and lemon juice in a medium saucepan. Heat the soup on low heat for 10 minutes, until it just simmers. Remove from heat.

5 Stir in the buttermilk. Season to taste with sea salt and pepper. Pour into preheated individual soup bowls and serve with seasoned Japanese rice crackers.

Cravings for carbohydrates

In the five or ten days before you begin your period, you may be especially hungry for breads of all kinds, chocolate cake, and any cookie you lay eyes on. Elevated insulin levels may be the cause. *Insulin* is the hormone that enables your body to store sugar in your cells for ready energy later. Excess insulin causes your cells to rapidly absorb the sugar. Once this sugar is inside the cells, your blood sugar drops, sometimes suddenly if you've eaten a lot of sugar quickly. You feel fatigued, dizzy, shaky, and faint and have a headache. This is the moment you decide that you can't live without lemon meringue pie.

You may also be craving carbs and sugar to self-medicate your menstrual anxiety. (See Chapter 14 on food and mood.)

When you crave sweets or carbs, have healthy ones such as a couple of whole-grain crackers topped with nut butter so that you give your system some protein and fat, along with the carbs. This helps steady blood sugar and even helps prevent weight gain. Also, sometimes a craving for sweets masks a craving for protein. Give yourself a little chicken breast and some vegetables and then notice whether you still have a strong urge for pie.

For carbohydrate cravings, focus on foods that contain these nutrients: B complex, vitamin E, magnesium, and omega-3 essential fatty acids. (Look up specific ingredients at the end of the chapter.)

Fluid retention, swelling with associated weight gain, and breast tenderness

Forty percent of women with PMS experience some bloating. Reproductive hormones that are out of balance can hamper the kidneys' ability to manage sodium and fluid levels in the body. You can end up with swollen hands and feet or difficulty cinching your belt. High insulin levels and vitamin B6 deficiency can also cause fluid retention.

To reduce bloating, minimize your intake (or completely avoid) salt and concentrated sweets, including refined white sugar, honey, and maple syrup, as well as foods made with these. Increase foods rich in potassium, such as bananas, and take advantage of the diuretic properties of certain foods such as parsley. (See Chapter 20 for more on fluid retention.)

These three nutrients are especially helpful: Vitamin B6, magnesium, and omega-6 essential fatty acids. (Find out the foods you need to eat at the end of this chapter.)

Feeling blue, depression

In this group of symptoms, related to depression, other possible complaints can include weepiness, confusion, insomnia, and forgetfulness. Such problems are again the result of hormone imbalance — in this case, a predominance of progesterone, which can act as a depressant. Low levels of certain neuro-transmitters in the central nervous system and low blood sugar can also cause these problems.

Like your mother said, eat breakfast and regularly scheduled meals to keep your blood sugar steady. (See Chapter 20 for other recommendations.)

You need these special nutrients to help decrease depression, plus phyto-estrogens and flavonoids: B complex, magnesium, potassium, and essential fatty acids. (For tips on what to eat, flip to the phytonutrient section of this chapter and the food list at the end.)

Treating menstrual problems

Even if you have virtually no troubling symptoms of PMS, other medical prob-lems can occur once menstruation begins. Like many women, you may experience abdominal cramping for the first few days of your cycle. Your menstrual flow may be particularly heavy or especially light. In these cases, too, a change in diet can greatly improve how you feel.

Cramps and lower back pain

Technically, cramps are not part of PMS because they do not occur "premen-strually," but only after menstruation begins. But cramps are a very common part of the package once you start having menstrual difficulties. Along with abdominal cramping, you may also feel pain in the inner thighs and lower back. In more severe cases, women also experience nausea, vomiting, diar-rhea, and heavy bleeding.

These symptoms can be caused by an imbalance in a particular group of hor-monelike compounds called *prostaglandins*. One sort of prostaglandin promotes expansion of blood vessels and muscles. Another sort, the Series II prostaglandin, promotes contraction. When Series II prostaglandins domi-nate, cramping can result as blood vessels within the uterus and the muscles surrounding the uterus contract. Sodium and fluid retention also do their share in causing menstrual pain.

Red meat and dairy foods promote the production of Series II prostaglandins. These foods contain *arachidonic acid,* which converts to the Series II prostaglandins. Beef contains the most arachidonic acid, lamb and pork somewhat less, and chicken and turkey the least of all. If you want to include meat in your meals, but are suffering from menstrual cramping, eat poultry rather than beef. If your cramps persist, go vegetarian for a few days before you start your period and during it.

Choose protein sources such as fish, beans, and whole grains rather than red meat. Avoid milk products and processed cheese, which are high in sodium (sodium promotes fluid retention and adds to your discomfort). Use nondairy nut and soy milks instead. Eat fresh fruits and vegetables for fiber. Avoid refined sugar.

Be sure to eat sufficient amounts of these nutrients, found in the foods listed at the end of the chapter: calcium, magnesium, and omega-6 essential fatty acids.

Heavy menstrual flow and related anemia

If your menstrual flow is infrequent or sporadic, you may experience heavy menstrual bleeding at times. This in turn may lead to anemia and iron deficiency, leaving you tired and pale. Other nutrients that are especially important are vitamin C and the flavonoids, both of which help strengthen fragile capillary walls and thus prevent excess bleeding. You may also benefit from including flax seed and flaxseed oil in your meals. Research shows that flaxseed can act as a menstrual regulator, restoring normal timing of the menstrual cycle.

Anemia can be a serious medical condition. If fatigue and pallor persist, consult a physician.

To replenish your blood supply, you need the following nutrients: vitamin A, B complex, vitamin C, copper, and iron. (See the end of the chapter for recommended foods that contain these.)

My general advice in this situation, if you are feeling tired, is to go with the flow. Slowing down a bit at this time of the month is normal, so if you are fatigued, plan some hours off, take on simpler tasks, and sneak in a catnap or a few moments of silence. I give you permission.

Eating for Two

There's no better time to begin eating quality foods than during pregnancy when what you eat also affects another's life. The first eight weeks of pregnancy are especially critical, when your baby's kidneys, heart, lungs, eyes, and mouth are beginning to form.

Begin by following these guidelines.

✔ You need protein, essential fatty acids, and complex carbohydrates. Eat natural, unrefined and unprocessed foods, including grains, beans, eggs, nuts, seeds, vegetables and fruits, and meats, poultry, and fish as free of toxins as possible. Organic foods should be the rule rather than the exception.

✔ Eat several smaller meals throughout the day rather than one or two large ones, which can be more difficult to digest.

✔ Avoid caffeine, including that found in sodas, teas, and chocolate, and avoid sugar. Eliminate all alcohol, tobacco products, and any over-the-counter drug (other than those prescribed by a physician) or illegal drugs. If you use these, a miscarriage or a birth defect in your child can result.

Getting the right amount of calories

When you're pregnant, you need about 300 more calories a day than you are used to. This is what a growing baby requires. Of course, the extra calories should not come from candy, chips, pizza, or ice cream. Increase your protein intake significantly to at least 100 g a day, well beyond the usually recommendation of 65 g a day. Protein is the building block of body tissue.

Most women gain between 20 and 40 pounds during pregnancy. If, by your fourth month, you have already gained 30 pounds, you may need to cut back on your eating. But never, under any circumstances, go on a low-calorie diet when you're carrying a child. Your baby could have a low birth weight and be weaker and more susceptible to disease. Delayed physical and mental development can also result, and such a diet can also leave you exhausted and unhealthy.

Always consult with your doctor before making radical changes in your diet while pregnant and before you begin nutrient and herbal supplements.

Calcium

During pregnancy, you need about 1,000 mg a day of calcium, but most prenatal vitamin supplements contain only up to 25 percent of that. You'll probably need to take a supplement, as well as eat calcium-rich foods including organic yogurt and other dairy products, almonds, and blackstrap molasses.

To increase your absorption of calcium, be sure also to consume foods that supply vitamin D, such as fatty fish and egg yolks. Or get 15 minutes of sunshine each day. Your body can use sunshine to manufacture vitamin D.

Folic acid

Folic acid helps prevent birth defects, especially those that affect the brain, spine, and nervous system. It also plays an essential role in the formation of DNA and RNA, the genetic material that controls cell division and replication and promotes the production of oxygen-carrying red blood cells. If you are pregnant or nursing, you need about 800 micrograms (mcg) of folic acid a day (1 microgram is a millionth of a gram). Fortunately, nature provides some delicious sources, which are listed at the end of this chapter.

You may also need to take a supplement, especially if before becoming pregnant, you used an oral contraceptive, which can deplete folic acid.

Artichokes, an excellent choice of folic acid, may look challenging, but they're easy to cook. Give it a try with this simple recipe.

Artichokes with Mediterranean Garlic Sauce

Artichokes contain a wide variety of nutrients important for female health — calcium, magnesium, iron, potassium, some zinc, and quite a bit of folic acid as well as other B vitamins. Even the process of slowly nibbling one of these thistles at the end of an anxious day can be quite soothing.

Preparation time: *15 minutes*

Cooking time: *20 minutes, plus time to cool*

Yield: *2 servings*

2 medium globe artichokes

1 quart filtered water

2 tablespoons red wine vinegar

3 cloves garlic, 1 clove minced

2 tablespoons commercial mayonnaise, preferably free of hydrogenated oil

2 tablespoons plain yogurt

1 teaspoon lemon juice

1 Snap off the artichoke's tough outer leaves. Using a paring knife, cut off the stem and trim the bottom to an even round shape with a flat base. Cut 1 inch from the top of the remaining leaves.

2 Sit the artichokes upright in a medium saucepan. Add the water, vinegar, and 2 cloves unminced garlic.

3 Cook, covered, on medium heat for 20 minutes or until a leaf can be easily pulled out. Remove from heat and let cool to room temperature.

4 In the meantime, combine the mayonnaise, yogurt, lemon juice, and 1 clove minced garlic in a small bowl; whisk until well blended.

5 Remove the artichokes from the cooking liquid and drain well. Place each artichoke on a serving plate. Dip each artichoke leaf into the sauce and relax while you enjoy the slow-paced ceremony of artichoke eating.

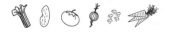

Fiber

The female hormone progesterone, essential for providing an environment in which the fetus can thrive, has a tendency to relax the bowel muscles during pregnancy, which can result in constipation. Don't take a laxative. Instead, rely on prune juice and high-fiber foods. Consult a doctor if that doesn't work.

A wide range of foods contain fiber: apples, barley, beans, bean sprouts, berries, broccoli, brown rice, buckwheat, carrots, corn, kale, lentils, mangoes, oats, okra, papaya, pears, peas, popcorn, prunes, and whole wheat.

Essential fatty acids (EFAs)

EFAs, the kind of fats that are good for you, are critical for the normal formation of membranes, the outer part of every cell in the body. The brain of a growing fetus also requires EFAs, as they make up about 60 percent of brain tissue. An estimated optimal dose of omega-6 fatty acids is 9 g a day, and 6 g a day of omega-3 fatty acids. A diet high in plant foods including nuts, seeds, and unrefined vegetables oils can provide what you need, and taking 1 to 2 tablespoons a day of flaxseed oil, especially high in the omega-3 fatty acids, is a good way to increase your intake. (See Chapter 10 for more EFA info.)

As you increase your intake of EFAs, be sure to also increase your intake of antioxidants. (Chapter 6 has information on these.)

Iodine

Pregnancy requires at least 175 mcg of iodine a day. (Take a look at the list at the end of the chapter for food sources.) You can eat seafood and seaweed to obtain this — but during pregnancy, limit your salt intake to 1 teaspoon a day.

Iron

The requirement for iron during pregnancy is 30 mg a day. (Check the end of the chapter for foods that contain iron.)

Avoid drinking coffee and tea, caffeinated and decaffeinated, which increase urination and flush iron out of the system.

Magnesium

The recommendation for magnesium is about 350 mg a day. (The food list at the end of the chapter tells you what foods.)

All green vegetables contain magesium.

Medicinals for morning sickness

Ginger works as well for morning sickness as it does for seasickness. Grate a half-inch of ginger root into a cup filled with boiling water. Steep for 5 minutes before drinking. Have this tea every morning before breakfast. Eating little snacks throughout the day can also help a queasy stomach.

Zinc

During pregnancy, you require 15 mg zinc. (Turn to the end of this chapter and write your shopping list for zinc foods.)

Oysters are far and away the richest source of zinc. Enjoy these cooked.

Foods to avoid during pregnancy

Certain foods that are relatively harmless when you're not pregnant can pose serious dangers to your body when you are. Stay away from foods that may carry various bacteria or parasites, such as

- Raw fish, including sushi and seviche
- Runny eggs
- Pâtés and soft cheeses such as blue cheese
- Unpasteurized milk, cheese, and juice

Also avoid garlic, onions, cabbage, red peppers, chilies, and other spicy or gas-forming foods if you're already sensitive to them.

In general, stay away from all herbal teas. Many can interfere with pregnancy.

After the baby arrives

Mother's milk is far superior nutritionally to baby formula. However, if you're nursing, you need to watch what you eat. It's a good idea to continue avoiding the foods, chemicals, and other substances that were dangerous for your fetus. Some of everything you eat or take into your body goes into your breast milk, and eventually into your baby.

As a nursing mother, you will need to increase your calorie intake by about 500 calories a day compared with before you were pregnant. And certain nutrients are especially important — all the B vitamins, including thiamin, riboflavin, and niacin, as well as calcium, iodine, and essential fatty acids.

Munching Your Way through Menopause

Women who enter menopause with adequate reserves of vitamins, minerals, and other essential nutrients pass through this transition with fewer symptoms than do women who reach midlife physically depleted and poorly nourished. Even if menopause is years away, you'll thank yourself later if you improve your eating habits now.

Symptoms of menopause are most dramatic during the year or two leading up to menopause, the phase called *perimenopause.* As in PMS, symptoms are the result of hormone imbalances. You may have abnormally high levels of estrogen as compared with progesterone or vice versa. Symptoms such as irritability, anxiety, depression, and "menopausal rage" can occur. Lowered estrogen levels can also affect memory. In addition, the body's ability to regulate temperature may go on the fritz like a broken thermostat, triggering hot flashes.

Food is a powerful tool for dampening and even preventing these annoyances. And what you decide *not* to eat is just as important.

Special nutrients for menopause

Vitamin E, taken in through diet or as a supplement, is one of the most important vitamins for menopause. (Be sure to take the "natural" form.) But the B vitamins and vitamins A and C, as well as a variety of minerals, are also essential. (You can find their food sources at the end of this chapter.)

Natural foods also provide other active compounds that recent research is showing are also vital for your health. These include flavonoids and the group of compounds called phyto-estrogens, which function like hormones and help balance your own.

Phyto-estrogens

Phytohormones, popularly called *phyto-estrogens,* are found in dozens of plant foods. They work in several ways to help *balance* hormones. When necessary, they mimic estrogen and *increase* estrogen levels, but when estrogen is high, phyto-estrogen can in effect *decrease* estrogen activity in your tissues.

They block estrogen receptor sites in tissues such as the breast. Phyto-estrogens may also promote the breakdown of estrogen and decrease its production.

Phyto-estrogens help prevent symptoms of PMS and menopause that stem from the dramatic rise and fall of hormones. Soybeans contain especially potent phyto-estrogen, but many everyday vegetables, fruits, legumes, whole grains, and nuts exhibit some estrogenic activity. In some cultures, such plant foods may contribute as much as 50 percent of calories. According to a 1990 study in the *British Journal of Medicine,* intake of phyto-estrogens at this level could potentially diminish menopause symptoms.

The phytohormones in soy are the isoflavones, specifically genistein (one of the most potent of phytohormones) and daidzein. Fresh soybeans provide the most genistein, but processing the soybeans lowers the amount. Tempeh and miso come in second place, while highly processed soy products provide the least. (See Chapter 5 for more on soy.)

Here are some foods to put on your shopping list to help you increase your intake of estrogenic compounds:

- **Vegetables:** Carrots, beets, potatoes, cabbage, fennel, broccoli, cauliflower, onions, celery, radishes, and parsley

- **Fruit:** Apples, cherries, citrus, and pomegranates

- **Legumes:** Soybeans, chickpeas, red beans, and split peas

- **Whole grains:** Barley, oats, rice, rye, wheat, and corn

- **Flavorings:** Licorice, anise, and garlic

- **Seeds:** Sesame and flax seed

- **Oils:** Extra-virgin olive oil, cold-pressed oils, and flaxseed oil

Flavonoids

Flavonoids are a group of vitaminlike compounds with a chemical structure and activity similar to estrogen. Flavonoids help minimize estrogen highs and lows. (See Chapter 6 for food sources of flavonoids.)

Buckwheat, which contains flavonoids, makes a good salad. In this recipe, it substitutes for bulghur wheat in the traditional Middle Eastern dish tabbouli.

Turkish Buckwheat Salad

Buckwheat groats supply iron, thiamin, and niacin, nutrients that help you feel energized. Buckwheat is a source of flavonoids that help balance hormones.

Preparation time: *10 minutes*

Cooking time: *15 minutes, plus at least 1 hour to blend flavors*

Yield: *4 large servings*

2 cups unfiltered water

1 cup unroasted whole buckwheat grouts

2 scallions, chopped

1 bunch fresh parsley, stems removed (1 cup), leaves chopped

2 sprigs fresh mint, stems removed, leaves chopped

1 teaspoon ground cumin

3 tablespoons fresh lemon juice

2 tablespoon extra-virgin olive oil

Salt and freshly ground black pepper to taste

1 In a large saucepan, bring the water to boil over high heat.

2 Stir in the buckwheat grouts and immediately lower heat to simmer. Cook, covered, for 15 minutes, or until all the water has been absorbed. Remove from heat and set aside.

3 Spoon the cooked buckwheat into a large bowl. Add the scallions, parsley, mint, cumin, lemon juice, oil, and salt and pepper.

4 Gently toss salad ingredients together until well blended. Cover and refrigerate for at least 1 hour to blend flavors. Serve as a side dish with grilled meats, such as lamb chops, and a cucumber-yogurt salad.

Healing foods for menopausal symptoms

What you choose to eat and — equally important — the foods you do not eat have a powerful effect on how you feel as you pass through menopause. Whether or not you are taking hormones, you still need to give yourself good nutrition at every meal to prevent and ease symptoms.

Menopause involves far more than changes in hormone production. It is a shift in body chemistry that affects the adrenal glands, the nervous system, the skeleton, and the brain. You need to nourish your body with sustaining foods as your body adjusts. Foods that contain phyto-estrogens are especially important to include in your meals. Many symptoms of menopause are triggered by rapid changes in estrogen levels, and these phytonutrients help you avoid the extremes.

Choosing foods so that your blood sugar remains steady is essential. (Turn to Chapter 20 for ways to do this.) Many of the symptoms of low blood sugar, including sweating, irritability, mood swings, and fatigue, are also typical of menopause.

Perimenopausal PMS

As your period becomes more irregular during perimenopause, you may experience PMS even if you did not when you were younger. You may also experience heavy menstrual bleeding. Follow the dietary advice for these conditions, earlier in this chapter.

Hot flashes

If it suddenly feels like you're living in the tropics, you're having a *hot flash*. A small burst of heat begins in the chest area and quickly expands to the face and arms. You sweat and then feel quite chilled as the perspiration evaporates and your body temperature quickly drops. You may also feel some anxiety.

Avoid stimulating and warming foods such as caffeinated coffee and tea, chocolate, spicy foods, and alcoholic beverages, including beer. A large dose of sugar, such as a slice of pecan pie, can also bring on a flash.

These special nutrients help with hot flashes: vitamin E, magnesium, and selenium. Vitamin E is considered the prime menopause nutrient, and selenium works with vitamin E to maximize its effectiveness. (You can find food sources at the end of the chapter.)

Flavonoids and phyto-estrogens are also important nutrients, because they both help balance hormones.

With all that sweating, hot flashes can leave you thirsty and depleted of minerals such as potassium, sodium, and magnesium, which you lose through the skin when you perspire. The same is true for *night sweats,* surges of heat that wake you from your sleep. At breakfast, replenish what you've lost with plenty of fresh filtered water and a mineral-rich fruit and nut compote. Start with this recipe.

Hot Flash Fruit Compote

Having a hot flash triggers your body to perspire in an effort to cool down. In the process of sweating, you lose fluids and several important minerals — sodium, potassium, and magnesium. Select from the following ingredients and assemble a fruit compote, making sure to include some juicy chunks of melon!

Preparation time: *10 minutes*

Cooking time: *None*

Yield: *4 servings*

4 cups fruit (cantaloupe, honeydew melon, bananas, apricots, cherries, black currants, dates, guava, kiwi, mango, papaya, and pears)

3 tablepoons pumpkin seeds

3 tablepoons nuts (almonds, cashews, and pistachios)

Sea salt (optional)

2 tablespoons yogurt (optional)

Unsulphured blackstrap molasses (optional)

Chopped fresh mint leaves (optional)

1 Cut the fruit into bite-sized pieces. Put the fruit in a bowl and combine with the seeds and nuts.

2 Sprinkle the fruit with a pinch of sea salt.

3 Spoon fruit mixture into individual serving bowl and top with yogurt and molasses. Dig in!

Fatigue

Fatigue is the most commonly reported symptom of menopause. Hot flashes can be draining. Anemia due to heavy bleeding may also cause fatigue, and iron-rich foods are needed.

Monitor how you feel after eating such potentially allergenic foods as wheat and milk. (See the section on food allergies in Chapter 20 for more information.)

These special nutrients help reduce fatigue: B complex, vitamin C, and iron. (I list food sources at the end of the chapter.)

Observe the *-pause* in menopause. If you are tired, rest!

Weight gain

With menopause, you may develop a rounded belly, due to changes in your output of reproductive hormones. It is here, in the lower abdominal tissue, that you make some of your postmenopausal estrogen as production in your ovaries diminishes. Gaining about 5 to 10 pounds at menopause is normal. Fluid retention can also lead to a temporary increase in weight.

Resist going on a crash diet, which will rob you of needed vitamins and minerals. Instead, have moderate portions of whole foods. And avoid refined sugar, which is all calories and no nutrients.

Memory

Research has shown that estrogen improves verbal recall and the ability to acquire and remember newly associated thoughts. Estrogenic foods, essential fatty acids, antioxidants, lecithin, B vitamins, and the minerals potassium, magnesium, phosphorus, and boron all promote mental alertness. In addition, maintaining stable blood sugar levels, as well as getting sufficient rest, and regular exercise to increase your oxygen supply can also help.

These special nutrients maintain memory: B complex, lecithin, beta-carotene, vitamin C, vitamin E , boron, magnesium, phosphorus, selenium, and essential fatty acids. (At the end of this chapter is a list of food sources.)

Mood swings, irritability, depression

Follow the nutrient and food recommendations given for these symptoms earlier in this chapter under the sections on irritability and depression. Phyto-estrogens can also help balance hormones and steady mood swings. Avoid refined and processed foods, caffeine, and alcohol.

Sexual problems

While sexuality does certainly continue postmenopause, there is also no denying that as your supply of reproductive hormones declines, your sexual energy can alter and diminish. Vaginal tissue also goes through changes. However, there is a way of eating that can help you restore a once-vital sex life.

First, make a special effort to avoid symptom triggers such as caffeine, white sugar, and nutrient-depleted refined foods. Then boost your intake of whole foods such as seasonal fresh fruits and vegetables, whole grains, seafood, nuts, and seeds. These foods supply nutrients that maintain vaginal health, keep tissues firm through the manufacture of collagen, and increase sexual response.

These special nutrients help maintain healthy vaginal tissue: vitamin A, vitamin B6, vitamin C, vitamin E, copper, and essential fatty acids. These special nutrients help you maintain vaginal lubrication and sexual vitality: niacin, folic acid, and zinc.

Menopause and degenerative disease

Although you often hear osteoporosis and heart disease lumped together with the symptoms of menopause, these degenerative diseases are not inevitable consequences of passing through the change-of-life. Lowered hormone levels can be a risk factor, and the likelihood of developing these diseases can increase as you pass middle age, but eating the right foods is a good way to help prevent these diseases. Please see Chapters 15 and 20 for details.

Top Nutrients and Best Foods

As a woman, you need certain nutrients in particular for hormonal health and normal reproductive function. I list both animal and plant food sources of these nutrients, because some conditions are best treated with a vegetarian diet. These ingredients give you a wide range of choices for everyday good eating.

- ✔ **Vitamin A and beta-carotene:** Both orange and dark green fruits and vegetables, such as butternut squash and collard greens, and organic liver

- ✔ **B-complex:** Meats, fish, and grains such as brown rice and oats

- ✔ **Niacin:** Meats, poultry, fish, peanuts, brown rice, and dates

- ✔ **Vitamin B6:** Meats, seafood, beans, peas, lentils, whole grains, and kale

- ✔ **Folic acid:** Pork, organic liver, trout, yogurt, lentils, peas, avocado, asparagus, artichokes, beets, boysenberries, cantaloupe, and pistachios

- ✔ **Choline:** Egg yolks, organ meats, whole wheat, fish, and legumes

- ✔ **Inositol:** Whole grains, citrus, blackstrap molasses, fish, and legumes

- ✔ **Lecithin:** Egg yolks, organ meats, whole wheat, citrus, and nuts

- ✔ **Vitamin C:** Sweet peppers, papaya, citrus, kiwi, alfalfa sprouts, and cantaloupe

- ✔ **Vitamin D:** Fatty fish, such as salmon, sardines, and herring, and egg yolks

- **Vitamin E:** Extra-virgin olive oil and other unrefined vegetable oils, whole grains, eggs, sweet potatoes, leafy green vegetables, nuts, and seeds

- **Boron (a trace mineral):** Apples, pears, dates, almonds, hazelnuts, broccoli, legumes, and honey

- **Calcium:** Yogurt, kale, kidney beans, canned salmon and sardines with the bones, and chicken soup cooked with the bones

- **Copper:** Organic liver, seafood, beans, and collards

- **Iodine:** Seafood, seaweed, and iodized salt

- **Iron:** Organic liver, oysters, clams, seaweed, blackstrap molasses, legumes, beets, raisins, seeds, and nuts

- **Magnesium:** Shrimp, halibut, whole grains, kale, lima beans, black-eyed peas, eggs, almonds, beets, plantains, bananas, and pumpkin and sunflower seeds

- **Phosphorus:** Fish, meats, poultry, eggs, legumes, whole grains, and nuts

- **Potassium:** Meats, whole grains, legumes, bananas, and sunflower seeds

- **Selenium:** Brazil nuts, seafood, meats, eggs, whole grains, and sesame seeds

Chapter 18

Healing Foods for Men

*T*his chapter features health issues that are unique to men and that can be affected by diet — enlarged prostate, prostate cancer, impotency, and faltering libido. Males are also particularly subject to heart disease, the primary cause of death in men, and stress-related ailments. I cover these topics in Chapters 15 and 20.

The general way of eating that is recommended for all these conditions is the same. Build meals based on natural, unrefined, and unprocessed whole foods. Avoid added hormones and toxins. Enjoy a wide variety of ingredients, from meats, poultry, and seafood to fruits of the field.

Prostate Problems

The prostate is a small, walnut-shaped gland that sits at the base of the bladder. Its job is to produce part of the fluid that makes semen. With the first contractions of orgasm, prostatic fluid begins to flow. The gland also metabolizes the male hormone, testosterone.

Time was when no one much thought about the prostate gland. But now that prostate tumors are the most commonly diagnosed form of cancer in men, (excluding skin cancer) and the second leading cause of death among males, prostate disease is a common concern. Talking about your prostate has even become acceptable dinner conversation, along with menopause and cholesterol levels.

One such condition is benign prostatic hyperplasia (BPH). About 60 percent of all men between 40 and 59 years of age have *benign prostatic hyperplasia (BPH),* or an enlarged prostate. The incidence has increased tremendously in the last few decades. Depending upon what portion of the prostate becomes enlarged, the gland can place pressure on the bladder, causing typical BPH symptoms. At first, a man may find he needs to urinate more frequently. Then, as BPH progresses, symptoms can include greater urgency of urination, increased frequency, especially at night, and difficulty completely emptying the bladder.

Risk factors

Following are the risk factors associated with BPH.

- ✔ Hormone imbalances that occur with age appear to be at the core of the problem.

- ✔ Elevated cholesterol levels play a role in the degeneration of prostate tissue and the gland's change in size.

- ✔ Exposure to pesticides and environmental toxins leads to hormone imbalances, which are a risk factor.

- ✔ Carrying excess weight in the abdomen can worsen symptoms because a portly belly may put pressure on the bladder.

Pumpkin seeds — Munchable medicine

Pumpkin seeds are an excellent source of zinc, essential fatty acids, and certain amino acids, all helpful in reducing symptoms of BPH. These are not the pumpkin seeds you find in the kind of pumpkin you carve and put a candle in for Halloween. These pumpkin seeds are long, flat, and dark green. They are sold in natural-food stores and in Latin markets where they are called *pepitas*.

Healing foods for prostatitis

In *prostatitis,* the prostate gland is infected, due to a urinary infection, a blood-borne infection or venereal disease. If you have this condition, avoid spicy foods and refrain from caffeine, alcohol, and cigarettes, all of which are potential irritants of the prostate gland. Also avoid sugar.

Just as women's hormone production alters after about age 50, men produce less testosterone, but higher amounts of other hormones, including the principally female sex hormones prolactin, *estradiol* (a form of estrogen), and two hormones that abruptly rise at ovulation, luteinizing hormone and follicle-stimulating hormone. One consequence of changing hormone production is an accumulation of a very potent form of testosterone, *dihydrotestosterone,* within the prostate. This hormone can promote the overproduction of prostate cells.

Special nutrients for BPH

To combat BPH, you need to take advantage of several nutrients. (See the end of this chapter for foods that contain these nutrients.)

- ✔ Both **zinc** and **vitamin B6** play a role in the complexity of processes and chemical reactions that lead to hormone balance.
- ✔ **Vitamin E** and **selenium** are also essential nutrients for prostate health.
- ✔ **Essential fatty acids** have been used clinically to successfully reduce symptoms of BPH. Have the equivalent of 1 teaspoon of essential fatty acids or 4 g day. Avoid processed and hydrogenated oils and lower your intake of saturated fats.

Recent studies show that the herb saw palmetto can significantly improve the urinary difficulties associated with BPH and is useful in the prevention of BPH. Other herbal treatments include flower pollen, prescribed in Europe, and ginseng, which is used in China.

Fish is an excellent source of essential fatty acids. An easy-to-make fish sandwich for lunch is a great way to increase your intake.

Contaminants that can upset hormone balance

Pesticides and other contaminants, present in food, some products, and the environment, break down into compounds that behave like hormones. These substances include dioxin, polyhalogenated biphenyls, hexachlorobenzene, dibenzofurans, and diethylstilboestrol (DES). Such compounds may contribute to hormone imbalance in males. In one animal study, DES caused prostate changes similar to BPH.

Here's a good reason to eat only organic foods. (Take a look at Chapter 4 for more on these.) And remember, nutrients such as carotenes, flavonoids, chlorophyll, magnesium, calcium, selenium, and zinc, as well as fiber, support the body's ability to rid itself of these contaminants.

Two-Fisted Tuna on Toast

Choose a fatty fish such as tuna, salmon, or sardines, which gives you an extra dose of healing omega-3 essential fatty acids, important for prostate health.

Preparation time: *10 minutes*

Cooking time: *2 minutes for the toast*

Yield: *1 hefty sandwich*

1 6-ounce can tuna, packed in water

⅓ cup diced onion

1 tablespoon red wine or balsamic vinegar

2 slices crusty whole grain bread, toasted

2 slices tomato

4 anchovies

Freshly grated pepper to taste

1 In a small bowl, mix together the tuna, onion, and vinegar.

2 Lay the 2 pieces of toast on a work surface. Cover 1 slice with the tomatoes and spread the tuna mixture on top of this. Arrange the anchovies on the tuna. Season with pepper. Top with the second piece of toast.

3 With a sharp knife, cut the sandwich in half. Wolf down with potato salad and a glass of fruit juice mixed with club soda.

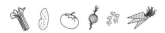

Fiber helps rid the body of toxins that can disturb hormone balance and also lowers cholesterol. Okra is a great source of various kinds of beneficial fiber, both insoluble and soluble, in the form of pectins and gums.

Protective nutrients for prostate cancer

Age, family history, and race affect your risk of prostate cancer. African-American men have an especially high rate. Prostate cancer is related to diet in only about 10 to 20 percent of cases. However, recent research is discovering some nutrients that may be beneficial in lowering your risk.

✔ Taking a daily supplement of 400 IU vitamin E, an antioxidant, can help reduce the incidence of prostate cancer.

✔ Selenium, another antioxidant, is almost as effective as vitamin E in reducing the risk of prostate cancer. This mineral may block cell damage, as well as protect the prostate from environmental carcinogens. (Nearly half the selenium a man carries in his body is in the testes and seminal ducts adjacent

to the prostate gland.) Unfortunately, selenium deficiency is common. In addition, men lose selenium in their semen.

✔ Vitamin D appears to inhibit the spread of cancer. Sunlight allows the body to synthesize this important nutrient.

✔ Lycopene, a phytonutrient in tomatoes, is associated with a lower risk of aggressive prostate cancer. (See Chapter 6 and Appendix A for more on this.)

In addition, regular consumption of red meat and dairy products is a risk factor. The Japanese, who consume a lowfat fish and vegetable diet, have the lowest incidence of prostate cancer in the industrialized world.

Quick and Easy Cajun Okra

You may stay away from okra because of its odd, slightly slimy texture, but that texture is just the reason you should be eating okra more than once every five years. In this recipe, the okra is cooked with tantalizing Cajun spices. Enjoy this dish with Dixieland red beans and rice.

Preparation time: *5 minutes*

Cooking time: *20 minutes*

Yield: *4 servings*

½ pound young okra, stems removed and cut into 1-inch lengths if the pods are large

1 teaspoon unsalted, organic butter

1 tablespoon prepared Cajon Creole Seasoning*

Salt to taste

1 Fill a medium pot with water to about 1 inch from the top. Bring to a boil and add the okra.

2 Simmer, covered, on medium-low heat, until okra is tender, about 10 minutes.

(continued)

3 Meanwhile, in a saucepan, melt the butter. Add the Cajun Creole Seasoning and heat over low heat for 1 minute to develop seasoning flavors. Add the okra. Using a wooden spoon, toss the okra in the seasoned butter to evenly coat. Cook for 2 to 3 minutes to combine flavors. Salt to taste and serve.

One brand that includes this spice mix in its line is Spice Hunter.

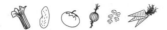

Nourishing your Sexuality

What you eat affects your sexual and reproductive anatomy just as much as any other part of your body. Problems such as impotence and lack of interest in sex can in part be brought on by poor food choices. The pituitary and testes produce sex hormones, and even the adrenals produce small amounts. These glands require specific nutrients to function properly. A change to eating healthier foods that supply certain vitamins, minerals, and healing fats can often help correct these conditions.

Erectile dysfunction (impotence)

The inability to achieve or maintain a full erection is known by the medical term *erectile dysfunction* (ED). If you have ever experienced ED, you are not alone. An estimated 30 million men in the United States — the majority over age 65 — have some degree of ED. (No, ED does not affect sexual drive or the ability to achieve orgasm.) Medications, stress, emotional problems, infection, and anatomical abnormalities can cause ED. In addition, certain medical conditions are often part of the picture.

Normal sexual function depends upon having healthy arteries and nerves. Diseases that cause damage to these in the trunk of the body and limbs can also do harm in the genital area. Forty percent of men diagnosed with diabetes also experience some degree of impotency. High blood sugar levels, which occur in diabetes, limit the amount of oxygen the blood is able to transport to body cells. Sexual difficulties can result, especially because tissues in the penis need more oxygen than usual during sexual intercourse. In advanced diabetes, nerve damage occurs, which can affect sexual activity.

The arteries in the penis are vulnerable to *atherosclerosis,* or narrowing of the arteries, preventing enough blood from entering the penis to cause sufficient hardness. Vascular disease can interfere with the delivery of oxygen and nutrients to cells. Hypertension, high total cholesterol, and low levels of HDL cholesterol are also risk factors for impotency.

Medications that promise to improve erection cannot function if the blood vessels themselves are nonresponsive due to degenerative disease.

Follow this way of eating to keep it all in tip-top condition:

- ✔ Follow a heart healthy diet to normalize cholesterol levels, help prevent hypertension, and keep the vascular system healthy. (Also see Chapter 15.)

- ✔ Avoid refined white sugar. When eating sweets such as desserts, have only small portions. Eat regular meals, and when having a carbohydrate, also eat some protein — for example, apple pie and cheese.

- ✔ Limit alcoholic beverages. A small amount stimulates blood flow, but alcohol also acts as a depressant and can be a downer. Caffeine can also interfere with performance.

- ✔ Avoid estrogens and growth hormones in meat that may interfere with your own hormone balance and reproductive health. Eat only meats that are free of hormone residues.

Take advantage of the special nutrients for potency. All the antioxidants — beta-carotene, vitamin C, vitamin E, and selenium — protect cells from free radical damage and help prevent tissues in the testes from degeneration. Zinc and the B vitamins are essential for the production of testosterone. Magnesium helps reverse hardening of the arteries in the penis. And manganese is typically low in body tissues of men who are impotent. (At the end of this chapter is a list of the top food sources for these nutrients.)

Feeding your libido

Sexual drive, or *libido,* requires one nutrient in particular — zinc. If you want to boost your reserve, you'd best like oysters. These crustaceans are by far the most concentrated food source. While crab is a good source of zinc (3 ounces supply 5 mg of zinc), six medium oysters contain an extraordinary 76 mg! Oysters have long been used as an aphrodisiac, and now you know why!

To get your daily dose of zinc, try this recipe for oyster stew.

Zinc and the mineral copper need to be kept in balance. Oysters also contain some copper, as well as small amounts of calcium and phosphorus, all minerals, which increase the effectiveness of zinc.

Don Juan's Oyster Stew

An easy way to cook oysters is to make a quick oyster stew. This recipe is delicious because it's buttery, the way oyster stew used to be made. If you care only about what the oysters can do for you and you're watching your fat intake, skip the cream and make it just with milk.

Preparation time: *10 minutes*

Cooking time: *10 minutes*

Yield: *4 servings*

2 dozen fresh, shucked oysters*

2 tablespoons organic, unsalted butter

1 cup oyster liquor or clam juice

½ teaspoon grated onion, or ½ cup sliced cooked celery

1½ cups milk, preferably without added hormones and organic

½ cup cream, preferably without added hormones and organic

Paprika, for garnish

1 Fill the lower portion of a double boiler with water and bring to a boil, making sure that the top pan does not touch the water. Put the oysters, 1 tablespoon butter, oyster liquor, and onion in the top half. Stir briskly and constantly until oysters are just beginning to curl, about 1 minute.

2 Add the milk and cream and continue stirring briskly, just to a boil, making sure not to boil.

3 Pour the oyster stew into warmed individual soup bowls, dividing the oysters evenly.

4 Serve the stew piping hot and garnish each serving with some of the remaining butter and a dash of paprika.

*If you feel accomplished shucking your own oysters, buy them in the shell, which should be undamaged and shut tight. Or have someone at your fish store shuck the oysters and make sure that he also gives you the juice from the oysters (the oyster liquor). Or buy oysters that are shucked, packaged, and marked with a "sell by" date.

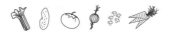

Smoking contributes to impotency

If you smoke, quit! Smokers, as compared with nonsmokers, are twice as likely to be impotent. Smoke injures arteries and disrupts blood flow. If a man smokes two packs of cigarettes a day, by the time he is 30, he will probably experience some problems. By stopping smoking, when impotency is only in the early stages, potency can be somewhat restored. But if the condition has continued for five to ten years, even quitting smoking will not restore function. Secondhand smoke can also cause impotency. Smoking also may hinder arousal and orgasm in women.

Nutrients for sperm production

Eggs are full of nutrients needed to launch new life, so it should be no surprise that sperm, too, are packed with vitamins and minerals. Sperm contains calcium, magnesium, zinc, and sulfur plus vitamin B12, vitamin C, and inositol, part of the B complex of vitamins. Whole grains, legumes, nuts, meats, liver, shellfish, and citrus are sources.

Zinc in particular is essential for the production of sperm. Low levels can result in sperm that are infertile.

If you'd rather take a nap

Besides desire, sex requires energy. If you've been overstressed and are not eating particularly nourishing foods, you risk adrenal exhaustion. Your body's stress coping mechanisms say, "No more." The adrenals cut back on energy production and insist that you rest. When these glands become exhausted, you're less likely to participate in your normal activities, including sex.

Help your adrenals revive by staying away from sugar and caffeine. Increase your intake of foods that supply B vitamins and vitamin C.

You may also lack the desire and strength for sex if your thyroid gland is not receiving essential nutrients. Your thyroid controls the rate at which you convert food to energy. A sluggish thyroid, or *hypothyroidism,* can also dampen desire. Foods that contain iodine, B vitamins, and especially thiamin, plus vitamin E are required.

Enjoy all sorts of seafood, whole grains, nuts, and unrefined oils to maintain your zest for life.

The Healthiest Foods to Eat and Order When You're Out

Many of the same nutrients are recommended for various aspects of male reproductive health. Check out the following list of nutrients you especially need and the foods that contain them.

- **Vitamin A:** Liver, eggs, sweet potatoes, carrots, winter squash, and cantaloupe

- **B1 (thiamin):** Pork, duck, lobster, egg yolks, pinto beans, potatoes, beans, grapes, and pistachios

- **B6 (pyridoxine):** Beef, chicken, tuna, brown rice, navy beans, broccoli, mangoes, walnuts, and sunflower seeds

- **PABA:** Organ meats, whole wheat, yogurt, blackstrap molasses, and kale

- **Folic acid:** Beef, chicken, trout, beans and lentils, whole grains, asparagus, beets, avocados, boysenberries, and pistachios

- **Vitamin C:** Citrus, cantaloupe, strawberries, broccoli, and green peppers

- **Vitamin E:** Unrefined oils, eggs, whole wheat, organ meats, sweet potatoes, kale, and cabbage

- **Magnesium:** Shrimp, oysters, halibut, egg yolks, beans, whole grains, figs, plantains, avocados, Brazil nuts, cashews, walnuts, and seeds

- **Manganese:** Clams, bass, trout, lima beans, beans and lentils, whole grains, okra, pineapple, bananas, hazelnuts, almonds, and maple syrup

- **Selenium:** Brazil nuts, shellfish, tuna, herring, chicken breast, beef, lamb, whole wheat, carrots, cabbage, and mushrooms

- **Zinc:** Oysters and other shellfish, sardines, pumpkin seeds, sunflower seeds, mushrooms, beef, lamb, and cheese

- **Essential fatty acids:** Unrefined vegetable oils, flaxseed, walnuts, organic eggs, and fatty fish such as sardines, tuna, and salmon

Chapter 19

Feeding Children Healing Foods

- -

In This Chapter

▶ Starting out life with quality foods

▶ Junking junk foods

▶ Treating common ailments with nutrition

▶ Reducing obesity to help prevent disease

▶ Managing eating disorders and attention deficit hyperactivity disorder (ADHD) with diet

- -

Children require basically the same healthy, unrefined and unprocessed, natural foods as adults. Parents who eat nutritious meals set the example. By feeding children wholesome foods, parents give kids a chance to develop a preference for good foods from an early age. Granted, serving boxed, bagged, canned, and frozen foods is easier and timesaving, but such foods are not particularly nutritious and can even undermine health.

Children in their growing years particularly need nourishing foods as the skeleton is developing and the body is maturing. What a child is eating often plays a role in their childhood ailments and can also sow the seeds for future medical problems. Among the younger population, obesity, heart disease, and diabetes are on the rise, all with clear links to diet.

In this chapter, you find out about the best foods to feed growing children. And if your child is under the weather, you can turn to the section on common childhood ailments like tummy upset and a runny nose. I also take a look at the growing incidence of obesity among children today and related disease and give parents some suggestions on how to care for children with eating disorders and attention deficit hyperactivity disorder (ADHD). You can make a great difference in your children's health by feeding them the right foods.

Feeding Baby

The perfect food for infants is human breast milk. Compared with other forms of milk, such as cow's milk, mother's milk has an ideal protein ratio for babies, more polyunsaturated fatty acids, less sodium, more antibodies to strengthen a child's immune system, and is better digested. It also contains 1 mg iron per liter, which is easily absorbed and critical for building blood.

Caffeine, alcohol, and most drugs are transmitted to infants in breast milk. If you're nursing, avoid these and refrain from smoking cigarettes, which reduces the amount of milk produced.

And when it's time to advance to solid foods, at about 4 to 6 months, feed baby *organic* ingredients! All major brands of baby food contain low levels of pesticides. Exposure to excessive amounts of these chemicals can damage the progress of developing organs and nerves in children. Children are vulnerable to pesticides because they consume more food per unit of body weight than adults do and far fewer types of foods than adults. Animal studies show that pesticides can cause such adverse effects as lower brain weight, behavioral problems, and learning disabilities. Shop in natural-food stores for organic baby food (see Chapter 4 for special brands) or buy organic ingredients and make your own baby food.

Feeding Growing Children

Giving a child a variety of fresh and natural foods helps ensure that they receive a wide range of vitamins, minerals, and phytonutrients. Having the correct mix of carbohydrates, protein, and fats is also important.

Complex carbohydrates

Complex carbohydrates are whole grains, such as whole wheat, oats, brown rice, whole barley, and millet, full of nutrients and fiber. The B vitamins and minerals they provide are essential for converting foods into energy, maintaining healthy nerves, building strong bones, and having good health in general. Avoid overly processed carbs like white bread and white rice because they have been stripped of much of their nutritional value, even if they have been "enriched."

Other sources of wholesome carbohydrates are fruits and vegetables (especially green leafy ones because they're packed with calcium, iron, and vitamins) and legumes.

Proteins

Growing children need protein to build body tissues and support the normal functioning of the body, including regulating hormones and controlling body temperature. No more than 25 percent of the child's diet should include proteins because there is a possibility of high cholesterol from the animal foods that the American diet relies on for protein. Best sources of high-quality protein are beef, poultry, fish, cheese, milk, eggs, pork, yogurt, and butter. The healthiest meats and poultry are organic and free of antibiotics and hormones. Small portions of lean meats provide plenty of nutrients, but less cholesterol.

Fats and oils

Be sure to include quality fats in your child's meals (Take a look at Chapter 10 for details.) A child's diet must contain monounsaturated fats found in olives, avocados, and nuts such as almonds, as well as the polyunsaturated fats present in nuts, seeds, and fish. The polyunsaturated essential fatty acids (EFAs) help regulate cholesterol and control blood pressure. A lack of EFAs retards the growth of a child's hair, skin, and nails. They also supply the means for fat-soluble vitamins to make their way to various tissues in a child's growing body.

Quality essential fatty acids are in the oilier fish such as salmon and tuna, as well as in walnuts, flax seeds, and sunflower, pumpkin, and sesame seeds.

Kids on caffeine

Kids are doing caffeine. Most get their buzz from carbonated beverages and chocolate. Research shows that when children consume caffeine, their performance on attention and dexterity tests improves. However, a recent study published in the *Journal of the American Academy of Child and Adolescent Psychology* found that there was a trade-off for the increased alertness. The same children were also more nervous and anxious.

When thirsty teenagers guzzle down caffeinated colas, they also sabotage their calcium reserves, which, over time, may result in poor bone development and osteoporosis later in life. (Turn to Chapter 20 for more on this connection.)

Lots of over-the-counter medications contain caffeine as well. Read labels carefully before administering medications to children, especially to children who are highly active.

Fluids

Children should drink fluids regularly throughout the day — not just a glass of milk or juice with each meal. If not, they could become dehydrated.

Signs of dehydration include dry mouth or skin, dark circles under the eyes, and dark urine. A lack of water begins to affect body function long before these symptoms appear.

In daily meals, include a variety of fluids, starting with water.

- ✔ **Water, fresh, filtered, tap water, or bottled, preferably not iced, which hinders digestion.** Assigning children their very own water bottle and keeping it full of water and within easy reach allows the child to help himself when thirsty.

- ✔ **Herbal tea made with chamomile, peppermint, and other gentle herbs.** As an introduction to the different teas, make a fuss about the special ceremony of brewing. Then serve it hot or chilled, invite the children and their dolls, and have a tea party!

- ✔ **Homemade fresh vegetable juices.** Vegetable juice is preferable to fruit juice, which supplies large amounts of sugar. Better to have whole fruit. If you do give fruit juice, dilute it with water.

- ✔ **Soups with a child's favorite noodles.** These soups provide both liquid and carbohydrates. Instead of canned soups, which are very high in sodium, make your own or search out brands that have a lower salt content.

- ✔ **Milk, which provides calcium and vitamin D, nutrients necessary for growing bones.** If you choose not to give your child milk, be sure that she gets good sources of calcium elsewhere, such as in green, leafy vegetables, beans, nuts, and blackstrap molasses. A quarter hour in the sun every day provides sufficient vitamin D, but it isn't always possible to do that. Food sources include mushrooms, fish, egg yolks, and liver.

- ✔ **Avoid sodas and packaged drinks.** Caffeine is not recommended. (See the sidebar "Kids on caffeine.") Sodas are also loaded with sugar, which causes tooth decay and leads to weight gain.

Fast food

Hopefully if you're feeding your child real food at home, the fast food now offered in schools and everywhere in town won't be quite so appealing. Although you can't control every move your child makes, explaining the consequences of eating fast food in terms of what's important to them — for example, feeling energized rather than sluggish, looking fit rather than overweight, or having nice-looking skin rather than breaking out in zits! — may have some impact.

Sugar and behavior

Some children are sensitive to sugar and experience a drop in blood glucose a couple hours after downing two or three sugary colas or eating a fistful of candy. This can happen especially if they eat these foods on an empty stomach. With the drop in blood sugar, adrenaline levels rise, potentially triggering a range of symptoms. A child may become shaky, weak, and headachy and experience a pounding heart. A child's thinking process can slow down, and he may have trouble concentrating. If these problems trouble your child, monitor what your child eats and, when an episode occurs, check whether your child had sugar in the hours just before. You may find a link between sugar intake and these problems.

Another good reason to keep your child off sugar is that the more sugar he eats, the less protein, carbohydrates, vitamins, calcium, and other minerals he consumes. By filling up on high-sugar treats, he loses his appetite for the good stuff.

Sweets

Get children started on naturally sweet foods such as sweet potatoes and all sorts of fruit. Use these foods to replace cookies and sugary toaster tarts. If you're making a dessert, cook with sugars that also provide some degree of nutrition such as maple syrup and blackstrap molasses.

For a healthy dessert, concoct a fruit cobbler with whole grains, nuts, and seeds. The protein and fat in these ingredients slows the absorption of the fruit in the sugar and helps keep blood sugar levels steady. Having a small serving of this sort of dessert can be considered a little meal.

Apple and Almond Cobbler

This cobbler is health food that looks and tastes like dessert. If you want something sweet for breakfast, have some of this nutritious dish instead of donuts or a Danish.

Preparation time: 15 minutes

Cooking time: 45 minutes to 1 hour

Yield: 9 servings

(continued)

¾ cup ground almonds

6 tablespoons ground sunflower seeds

¾ cup whole-wheat pastry flour

2 teaspoons cinnamon

⅜ teaspoon cloves

¾ teaspoon ginger

¼ teaspoon salt

1 tablespoon unrefined safflower oil

3 tablespoons maple syrup, plus ½ cup

5 apples, preferably organic, cored and sliced, or fruit of choice

¼ cup arrowroot

1 teaspoon vanilla extract

2 tablespoons blackstrap molasses (optional)*

½ cup water

1 Preheat oven to 350°. Using a food processor fitted with a blade, grind almonds and sunflower seeds.

2 In a medium bowl, mix the whole-wheat pastry flour with the nut and seed mixture, cinnamon, cloves, ginger, and salt. Drizzle with oil and 3 tablespoons maple syrup and toss until evenly distributed. Set aside.

3 In a large saucepan and using a wooden spoon, mix together the sliced apples and the arrowroot until the fruit is coated. Stir in the vanilla, remaining ½ cup maple syrup, blackstrap molasses, and water.

4 Cook the apple mixture over medium heat, stirring constantly, until it comes to a boil. Continue boiling for 30 seconds. Pour into an oiled 9-inch baking pan.

5 Using your fingers, crumble topping and sprinkle it over the fruit. Bake cobbler until topping is golden and fruit is cooked, about 35 to 40 minutes.

*Adding a bit of nutrient-packed blackstrap molasses here and there to the foods you are cooking is an excellent way to increase your intake of minerals, including calcium, iron, and potassium.

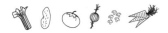

Childhood Obesity

Obesity in children has risen dramatically in the past several decades and is reaching epidemic proportions. Twenty-five to 30 percent of children in the United States are affected by obesity, but researchers believe that is a low estimate. A child is considered obese if he weighs 20 percent more than the expected norm, based on age, sex, height, and body build.

Hormonal and genetic causes are rare. Consumption of junk foods, convenience foods, and an overabundance of simple carbohydrates is usually the cause. Exercise is also a very important factor. Exercise also reduces appetite and increases the metabolism so more calories burn faster.

Weight gain left unchecked in children can lead to heart disease and diabetes at an early age. Sadly, more than 600,000 of America's children are diagnosed with some form of heart disease. Obesity has tripled the incidence of type 2 diabetes among children. This is the type of diabetes that typically afflicts middle-age adults and can result in poor circulation, kidney failure, and even blindness.

One surefire way to help most kids attain optimum weight is to feed them only high-fiber whole grains, fresh fruits and vegetables, and smaller portions of animal protein. Other tips include

- Drink ample filtered water appropriate to a child's body size. It fills up the tummy, is good for eliminating toxins, and is great for overall body chemistry.

- Eat lean beef or fish and the white meat of turkey and chicken.

- Steam vegetables or eat them raw.

- Avoid all processed or refined foods, including canned and boxed foods, fast foods, and sweets.

- Forget about desserts unless it comes in the form of fresh fruits.

- Eat slowly and chew food well. Make up games with kids to help them count the number of times they chew before swallowing.

- Reduce the intake of fatty foods, but don't try to eliminate all fat. A moderate amount of healthy fats do belong in the diet.

- Avoid diet sodas and sugar substitutes. Instead, turn to fresh fruit to satisfy sweet cravings and experiment with herbal teas. Artificial sweeteners can cause side effects such as headaches, dizziness, and nausea.

- Neither young people nor adults should go on a very restricted calorie diet for longer than about a week. After two weeks of calorie restriction, the rate at which calories are burned slows down, making it more difficulty to lose weight. This slowdown continues for about six months, even though food intake returns to normal. For this reason, most people who go on crash diets are actually heavier one year later.

Shape up your own diet. Eating habits within the family can also be a deciding factor on whether or not a child becomes obese.

One way to cut back on calories while providing children with the protein they need is to use more lowfat sources of protein, such as turkey and beans. You guessed it — turkey chili!

White Chili

You can make this turkey chili just as tasty as the red meat and tomatoes version. Adults will like it garnished with chopped cilantro, chunks of avocado, and a wedge of lime.

Preparation time: *20 minutes*

Cooking time: *1 hour, 45 minutes*

Yield: *6 to 8 servings*

3 cups Great Northern beans, washed, picked over, and soaked overnight

Filtered water

1 whole onion, unpeeled, plus 1 small onion, finely chopped

Salt and freshly ground black pepper to taste

2 tablespoon extra-virgin olive oil

1½ pounds ground turkey meat, half light meat and half dark meat

1 tablespoon chili powder

3 cups chicken stock

3 large cloves garlic, minced

2 fresh or dried chilies, stem and seeds removed, and minced

2 teaspoon ground cumin

1 teaspoon dried oregano

1 Place the soaked beans in a large pot and cover with filtered water. On high, bring to a boil, skimming off the foam. Add the whole onion. Lower the heat, cover loosely, and simmer the beans.

2 Continue cooking, stirring occasionally, until the beans are tender but the skins are still intact, about 1 hour, 30 minutes. When the beans are somewhat soft, add the salt and pepper. If necessary, add additional water.

3 In the meantime, put the oil in a large skillet and cook the turkey over medium heat, stirring occasionally, until meat is no longer pink. Season with the chili powder and salt and pepper. Set aside.

4 Drain the liquid from the pot of cooked beans and discard the onion. Place 2 cups beans in a food processor and puree. Return pureed beans to pot with the whole beans.

5 Add the cooked turkey, chicken stock, garlic, chilies, cumin, and oregano to the beans and stir. Over medium heat, bring the chili to boil. Cover and reduce heat to low.

6 Cook the chili, stirring occasionally, until the beans are very tender and the flavors have mellowed, about 15 minutes. Adjust seasoning.

7 Spoon the chili into individual serving bowls and serve with Wild Western Corn Bread (see the recipe later in this chapter).

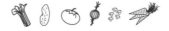

Unfortunately, when kids reach for a sweet snack, most likely it will also be high in poor quality fats. Studies show that children who are given healthy foods (fruits, vegetables, and yogurt) for snacks instead of the high-fat, super-sweet, nonnutritious ones are perfectly happy with the good stuff. Infants and babies adore the taste of fresh fruit, yogurt, applesauce, frozen juice pops, and other nutritious foods. Start children with these healthful foods as treats, and although they might ask for the empty-calorie treats, they will still associate good foods with a positive feeling and gratification.

For snacks, give your child crunchy raw vegetables with yogurt dip, popcorn, a piece of melon, a wedge of baked apple, or a piece of this corn bread.

Wild Western Corn Bread

If you're russlin' up some grub for the little ones, try this recipe for corn bread, with the added kick of chilies and cheese. One piece is a substantial minimeal, supplying complex carbohydrates, protein, and some fat to steady blood sugar levels and moods. It tastes great with White Chili (see preceding recipe), and leftovers make a nutritious midafternoon snack.

Preparation time: *15 minutes*

Cooking time: *25 minutes*

Yield: *8 generous servings*

1 cup yellow corn meal	*2 cups fresh corn kernels, cooked*
¾ cup whole-grain pastry flour	*1 cup buttermilk*
2 teaspoons baking powder, aluminumfree	*2 tablespoons organic, unsalted butter, melted*
1 teaspoon baking soda	*½ cup grated extra-sharp cheddar cheese*
½ teaspoon salt	*2 small green serrano chilies, seeded and chopped*
2 whole eggs	
1 egg white	

1 Preheat oven to 350°. In a large bowl, combine the corn meal, pastry flour, baking powder, baking soda, and salt.

2 In a medium bowl, beat together the eggs and egg white. Add the corn, buttermilk, butter, cheese, and chilies and stir. Stir this mixture into the corn meal mixture until just combined.

3 Butter a 9-inch-square baking pan and turn the batter into the pan and spread evenly. Bake the corn mixture until a toothpick inserted into the center of the bread comes out clean, about 25 minutes.

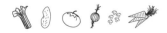

For information on diabetes, see *Diabetes For Dummies,* by Alan L. Rubin, M.D. (IDG Books Worldwide, Inc.).

Common Childhood Ailments

Common garden-variety ailments of childhood respond well to proper nourishment. I cover dietary recommendations for colds, bronchitis, and digestive problems in the sections on respiratory and digestive complaints in Chapter 20. I also give dietary advice for all these conditions in Appendix A. In addition, here are some special tips on treating these conditions in ailing children.

- ✔ **Acne:** Make sure that teenagers, especially boys who are more prone to this skin problem, stay away from all junk food. Keeping the face clean, with hypoallergenic soaps, is also very important.

- ✔ **Anemia:** Give teenage girls, who are menstruating and thereby losing some iron each month, iron-rich foods such as red meat, liver, figs, apricots, and blackstrap molasses. And explain that caffeinated soda, because of the caffeine, is a diuretic, triggering urination, which results in the loss of iron.

- ✔ **Bronchitis:** If your child has bronchitis, be rigorous about eliminating from your child's meals all foods that are mucus-forming, which includes sweets you may be tempted to give your child as a treat and fried foods.

- ✔ **Canker sores:** When your child has these painful ulcers on the surface of the mouth, cheek, or tongue, don't feed him sugar, citrus and citrus juice, or crunchy foods that can irritate the ulcer and cause pain.

- ✔ **Colds:** Putting a child on a regimen of drinking fruit juice, such as orange juice, all day long is not a good idea. Give them whole fruit instead and use water and herbal teas as a source of needed fluids. Avoid milk and all dairy products, including cheese, yogurt, and ice cream. Milk inhibits the normal release of secretions that water down mucus and make it easier to excrete.

- ✔ **Constipation:** Feed children a piece of fruit about an hour before and an hour after meals. Meals should consist of high-fiber foods such as vegetables and whole grains. Celery, wheat bran, pinto beans, and green leafy vegetables are good choices.

- ✔ **Diarrhea:** If a child has diarrhea for a day or two, be especially sure to avoid dehydration by giving your child filtered water, broth, fruit and vegetable juices, and teas. These also provide minerals as do electrolyte-packed drinks made especially for kids to help avoid dangerous mineral imbalances within the system.

If your child has chronic diarrhea, bloating, or abdominal discomfort, dairy foods may be the cause. By the time children are 7 years old, they may begin to lack the enzyme needed to digest milk. A lactose challenge test can determine whether this is the cause of the diarrhea. Lactose intolerance is especially seen among Asians and black children.

A potassium broth is a wonderful antidote for diarrhea, replacing lost minerals. Put a cup each of parsley, potatoes, beets with their tops, celery, carrots, and kale in a large pot of salted, filtered water. Simmer, covered, over low heat, all day, adding more water if needed. Strain the broth and sip this mineral-rich elixir.

✔ **Motion sickness:** Riding in a car can bring on motion sickness. Symptoms of dizziness, headache, and nausea can last for hours after the ride is over. It's best to prevent motion sickness because arresting it is more difficult. Some trial and error is necessary. You'll have to decide whether your kids travel better on a full or empty stomach. Use ginger, a tried-and-true remedy, in the form of tea (see Chapter 20 for Motion Potion recipe), gingersnaps, or ginger candy. Or there are ginger tinctures and capsules. Feed ginger to your child before and during the trip. Ginger ale doesn't work because real ginger isn't usually in it. Health-food stores are the best place to shop for authentic ginger products.

If you do give your child something to eat, stay away from greasy or fried foods that are more likely to upset the stomach.

Special Problems

Eating disorders, autism, and attention deficit hyperactivity disorder (ADHD) are medical problems that have a psychological and behavioral component. Developing healthy eating habits can play a role in lessening symptoms and helping a child to heal.

Eating disorders

In the United States, seven million people age 15 to 35 have an eating disorder. Most people who have eating disorders feel a loss of control over their lives and try to make up for it by controlling what and how they eat. Low self-esteem and a distorted body image are also usually involved.

One form of eating disorder is anorexia, which is characterized by severe dieting and excessive exercise. Girls who starve themselves and weigh 15 percent less than the expected norm for their height are defined as having an eating disorder. Girls with anorexia often cut their food into tiny pieces before eating what little they consume. They typically become hyperactive and hypothermic and cease having periods. Parents should pay close attention to a dieting daughter's physique, especially if she dresses in baggy clothes.

Bulimia also involves diet and exercising excessively, but rather than eating miniscule amounts of food, a bulimic goes through binges of eating huge amounts of food and then either induces vomiting or takes diuretics to eliminate the food.

Girls can become so malnourished that they need to be hospitalized. Many can die if their conditions go undetected. Contact a health-care professional immediately if you suspect your child is suffering from one of these disorders.

Attention deficit hyperactivity disorder

Attention deficit hyperactivity disorder (ADHD) is a behavior disorder whose diagnosis is based on a child having symptoms of inattention, hyperactivity, and impulsiveness to such an extent that the child has difficulty functioning. These kids simply cannot sit still long enough or pay attention long enough to learn what they need to know in school. Approximately 3 to 5 percent of children in the United States are diagnosed with ADHD, and the problem is more common in boys than girls.

Some physicians are concerned that not only is the diagnosis being applied too freely, but that drugs such as Ritalin are being prescribed too liberally while treatments such as diet are being overlooked.

Substances that worsen ADHD symptoms

Evidence continues to accumulate that additives in food can aggravate hyperactivity. The Feingold Diet, developed by the late Benjamin Feingold, M.D., eliminates all foods that contain artificial food colors, flavors, and preservatives. This diet is effective in treating symptoms in about 30 percent of patients with ADHD. Other substances in food, including sugar, chocolate, caffeine, and the flavor enhancer monosodium glutamate (MSG), can also trigger symptoms. The kind of whole foods eating recommended in this book contains none of these.

Foods that can provoke an allergic response may bring on an episode of hyperactivity, anger, and confusion. Notice whether your child's behavior changes after eating apples, oranges, grapes, wheat, corn, oats, eggs, tomatoes, peanuts, soy products, or fish.

In addition, foods that contain *salicylates,* a chemical found in a very wide range of natural foods and food products, can exacerbate ADHD in some individuals. Foods that contain salicylates include many fruits, such as apricots, berries, raisins, and prunes, as well as cucumbers, tomatoes, processed meats, and such items as self-basting turkey and fish sticks.

Children should be given an elimination diet as it is critical to determine which foods adversely affect each individual child.

Recommended foods

The best diet for ADHD kids includes the following foods:

- Natural cereals free of additives and artificial colorings
- Homemade baked goods
- Wheatless bread
- Poultry, meats, and fresh fish that do not contain salicylates
- Plain yogurt with fresh fruit
- Grapefruit and pineapple juice
- Milk
- Natural white cheese

A recent study showed improved behavior in children taking magnesium supplements. Green vegetables are an excellent source of this mineral.

Chapter 20

Food Remedies for Common Problems

In This Chapter

▶ Treating respiratory problems

▶ Maintaining good digestion

▶ Dealing with kidney-related problems

▶ Steadying blood sugar

▶ Dealing with food sensitivities

▶ Helping prevent arthritis and osteoporosis

▶ Managing stress to bolster immunity

In this chapter, I tell you how to treat a number of ailments, including colds and flu, sore throat, bronchitis, hay fever, asthma, indigestion, ulcers, fluid retention, urinary tract infection, low blood sugar, food allergy/sensitivity, arthritis and joint ailments, osteoporosis, skin conditions, and stress.

Treating Colds and Flu

When you come down with a cold or have the flu, your respiratory system has become infected, usually with a virus. Your immune system response to the infection triggers inflammation of the air passageways and the production of mucus. With a cold, you may have chest congestion, a stuffy nose, painful sinuses, and a sore throat. Flu symptoms are more severe and varied, but can include aches, pains, and fever.

Certain foods, herbs, and spices can help prevent these ailments and speed your recovery. Their primary function is to strengthen your own immune system so that it can effectively do its job of healing. With an adequately functioning immune system, a cold should not last longer than two to three days.

Drinking plenty of fluids

Breathing through your mouth, which happens when you have a stuffy nose, dehydrates mucus membranes. A virus thrives in such an environment. When you are down with a cold or flu, drink eight glasses of liquid throughout the day and evening. Mostly drink filtered water. If you do crave fruit juice, drink it in a highly diluted form. Better yet, enjoy juicy whole fruit such as melons.

When a fluid is hot, it is even more effective in inhibiting viruses. Enjoy soothing broths made from fresh and substantial ingredients, such as root vegetables, beef bones, and pieces of chicken. Mint and other herbal teas are also good choices.

One of the body's defenses against a virus is fever. For this reason, you should not try to suppress it unless it is over 102°F. If you start out with a normal temperature that rises above this mark, you need to deal with your fever more vigorously. Fever causes sweating, so you need to drink plenty of water to replace fluids you lose in perspiration.

Foods with medicinal properties

Food may have a more subtle effect than medication, but can be an effective treatment tool when used to arrest a cold or the flu at the first sign of symptoms.

- **Garlic** has both antibacterial and antiviral properties and is a potent immune enhancer. If you feel like you're coming down with something, cut one or two cloves of raw garlic into bite-size pieces and swallow like pills.

- **Onions** fight bacteria and viruses. In addition, onions trigger the release of fluids that dilute mucus so that it can move through the lungs and into the throat from where it can be coughed up. While raw onions are the most beneficial, cooked onions are also therapeutic. Half an onion a day is considered an ample dose.

- **Watercress** helps clear up phlegm and is high in healing minerals.

- **Sea vegetables, or seaweed,** supply abundant minerals, which support the healing process. Add these to a cucumber salad or miso soup.

The medicinal herbs echinacea and goldenseal, which you can take as teas, provide powerful immune function support.

If you feel under the weather, treat yourself to a medicinal cup of garlic soup.

Sopa de Ajo

Sopa de Ajo, garlic soup, is a classic dish of Spain. Made with chicken broth, it becomes a delicious remedy for colds, as garlic has therapeutic properties. If you want an even more potent brew, add some hot chilies. These also help clear congestion.

Preparation time: *5 minutes*

Cooking time: *5 minutes*

Yield: *2 servings*

3 cloves garlic   *2 cups organic chicken broth, fresh-made or canned*

1 With the side of a broad knife, and using a cutting board, firmly press down on each garlic clove and crush to release juices. Mince garlic. Transfer garlic to a small plate and let rest 15 minutes, to develop its therapeutic properties.

2 Heat the chicken broth in a small saucepan. Add the minced garlic and cook, covered, over medium heat for 5 minutes. Pour into a mug or oversized coffee cup and quietly sip. (Spooning it from a soup bowl is too much work.)

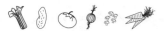

Foods high in nutrients that fight infection

Vitamin A, or beta-carotene, vitamin C, and zinc support your natural immune response. Let the following foods inspire your menus. Have a little meal of baked acorn squash along with mushrooms on toast. Make some hummus with chickpeas (see Chapter 24 for Chickpeas in Disguise). Nibble on cashews. Have a cup of rose hips tea.

- ✔ **Vitamin A:** Sweet potatoes, carrots, winter squash, cantaloupe, and greens
- ✔ **Vitamin C:** Sweet peppers, broccoli, papayas, kiwis, rose hips, and mangoes
- ✔ **Zinc:** Oysters, pork, beef, pumpkin seeds, chickpeas, cashews, oysters, and mushrooms. Beef liver is also loaded with vitamin A, selenium, and zinc, but only eat organic liver.

Warming condiments for congestion

When you have congestion, use these flavorings in your cooking to benefit from their medicinal powers.

- ✓ **Chili peppers stimulate circulation and thin mucus.** This reduces congestion and can relieve headaches that sometimes can occur along with colds and flu. Cayenne is made from chili peppers. If you have chest congestion, put a pinch of cayenne in a cup of hot water and sip away. Tightness in the chest will seem to melt away.

- ✓ **Ginger also helps to clear up mucus and makes it easier to cough up.** Enjoy Motion Potion, later in this chapter, or add an ounce of powdered ginger to a bathtub filled with very warm water and soak in it. The ginger will help you to perspire and eliminate toxins. After your bath, wrap up in a warm robe, crawl into bed, and have a deep and restoring sleep.

- ✓ **Fennel seeds are warming and have a relaxing effect.** If you have a dry cough, munch on some crushed fennel seeds. You can also buy fennel tea.

Fruit can be a cooling and soothing food when you have a cold and congestion. Spike it with pepper for an added benefit.

Tropical Tamer for Congestion

In this recipe, mineral-rich melons and tropical fruit are seasoned with cayenne. The mix of ingredients in this recipe is inspired by the fruit snacks I sometimes buy in Los Angeles from street vendors who are from Central America.

Preparation time: *10 minutes*

Cooking time: *None*

Yield: *4 servings*

2 cups melon chunks (cantaloupe, crenshaw, honeydew, watermelon, or a mixture).

1 mango, peeled, sliced, and cut into chunks

1 papaya, halved, seeds removed, and cut into chunks

Juice of 1 small lime

½ teaspoon cayenne pepper

1 In a serving bowl, put the melon, mango, and papaya and combine.

2 Distribute the mixed fruit in 4 individual serving bowls.

3 Top each serving of fruit with a squeeze of lime juice and a sprinkling of cayenne. Take a rest and enjoy this juicy little meal.

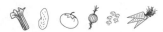

Foods that increase congestion

Various common foods promote the accumulation of viscous phlegm. To reduce mucus, cut back on your intake or eliminate sugar, eggs, potatoes, and turnips. Grains also increase mucus, especially those high in gluten, such as wheat, barley, oats, and rye. Also cut out milk and diary products. Milk inhibits the normal release of secretions that water down mucus and make it easier to excrete. In addition, many people report that once they stop eating dairy foods, their sinus conditions greatly improve.

Dealing with a Sore Throat

If you have a sore throat, gargling with warm salt water is an instant, although short-lived, cure. To keep a sore throat at bay, eat lightly and keep meals vegetarian. Have fresh vegetables, tropical fruit such as mangoes and papayas, whole grains, legumes, and other mineral-rich foods. Zinc is especially beneficial. Sucking on zinc lozenges has proven to be an effective therapy.

A time-honored remedy for a sore throat is to have a cup of tea sweetened with honey, which has antibacterial properties, especially if it's raw honey. Honey is used to soothe and coat throat tissue. This may help you feel better in the short term, but having a lot of honey can actually make your sore throat worse. A better choice is unsweetened tea made with slippery elm bark, and try some licorice tea, which can relieve pain.

For nutrition information for cold sores, take a look at Appendix A.

Warding off Bronchitis and Sinusitis

A cold can develop into *bronchitis,* an infection in the tubes leading to the lungs, or *sinusitis,* in which the sinuses at the sides of the nose and around the eyes become infected. In bronchitis, the trachea and large *bronchi,* passageways to the lungs, become inflamed. This ailment can be caused by bacterial or viral sources or provoked by a reaction to allergens in the environment. Symptoms include coughing, chills, fever, and fatigue. The cough may become a hack. Bronchitis can even develop into pneumonia.

Many of the same foods, drink, herbs, vitamins, and minerals good for treating colds and flu benefit bronchitis and sinusitis. The diet should support the immune system and stimulate drainage of congested areas. A good expectorant is comfrey. Ginger tea also helps the body cough up phlegm.

Coping with Hay Fever and Asthma

Both hay fever and asthma are allergic disorders. *Hay fever* is seasonal, caused by grass and tree pollens that are in the air, while *asthma* is an ongoing condition with recurrent attacks. To counteract symptoms, increase your intake of garlic and onions, which are anti-inflammatory, horseradish, cloves, cinnamon, ginger, rosemary, and thyme to help clear sinuses. Avoid red meats and mucus-forming foods and increase your intake of vitamin C and omega-3 fatty acids, which counteract inflammation.

A folk remedy for hay fever is honey from local hives, which contains pollen from plants that may be triggering your symptoms. Eating honey may act like an allergy shot. Be sure to use honeycomb or unfiltered, cold-pressed regular honey.

Asthma can be brought on by an allergic reaction to food, eating certain food additives — the preservatives sulphur dioxide and benzoate, and the dye tartrazine — and, in some cases, low stomach acid. Common food allergens that cause an immediate asthmatic reaction are (in decreasing order of frequency) eggs, fish, shellfish, nuts, and peanuts. Milk, chocolate, wheat, citrus, and food colorings usually cause a delayed reaction. (Also see the section "Food Sensitivity and Allergy," later in this chapter.) Treating asthma with diet may require the elimination of all animal foods, as well as supplementation with vitamins and minerals, in particular, magnesium. Increase magnesium-rich foods, including green vegetables. A traditional remedy for asthma is licorice, a powerful anti-inflammatory, which you can drink as tea.

Black and green tea contain theophylline, which dilates the bronchial passageways that become constricted in an asthmatic attack. Use tea in concentrated form to counteract an attack.

Dealing with Indigestion

You are not what you eat. You are what you digest and absorb. For you to be well nourished, your digestive system must be able to break down food so that it can pass through the intestinal walls, enter the bloodstream, and eventually feed the cells. If the digestive function is impaired, you may be receiving sufficient calories but not nutrients. Symptoms such as bloating, gas, abdominal pain, a burning sensation, and nausea can occur.

For good digestion, you need adequate digestive juices and enzymes. Individuals, as they age, may produce insufficient stomach acid and need to take hydrochloric acid supplements. Many people also take enzyme supplements to aid in the digestion of carbohydrates, proteins, and fat.

To stop indigestion, antacids are not the answer. Here are better ways to prevent indigestion (and, yes, they include some things your mother told you).

✓ Chew your food well, but not with your mouth open. Don't talk while you're chewing.

✓ Slow down. Dine. Don't gulp.

✓ Eat smaller meals.

✓ Don't drink a lot of fluids with meals.

✓ Add foods to your meals that are also digestive aids, such as celery, asparagus, parsley, horseradish, oats, fennel, ginger, and cinnamon.

✓ Limit your intake of high-protein foods, such as meat and dairy products, which increase the amount of acid the stomach produces. Avoid hard-to-digest fatty foods.

✓ For dessert, have fresh papaya and pineapple, which contain food-digesting enzymes. (You can also supplement with digestive enzymes, specifically amylase, protease, and lipase.)

✓ Finish your meal with peppermint tea to relax tense muscles in the stomach and intestines.

Taking antibiotics can kill off the friendly bacteria in your gut and cause intestinal upset. Active bacteria yogurt can remedy this because it replenishes the beneficial bacteria. But don't take the yogurt with the antibiotic. Wait two hours so that the antibiotic and yogurt don't combine in your stomach. Milk products, including yogurt, inactivate most antibiotics.

Nausea and vomiting can result from eating rich food, drinking too much alcohol, and having the flu, and experiencing motion sickness and morning sickness.

Try these tips to settle your stomach.

✓ Ginger calms nausea. The crystallized chunks of ginger are delicious, or you can drink ginger tea. Peppermint and chamomile teas are also good for settling the stomach.

✓ If nausea results in vomiting, replenishing lost fluids is of first importance. Drink herbal teas and sip these slowly to treat your stomach gently. If the body asks for salt, be sure to have some to replace minerals that are lost along with the fluids. A salty broth may taste good. Fluids are especially important for babies and young children, who can quickly become dehydrated.

Fruit juice, especially orange and grapefruit juice, is highly acidic and can irritate the stomach. Coffee and black tea too are highly acid.

✓ When you feel like eating again, begin with easily digestible foods, such as bananas, rice, and dry toast.

✔ When nausea occurs, supplementing with vitamin B6 can be useful. Treatment with a combination of vitamin K and vitamin C has also been very effective.

If you have nausea and vomiting but you don't know why, immediately seek medical advice to rule out a more serious health condition.

Ginger is given on cruise ships to quell sea sickness, but ginger tea is also a reliable home remedy. It's so tasty, it's good anytime.

Motion Potion

In motion sickness, what the eye sees doesn't jive with the messages the brain is receiving. You suddenly feel dizzy, faint, and sick to your stomach. What you need is a cup of hot ginger tea! If you're drinking the ginger tea to prevent feeling queasy from a car ride or a boat trip, drink the tea as close to departure time as possible and bring some along in a thermos.

Preparation time: *3 minutes*

Cooking time: *12 minutes*

Yield: *2 servings*

1-inch length of ginger root

3 cups filtered water

2 teaspoons raw honey

1 Grate the ginger root and set aside.

2 Boil the water and pour into a large mug. Add the grated ginger root and honey.

3 Cover the top of the mug with a saucer to hold the heat and allow the ginger tea to brew for about 10 minutes. Give yourself a quiet moment and enjoy a cupful.

Easing Diarrhea

Diarrhea has many causes — bacterial and viral infection, parasites, antibiotics, exposure to toxins, food allergy, a deficiency of the enzyme that digests milk, and consuming large quantities of the low-calorie sweeteners mannitol and sorbitol. Because most cases of diarrhea are due to only mild infection or are a reaction to something you've eaten, it's usually best to simply let nature take its course. Diarrhea usually abates after a day or two. However, you do need to drink plenty of fluids, especially diluted vegetable and fruit juices, to restore minerals. You can also have consommé. In the acute phase, no food should be eaten.

When food is resumed, begin with simple foods, such as nutritious soups, stewed fruits, and steamed rice with a little added salt. Have bananas, true comfort food, which replenish potassium, provide fiber, and are easy to digest. Live culture yogurt restores normal intestinal flora. Whole grains and legumes provide bulk. Apples, beets, carrots, and potatoes are also therapeutic.

Handling Constipation

Constipation has no exact definition. Health professionals vary in their opinion of what constitutes the frequency of normal bowel movements. If you're eating a low-fiber diet of processed and refined foods and doing little exercise, you may have only three bowel movements a week. A more natural, high-fiber diet of whole grains, legumes, fresh fruits and vegetables, nuts, and seeds, coupled with regularly exercising, can result in two to three bowel movements a day.

Besides discomfort, constipation is the No. 1 cause of hemorrhoids. Slow passage through the GI tract also increases the body's exposure to potential carcinogens. In addition, bowel bacteria may be related to such conditions as ulcerative colitis and other medical problems. Constipation is also a sign of an unhealthy diet high in refined and processed foods.

Adding fiber to the diet is the primary treatment for constipation. In particular, insoluble fiber such as cellulose passes through the intestine intact, carrying other matter along with it. Cellulose also draws water to it, increasing stool weight and consequently speeding transit time.

To help with constipation:

✔ Eat bran, which contains cellulose. The dosage is 1 to 1½ cups bran a day. The most effective is corn bran, while the least irritating is oat bran. For best results, be sure to drink plenty of water.

✔ Common herbal laxatives include senna, aloe vera, cascara sagrada, and psyllium seed husks. A standard dosage of psyllium is 2 rounded teaspoonfuls in a full glass of water after meals. These herbs should be used as treatments, but not relied upon habitually.

✔ Figs and prunes, like the medicinal herbs, are excellent laxatives. Eating these fruits or drinking prune juice can be therapeutic, but should not be used to compensate for a diet low in fiber.

Coping with Ulcers

Ulcers occur when the tissue lining the digestive tract is damaged by stomach acids and enzymes, and the production of protective mucus is not sufficient. The most common ulcers occur in the stomach *(gastric ulcers)* and in the duodenum in the uppermost portion of the intestines. Ulcers can cause gnawing pain, which occurs 45 minutes to an hour after a meal and during the night.

Spicy foods were once thought to bring on ulcers. In fact, the active ingredient, capsaicin, in chili peppers not only reduces pain, but it stimulates circulation in tissue lining the digestive tract. Another outdated theory is that high-fiber foods are irritating, but little evidence exists that soft-textured diets are actually beneficial. A study published in 1997, in the *Journal of Epidemiology,* found that individuals who had the highest intake of fiber, as compared with those who had the lowest intake, were only about half as likely to develop ulcers.

Milk and milk products were also a standard part of ulcer diets. Now it's known that the calcium and protein in milk and milk products stimulate production of stomach acids. At first, the milk soothes the tender tissue, but then makes the condition worse.

New research has now confirmed that infection with the bacteria *Heliobacter pylori* is the actual cause and can be treated with medication. However, you can still support the health of the tissues in your digestive tract by eating foods that contain vitamin A, vitamin E, and zinc, which help maintain the structure and function of skin tissue. Eating foods such as orange squash, unrefined vegetable oil, and seafood, which contains healing essential fatty acids, can protect against ulcers.

Beer, tobacco, and coffee (whether caffeinated, decaffeinated, or half-caff) can damage tissues lining the GI tract. In addition, a particular food may also cause an allergic reaction, which can lead to the development of an ulcer.

Ironically, taking antacids that contain calcium can promote ulcers. The calcium stimulates acid secretion.

The following foods can help when you're suffering from an ulcer:

- ✔ For effective and quick-acting pain relief, drink fresh, filtered water to dilute stomach acids. This remedy also works for pain due to inflammation of the stomach *(gastritis)* and the intestinal tract *(duodonitis),* as well as heartburn.

- ✔ Raw, fresh-made cabbage juice is an ulcer remedy long in use. One quart a day is recommended. Spring and summer cabbage is the most effective. Mixing the cabbage juice with some celery juice makes it more palatable.

✔ Licorice helps tissues heal and stimulates the secretion of mucus. The average licorice candy is flavored with anise, not licorice. Look for authentic licorice in health-food stores.

✔ New Zealand manuka honey, in studies, has been more effective than antibiotics in doing away with the suspect *Heliobacter pylori* bacteria.

✔ Herbs such as chamomile, goldenseal, sage, aloe vera, and slippery elm soothe and heal ulcerous tissue.

✔ Bananas and plantains, especially green plantains, are a traditional cure for ulcers in many countries. These foods help build tissue that is more resistant to acids by stimulating the production of protective mucus, and the growth of cells to thicken the stomach wall. And did I mention, cooked with garlic, they taste out of this world?

Banana from Havana

Both bananas and plantains, a type of banana, have been used traditionally to help prevent and heal ulcers of the stomach and upper intestine. (Plantains have a squashlike flavor and in South America, Africa, and India are eaten like potatoes.) While scientific results are mixed on whether bananas are actually protective, plantains are clearly proven to be an effective anti-ulcer food. Unripe, green plantains are especially therapeutic. I suggest fully ripe plantains for this recipe, which makes a sweet and garlicky accompaniment for black beans and rice, a classic Caribbean combo!

Preparation time: *5 minutes*

Cooking time: *25 minutes*

Yield: *6 generous servings*

4 ripe plantains	*3 cloves garlic minced*
1 to 2 tablespoon extra-virgin olive oil	

1 Preheat oven to 375°.

2 Peel the plantains and cut each lengthwise and then in half crosswise. Arrange in 1 layer in a baking dish.

3 Drizzle with olive oil and evenly distribute minced garlic.

4 Bake in oven until golden, about 25 minutes.

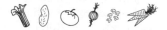

Reducing Fluid Retention

The kidneys and the large bowel normally regulate how much fluid is retained in the body or excreted. However, this balance can be disturbed and can be related to such conditions as PMS, heart disease, diabetes, enlarged prostate, and even food allergy.

The first step in treating fluid retention, or *edema,* is usually to restrict sodium intake. Sodium draws water to it. When your tissues contain a high level of sodium, they more readily retain fluid. The minimum amount of sodium you need for health is 500 mg a day, equivalent to ¼ teaspoon salt. (The average adult consumes just under 2 to 3 teaspoonfuls.) And here's a seeming contradiction: You also need to drink sufficient water, which stimulates the kidneys and promotes urination. Another way to treat edema is to increase your intake of potassium. Your kidneys require this mineral in order to excrete excess sodium and fluid.

Excellent sources of potassium include bananas, potatoes, all green leafy vegetables, artichokes, avocado, celery, parsley, dried fruit, oranges, meats, unsalted nuts, sunflower seeds, blackstrap molasses, mint leaves, and garlic. Before you turn to a medication to reduce fluid retention, try eating foods that do the same thing.

You can also treat edema by eating foods that function as diuretics, such as parsley in particular, as well as celery, onion, garlic, lemons, eggplant, endive, and cucumbers. An herbal diuretic is dandelion. If your lawn harbors dandelion, harvest the pale green inner leaves, which have a slightly bitter, tangy flavor. Add to salad greens or use the leaves to make some dandelion tea.

If you suffer from fluid retention but the cause has not been identified, your edema may be a symptom of food allergy. Notice whether you develop edema six to eight hours after eating a particular food and whether it subsides in a day. Likely allergens are wheat, milk, eggs, corn, coffee, tea, alcohol, yeast, citrus, and sugar.

Urinary Tract Infection

Urinary tract infection (UTI) most commonly involves the bladder, which becomes infected, a condition known as *cystitis.* Bacteria, which typically originate in fecal contamination or vaginal secretions, can ascend the urinary tract. The danger is that the infection will eventually extend into the kidneys at the top of the urinary tract. Urination becomes painful.

UTI is very common in women and can occur at least once every year. If infection continues, in more than half of cases, the problem will eventually involve the kidneys. In men, UTI is relatively rare.

Normally ample and free-flowing urine flushes the urinary tract, and the immune system fights off any potential infection — which means, when you have to go, you should go!

And when problems do occur, food and herbs can be used for treatment. The effectiveness of drinking cranberry juice, a well-known home remedy for cystitis, has been confirmed by science. Drinking cranberry juice can cut your rate of infection by nearly half and also greatly reduce your risk of reinfection. Blueberries work in the same way.

Cranberry's usefulness in treating cystitis was long thought to be due to its acid content. But according to new research, cranberries contain a compound that covers the lining of the bladder and urethra. This prevents bacteria from adhering and multiplying. This also allows bacteria to be more easily flushed from the system and the cystitis cured.

Almost all commercial cranberry juice is sold diluted with very sugary water. Although this cuts the tartness of the berries, sugar also weakens immunity and may slow the healing process.

Buy 100 percent cranberry juice concentrate at a natural-food store and dilute it yourself with filtered water.

Enjoy blueberries for breakfast, fresh and raw, or turned into a sauce for pancakes and waffles.

Fruity Flavonoid Syrup

Enjoy naturally sweet blueberries as a tonic for cystitis and benefit from their flavonoid content as well. Make a quick blueberry sauce and spoon over ready-made waffles.

Preparation time: 5 minutes

Cooking time: 15 minutes

Yield: 4 servings

1 pint (2 cups) fresh, sweet blueberries, rinsed and sorted

¼ filtered water, plus 2 tablespoons

1 tablespoon cornstarch

½ teaspoon grated lemon zest, preferably organic

4 Van's whole-grain frozen waffles

(continued)

1 In a small saucepan, put the blueberries and ¼ cup water and cook, covered, on medium heat until berries begin to soften, about 3 minutes.

2 Mix together the cornstarch and 2 tablespoons water in a small bowl. Add to blueberries. Continue cooking berries over medium-low heat until the mixture thickens, an additional 2 or 3 minutes. Remove from heat.

3 Stir in the lemon zest. Let sauce stand for at least 5 minutes.

4 In the meantime, toast the waffles and place on individual warmed serving plates. Pour sauce over waffles and serve immediately.

 In addition to cranberries and blueberries, the following foods and herbs help speed recovery from UTI:

- Garlic is known to fight types of bacteria that are associated with UTI.

- Parsley, celery root, and other foods that function as diuretics help flush infection from the urinary tract.

Steadying Blood Sugar

One of the most vital functions your body performs is keeping steady the level of *glucose,* a form of sugar, in your blood. Your brain is fueled by glucose, and having a steady supply is critical. When you eat, the food you absorb is metabolized, and the sugars make their way into your bloodstream. In particular, the simple sugars in candy rapidly enter your system and elevate your blood glucose levels. This sugar is quickly used for energy, stored, or turned into fat. As it is removed from the bloodstream, your blood glucose level drops.

If this decline occurs suddenly, symptoms can include anxiety, an increased heart rate, sweating, tremors, and hunger. If your blood sugar gradually declines, another group of symptoms occurs as the brain is starved for fuel. You may develop a headache, cloudy vision, dizziness, dulled thinking, confusion, or emotional highs and lows.

While hypoglycemia can be secondary to very serious health conditions such as tumors, the type most people describe is the low blood sugar that they experience some time after eating, from 1.5 to 5 hours later. This can occur especially if the meal is high in sweets and refined starches. And being under stress or suffering from alcoholism can increase sensitivity to sugar.

Eating for hypoglycemia

Whether or not you have been diagnosed with hypoglycemia or simply suffer from a tendency to have low blood sugar, these eating guidelines can help you keep your blood sugar on an even keel.

- ✔ Avoid sugar and concentrated sweets. These include jam, jelly, colas, all sweet desserts, dried fruit, fruit juice, and such concoctions as the sugar sauce on sweet and sour spare ribs.

- ✔ Substitute whole grains and whole-grain flour for refined grain and flour.

- ✔ Eat small meals and eat more frequently, every two to three hours.

- ✔ In each meal and snack, include a source of complex carbohydrates, protein, and fat. If you eat an apple, have a little cheese along with it.

- ✔ Snack on foods that supply some protein and fat. Munch on almonds.

- ✔ Eat foods high in vitamin C, because hypoglycemia interferes with the vitamin's metabolism.

Special nutrients for hypoglycemia

Both chromium and manganese play an important role in the metabolism of glucose. People with hypoglycemia are also often deficient in zinc. These minerals are present in many common foods.

- ✔ **Chromium:** Mushrooms, beets, asparagus, seaweed, potatoes, broccoli, prunes, grapes, whole wheat, brown rice, whole oats, bulgur wheat, clams, beef, turkey, and maple syrup

- ✔ **Manganese:** Lima beans, chickpeas, soybeans, navy beans, collards, okra, peas, pineapple, bananas, whole wheat, brown rice, buckwheat, Brazil nuts, hazelnuts, sunflower and pumpkin seeds, bass, and trout

- ✔ **Zinc:** Oysters and other seafood, egg yolks, lamb chops, liver, lima beans, mushrooms, and sunflower seeds

For more on handling hypoglycemia, as well as information on diabetes, check out *Diabetes For Dummies* by Alan L. Rubin, M.D. (IDG Books Worldwide, Inc.). Also take a look at Appendix A in this book.

An unusual food that helps lower elevated blood sugar is *nopales,* a form of cactus (the taste is similar to string beans). In studies, nopales has been shown to lower elevated blood glucose associated with diabetes. Nopales is sold fresh in markets in the Southwest and is widely available canned.

Food Sensitivity and Allergy

The definition and differences between food allergy, sensitivity, and intolerance is not generally agreed upon. The causes are many as are the symptoms, and it's a matter of degree. Something in food — a protein, the gluten in starch, additives such as food coloring, or sulfites — can trigger a response. The immune system may or may not be involved, but when it is, the food is treated as a dangerous invader as if it were bacteria or a virus.

Inflammation and congestion can develop as part of the healing process. Other symptoms, depending upon what area of the body becomes involved, can be as diverse as asthma, hives, arthritis, malabsorption, headaches, difficulty thinking, memory loss, and childhood hyperactivity. As much as 60 percent of the American population experiences symptoms caused by a reaction to food.

The great majority of food sensitivities occur because a food is eaten too frequently. Common foods are common allergens. You'll probably never become allergic to caviar, but you may have a problem with wheat. Eating a wide variety of food is the best defense against developing a food allergy. Possible food sensitivities include

- **Grain and grain fractions that contain gluten:** Wheat, rye, oats, and barley

- **Foods that contain sulfites:** Dried fruit that is brightly colored because it has been treated with sulfites, processed meats, wine, beer, and restaurant foods such as avocado dip, salads, and potatoes

- **Foods likely to cause a severe and rapid reaction:** Eggs, seeds, fish, shellfish, nuts, and peanuts

- **Substances likely to cause chronic vague symptoms or a reaction sometime in the 24 hours following ingestion:** Milk, chocolate, wheat, citrus, berries, soy products, food coloring

- **MSG (monosodium glutamate):** Often added in Asian restaurants to enhance the flavor of foods. Many people do not realize that MSG is also a component of many food additives.

Many food additives contain MSG: Hydrolyzed vegetable and animal protein, textured protein, glutamate, monopotassium glutamate, glutamic acid, calcium, caseinate, sodium caseinate, gelatin, yeast extract, yeast food, autolyzed yeast, and yeast nutrient. Many "natural flavorings" also contain MSG or create MSG during processing.

Identification of problem foods can be a complicated process. You may want to figure out your problem with the help of a health professional trained in treating allergies. A physician can order a variety of clinical tests to help identify your sensitivity and you may be placed on a rotation diet that can ease symptoms. Specific foods and groups of food such as melons, seafood, and squash are rotated in the diet and eaten only every few days.

Especially don't experiment with foods and self-diagnose if your symptoms are severe. Symptoms can be life-threatening.

However, if your symptoms are relatively mild, you can conduct your own investigation. By removing foods from your diet that you suspect are causing you problems, and then after a while reintroducing these foods one by one into your meals, you can figure out which ingredients are causing you problems. Here are the steps to take.

1. **Write down the following:**

   - Foods you eat almost every day

   - Foods that make you feel fatigued

   - Sugar, soy, corn, yeast, food preservatives, additives, and artificial coloring, if you eat a lot of processed foods

   - Foods that you crave and make you feel good. (If your allergic to a food, your body rewards you with a little high to keep you eating that food in order to prevent withdrawal symptoms. This is the adaptation stage of food allergy)

2. **Stop eating all the foods on your list for two to three weeks.**

3. **In the interim, eat only foods that are organic and drink filtered water to avoid possible allergens.**

4. **After two to three weeks, reintroduce a single food.**

   Have a large serving of this food for breakfast, with nothing else. If you have no symptoms, eat the same food for lunch.

5. **Keep a record of changes in your physical, mental, and emotional states and monitor how you feel for the next four days.**

   If you experience symptoms, you're probably allergic to the food you're testing. If you don't notice symptoms, keep this food as a standard part of your meals, but again, not too frequently.

6. **Repeat Steps 4 and 5 for all items on your list.**

A change in eating habits can help you restore your tolerance of a food.

   ✔ If you eat a particular food all the time and you begin to experience symptoms after eating it, to restore your tolerance, try abstaining from it for four months or more. You may again tolerate it if you eat it only occasionally.

- ✔ If you absolutely can't tolerate a certain food, you may likely never be able to eat it again. But sometimes such a food can be reintroduced after a long period of time.

- ✔ When the body is toxic from contaminants in food and pollutants in the environment, the liver can become overworked, increasing your risk of food sensitivity. It can be helpful to use herbs and clean food to cleanse the body.

If you eliminate a food, be sure to replace it with one that supplies similar nutrition — for example, you can replace calcium-rich milk with calcium-rich fruits and vegetables.

If you are gluten sensitive, you don't have to give up baked goods and pasta just because they normally are made with wheat. Lots of wheatfree baked goods products are now available, and pasta made with rice flour is a very acceptable substitute for regular wheat pasta. The Lundberg Family Farms organic brown rice rotini pasta is excellent. For a quick sauce, sauté chopped fresh tomatoes and garlic in extra-virgin olive oil until the tomatoes soften, add some chopped fresh basil, cook the mixture for 2 minutes more, and you have a salsa cruda, fresh tomato sauce for your rotini.

Coping with Arthritis and Ailing Joints

Arthritis involves most commonly the joints of the hand and weight-bearing joints such as the knees. Cartilage, which cushions joints, is damaged. Bone spurs develop, causing pain, limited motion, and some deformity. Morning stiffness can be a first sign, developing into a condition in which movement of the arthritic joint is painful.

Cartilage is a highly slippery substance that allows bones to slide across each other where they meet at the joints. The basic framework of cartilage is collagen, a protein that is elastic and allows your joints to absorb shock. Vitamin C is essential for the maintenance of collagen, as are flavonoids. Both nutrients are found together in citrus fruit. (Blueberries, blackberries, and cherries are particular good flavonoid sources.)

To help with arthritis, eat a diet high in complex carbohydrates and fiber, such as whole grains, as well as fruits and vegetables. You should also eat foods that supply essential fatty acids, found in fish and unrefined vegetable oils, which help normalize joint function. And cutting back on portion sizes can help you reach a healthy weight and lighten the load your joints must support.

Studies show that the antioxidants vitamin E and vitamin C, individually and together, help maintain cartilage and support its repair. Other nutrients essential for the synthesis and repair of cartilage are vitamin A and vitamins B5 and B6, plus copper and zinc. To find out the food sources of each nutrient, see Chapter 6 on fruits and vegetables.

Should you avoid the nightshades?

The nightshade family of vegetables includes tomatoes, eggplant, peppers, and white potatoes. Tobacco is also a nightshade. These contain alkaloids that, according to a controversial theory, can worsen symptoms of arthritis. The theory was developed by a researcher at the Department of Agriculture who noticed that cattle developed arthritis from eating nightshade plants. These foods are thought to inhibit normal repair of collagen in the joints and to promote inflammation. While science has not confirmed this theory, some individuals swear by the improvement in their arthritis that they have enjoyed once they stopped eating these foods. Some people may be more sensitive than others. If you're troubled by arthritis, avoiding these foods for a month or so and noticing how you feel may be worth the effort.

For treatment of rheumatoid arthritis, turn to Appendix A.

Many ethnic cuisines rely on flavorings that reduce inflammation. Curry is a good example.

Curried Chicken in Healing Spices

If you're troubled by inflammation associated with arthritis or rheumatoid arthritis cook up a curry using white meat chicken, less likely to cause inflammation than red meat, and flavor the curry with ginger and turmeric, both anti-inflammatory spices, and cinnamon, a sedative, which acts as a pain-killer.

Preparation time: 15 minutes

Cooking time: 1 hour, 20 minutes

Yield: 6 servings

6 large skinless chicken breasts, preferably organic and residuefree

4 teaspoons lemon juice

3 tablespoons butter

2 cups finely chopped onions

2 cloves finely chopped garlic

2 tablespoons finely chopped fresh ginger root

1 stick cinnamon

4 cardamom pods

4 whole cloves

1 teaspoon ground cumin

1 teaspoon ground coriander

1 teaspoon turmeric

1 large tomato, chopped

3 tablespoons almond butter

½ cup filtered water

2 tablespoons chopped fresh coriander

(continued)

1 Prick chicken all over with fork. Put in a bowl and rub with 2 teaspoons lemon juice.

2 In a large, heavy-bottomed sauté pan, melt the butter over medium-low heat. Add the onion and sauté over medium-high heat until golden, about 12 minutes. Stir constantly to prevent the onions from burning.

3 To the sautéed onions, add the garlic and ginger and cook 2 minutes. Add the cinnamon, cardamom, and cloves and cook an additional 2 minutes.

4 Lower heat to medium and add the chicken. Cook, turning frequently, until lightly seared, about 5 to 7 minutes. Add the cumin, coriander, and turmeric. Stir to distribute spices.

5 Add the remaining 2 teaspoons lemon juice, tomato, almond butter, and water. Bring to a boil. Lower heat and simmer chicken, covered, until fork-tender, about 50 minutes. Stir frequently during cooking to prevent sticking and burning. Add more water if needed.

6 Transfer to a heated platter and serve with Anti-inflammatory Papaya-Ginger Chutney (see next recipe).

Anti-inflammatory Papaya-Ginger Chutney

Both the living enzymes in papaya and active compounds, such as gingerol in fresh ginger, can lower inflammation associated with arthritis. Many studies show that powdered ginger, also can produce results, but the fresh spice may be even more effective. Medicine never tasted so good!

Preparation time: *20 minutes*

Cooking time: *1 hour to combine flavors*

Yield: *About 1½ cups*

1 papaya, peeled, seeded, and coarsely chopped

2 tablespoons minced, peeled fresh ginger

2 tablespoons finely chopped cilantro

2 tablespoons fresh lime juice

Cayenne

1 In a bowl, combine all ingredients except the cayenne and mix.

2 Cover the chutney with plastic wrap and chill for 1 hour or more. Season with cayenne and serve as a condiment with any Indian meal.

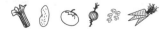

Osteoporosis

Some 25 million Americans have *osteoporosis* or porous bones, a degenerative disease that affects bone mass and bone strength. Nearly one-third of women with this disease will suffer a bone fracture. If this involves the hip, a woman may lose her ability to walk independently, and health consequences can even be fatal. Women begin to lose bone mass at about age 35, accelerating after menopause, while bone loss in men occurs gradually and to a lesser degree. However, osteoporosis in men can be severe.

Osteoporosis occurs at a higher incidence in America and other Western countries, in comparison with China, India, and developing countries where refined and processed foods do not dominate the food supply. The Western diet is full of acid-forming foods, which trigger the body to draw calcium along with other alkaline minerals from the bones to buffer the acids. (A far more sedentary lifestyle in the West is also a major factor. Your body is simply unable to build bone if you remain inactive.)

Staples of the typical American meal — red meat, white flour, sugar, colas, coffee, tea, caffeine, and salt — are all acid-forming foods. Mineral-rich fruits and vegetables, whole grains, and beans are alkalizing but usually in short supply on the average dinner table. These same plant foods are the mainstay of diets in less developed countries where osteoporosis is rare.

Colas are exceptionally high in phosphorus, which the body must keep in balance with calcium. They also can contain large doses of sugar and caffeine. Remember as you down your next cola that your body will quickly respond by drawing calcium from bones.

The most plentiful mineral in your bones is calcium. The current RDA is 1,000 mg for adults and 1,500 mg for women postmenopause. However, if you cut back on acidifying foods, you may need less than you've been told. The World Health Organization offers a general guideline for adults of 400 mg a day. Foods that contain calcium include cornmeal, whole wheat, brown rice, kidney beans, broccoli, dark leafy greens, okra, acorn squash, butternut squash, figs, papayas, hazelnuts, Brazil nuts, almonds, canned fish with their bones, blackstrap molasses, goat cheese, and yogurt. Another good source is chicken soup, made with the bones and a little vinegar, which helps pull the calcium from the bones into the broth. (Kale is a good plant food source of calcium. Sample the Leafy Greens with Garlic in Chapter 6.)

Using antacids that contain calcium to increase your intake can be counterproductive, because antacids decrease stomach acidity, contributing to decreased absorption of calcium.

Besides calcium, many other minerals are essential for bone strength. Leading the list is magnesium. The balance between magnesium and calcium is very important in lowering your risk of osteoporosis. Everyone has different needs, but magnesium deficiency is common. (Sample Magnesium Munchies in Chapter 10 and Puree of Green Soybean Soup, which includes lima beans, a great source of magnesium, in Chapter 17.)

If you use milk as your main calcium source, be aware that it contains only a trace amount of magnesium and is high in protein that promotes the excretion of calcium.

Boost your magnesium by eating whole grains, lima beans, Great Northern beans, chickpeas, beets and beet greens, broccoli, potatoes with their skin, figs, plantains, avocados, cashews, Brazil nuts, pumpkin seeds, and shrimp.

Bone-building also requires a host of other nutrients — boron, copper, manganese, silicon, strontium, and zinc, as well as vitamin B6, folic acid, vitamin C, vitamin D, and vitamin K. Be sure to eat a considerable variety of fruits, vegetables, nuts, and seeds. That way, you are more likely to consume this wide assortment of nutrients.

Skin Conditions

Your skin reflects the quality of food you've been eating. A diet that supplies such nutrients as zinc, vitamin C, and vitamin A as well as healthy oils helps keep the skin firm and supple. Being able to digest food properly to prevent toxins from accumulating in the system and avoiding toxic fats and chemicals in foods also helps maintain skin quality. The skin is the largest organ of elimination and substances that the body attempts to rid itself of can make their way to the skin. Treat yourself to a beautiful bod by shaping up your diet! For information on acne, turn to Chapter 19. For information on hair and scalp, check out Appendix A.

Eczema

Eczema is characterized by skin that is inflamed, dry, thickened, and itchy. Areas typically affected are the face, wrists, and insides of the knees and elbows. One form, *atopic eczema,* is triggered by allergy to food or a pollutant such as household dust. Stress can also cause or aggravate this condition. Atopic eczema is most often seen in infants, up to the age of 18 months, and runs in families. A person who has had eczema as a child is far more likely to develop this again as an adult and to have other allergic conditions such as asthma.

Contact eczema, or contact dermatitis, occurs in sensitive individuals if a particular substance comes in contact with the skin. Possible allergens include cosmetics, perfumes, wool, industrial chemicals, nickel found in jewelry, and plants such as chrysanthemums and poison ivy.

What to eat and not eat:

- Be sure to drink plenty of filtered water to keep your skin moisturized from the inside out.

- Having sufficient levels of zinc in body tissues is especially effective in helping prevent and treat eczema. Other important nutrients include vitamin A, beta-carotene, B-complex vitamins, vitamin C, bioflavonoids, vitamin E, and selenium, as well as healthy oils in vegetables, unrefined seed oils, fish, and flax seeds and flaxseed oil. These nutrients strengthen the immune system, provide antioxidants, reduce inflammation, and support the regeneration of healthy skin tissue.

  Certain foods such as onions contain phytochemicals that inhibit inflammation. In onions, the active ingredient is the bioflavonoid, quercetin.

- Avoid sugar, coffee, black and green tea, and alcohol.

- You may also want to try supplementing with evening primrose oil, which supplies healing essential fatty acids, and glycyrrhiza glabra, or licorice root, which reduces inflammation.

- For atopic eczema, avoid foods that are possible allergens, especially, eggs, milk, wheat, and chemical additives in food. (See "Food Sensitivities and Allergy," earlier in this chapter.) Eczema in infants is most commonly due to a milk allergy. If you find that a particular food triggers your eczema, you need to also eliminate all others in the same family, such as wheat plus rye, oats, rice, barley, and millet.

Psoriasis

In psoriasis, skin cells rapidly multiply. As they pile up, they begin to form a silvery scale. Mechanisms that control the rate at which cells divide become unbalanced. This condition is most likely to develop on the scalp and on the backs of the wrists, elbows, knees, and ankles.

Poor digestion and an accumulation of toxins are involved in the development of psoriasis. It appears that protein is not completely broken down, leading to an accumulation of toxic byproducts. Other toxins may originate in the gut. In turn, these toxins can overwork the liver. The following dietary suggestions for psoriasis are meant to counteract these tendencies.

✔ Restrict or avoid meat, dairy products, and animal fats to decrease toxins and aid the liver in its role of clearing these from the system, and to reduce inflammation. Avoid all organ meats.

Supplementing with the herb milk thistle, which contains the active compound silymarin, can improve liver function and slow the rapid multiplication of cells. Goldenseal is another useful herb.

✔ Eliminate all alcoholic beverages. Alcohol burdens the liver, which must break down this toxin before it can leave the body.

✔ Avoid sugar and chemical additives in food.

✔ Experiment with avoiding grains that contain gluten — wheat, rye, oats, barley.

✔ Each day, have some omega-3 fatty acids found in fish oils, flax seeds, and walnuts to reduce inflammation. Recent studies show that fish oil that contains these fatty acids is especially useful.

✔ Increase your intake of high-fiber foods such as sweet potatoes, cauliflower, whole wheat, dried beans and peas, and apples.

✔ Consume foods that supply zinc, chromium, vitamin E, selenium, folic acid, and vitamin A, and B complex.

If you have the opportunity, dine outdoors and let gentle sunlight fall on those areas of your body that have the psoriasis. Sunlight has proven to be extremely beneficial for healing this condition.

Managing Stress

Do you start eating when you're under stress? Cookies, chocolate, bits of last night's macaroni and cheese — anything will do. In a way, snacking is one way your body attempts to calm you down, at least if you eat carbohydrates. These help you produce more *serotonin,* a neurotransmitter that promotes a feeling of well-being. If you self-medicate with a nourishing slice of whole wheat bread from time to time, this would be fine. However, all too often stress eating does not take such a noble form.

What you eat can indeed prepare your body to withstand stress and help you through troubling times, but foods such as chocolate cake are not the answer long term. You need to eat foods that nourish the adrenal glands and avoid those which undermine your stress response.

Stress weakens immunity

Excessive emotional and physical stress can weaken your immunity. Being stressed increases the production of adrenal hormones such as catecholamines and corticosteroids. These inhibit white blood cells, which fight infection.

Under stress, the thymus gland, which produces some of your supply of white blood cells, begins to shrink. Any medical condition, including the common cold, psoriasis, and hypertension, tends to become worse with excessive stress.

Stress stimulates your sympathetic nervous system, which is in charge of the fight-or-flight response. The adrenal glands react to stress by producing hormones such as adrenaline and corticosteroids. Adrenal hormones trigger the release of stored glucose for quick energy and, in general, prepare the body to survive the crisis — be it losing your keys or having to ride out an earthquake. The stress response is a normal body function. You have an inborn ability to withstand a reasonable amount if you are eating foods that nourish the adrenal glands.

Adrenal function and the ability to produce hormones depends upon having adequate vitamin C, zinc, magnesium, and B-complex vitamins — in particular, vitamin B5 or pantothenic acid. The stress response also depends upon having sufficient magnesium, which stress depletes.

The following food sources of these nutrients can help you manage stress:

- ✔ **Pantothenic acid:** Whole grains, legumes, sweet potatoes, tomatoes, cauliflower, broccoli, avocado, sunflower seeds, liver, bluefish, salmon, and trout

- ✔ **Magnesium:** Green vegetables such as broccoli and beet greens, many beans including pinto, navy, black, and kidney beans, many whole grains such as buckwheat and whole rye, and millet, pine nuts, walnuts, egg yolks, oysters, halibut, and shrimp

- ✔ **Potassium:** Potatoes, avocado, lima beans, banana, cantaloupe, light-meat chicken, leg of lamb, flounder, salmon, and cod

Chinese or Korean ginseng, *Panax ginseng*, has long been a traditional tonic for stress. Other antistress herbs are chamomile, rose hips, valerian root, skullcap, passionflower, pau d'arco, and catnip.

You also should stay away from the following stressors:

✔ **Sugar:** Refined sugar does not contain vitamins or minerals. However, to convert sugar into energy, the body requires B vitamins and magnesium, nutrients your adrenals also need to properly function. Eating sugar robs the adrenal glands of these supporting nutrients.

✔ **Caffeine:** After prolonged stress, the adrenals automatically shut down in order to allow the body to rest and recover. Caffeine inhibits this self-protective response to stress. By making a pit stop for a cup of caffeinated coffee, tea, or a cola, you and your adrenals can keep on going. But if overstimulating your adrenal glands becomes a way of life, you risk reaching exhaustion.

The scent of certain plants is healing. The scent of roses is said to impart the aroma of love. In the Middle East, rosewater, a distillation of rose petals that tastes like garden roses smell, is added to tea and desserts such as the one that follows. How could you feel stressed out while eating fruit flavored with rosewater?

Oranges in Rosewater

Sliced oranges are an excellent source of vitamin C, which helps enable your body to manage stress.

Preparation time: *15 minutes*

Cooking time: *None*

Yield: *4 servings as a dessert*

4 navel oranges, peeled

4 large sprigs mint, stems removed, plus 4 sprigs for garnish

¾ cup plain active-bacteria yogurt, preferably organic

1 tablespoon honey

½ teaspoon rosewater

¼ cup pistachios

1 Slice the oranges and cut into chunks. Refrigerate while preparing sauce.

2 Using a cutting board, mince the mint leaves.

3 In a medium bowl, gently mix together the mint, yogurt, honey, and rosewater.

4 Remove the chilled oranges from the refrigerator. Reserve some for garnish. Mix remaining oranges with yogurt sauce.

5 Distribute the orange mixture evenly among stemmed glasses. Top with reserved oranges, sprigs of mint, and pistachios.

Chapter 21

Putting It All Together

Recipes in This Chapter

▶ Cod Cakes with Tomato Tarragon Sauce

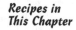

*F*inding out about all the healing foods that are good for your health is one thing. Figuring out what to eat for lunch is another! You may indeed be convinced that you need more foods that supply zinc or selenium, and you're ready to watch out for transfatty acids. But where do you start making changes? How should you plan your daily meals?

Planning Your Meals

When you take a little time to plan your meals, you have the chance to make sure that you include special foods you need. No more making do with whatever is in the fridge. You can spend your food dollars wisely and turn food shopping into a way to support your health.

First, determine to invest some time into shopping for new foods. These may be in your local supermarket, or you may find you need to search other neighborhoods for good sources of healing ingredients. Second, if you do have a special ailment, turn to Chapter 20. Begin your shopping list with the special foods recommended. Third, keep the following guidelines in mind:

✔ **Eat whole foods** — those that are natural, unrefined, and unprocessed. You really only need to remember this rule. Most of the nutritional advice in this book comes down to this simple guideline.

✔ **Avoid adulterated foods** that contain added sugars, preservatives, pesticides, added hormones, and foreign chemicals.

To help you picture how all this dietary advice translates into daily meals, I assembled the following week of menus. This eating calendar is meant to give you a general idea of how often to have certain kinds of food so that you eat a variety. For example, have at least five servings a day of fruits and vegetables and eat fish two to three times a week. To increase your intake of plant foods and lower your intake of saturated animal fats, I made the menus for the sixth day completely vegetarian and the third day semivegetarian.

This list of foods may look like a lot to eat, especially if you're concerned with weight. However, it's all a question of portion size. (See the sidebar "How much is a portion?") A portion size is probably smaller than you may have thought. Have moderate amounts of a variety of foods to make sure that you get the full range of vitamins and minerals you need.

- **Day 1:** *Breakfast* — Whole-grain pancakes, blueberries; *Lunch* — Beet and potato soup, yogurt with pistachios, pumpernickel bread; *Dinner* — Salmon, wild rice pilaf, asparagus, cucumber salad, fresh dill; *Snacks* — Popcorn.

- **Day 2:** *Breakfast* — Millet, oats, or other cooked cereal, stewed prunes; *Lunch* — Salad with sweet peppers, raw onion, tomato, feta, olives, chickpea hummus, and whole-grain pita; *Dinner* — Beef, pork, or lamb, mushrooms, artichokes, carrots, baked potato; *Snacks* — Brazil nuts, pumpkin seeds.

- **Day 3:** *Breakfast* — Poached eggs, whole-grain toast, sliced oranges; *Lunch* — Tuna sandwich, carrot and celery sticks, ginger cookies; *Dinner* — Vegetable enchilada, salad with avocado and flaxseed and extra-virgin olive oil dressing, fresh pineapple; *Snacks* — Melon.

- **Day 4:** *Breakfast* — Whole-wheat bagel, ricotta cheese, ½ pink grapefruit; *Lunch* — Bean soup, pear and cheese, whole-grain crackers; *Dinner* — Broiled chicken, acorn squash, lima beans, whole-grain dinner roll; *Snacks* — Sunflower seeds, currants.

- **Day 5:** *Breakfast* — Polenta, apricots, turkey sausage; *Lunch* — Chicken sandwich, papaya with lime; *Dinner* — Shellfish stew in tomato sauce, green salad with endive and watercress; *Snacks* — Plain yogurt and fresh fruit.

- **Day 6:** *Breakfast* — Eggs with salsa and corn tortillas; *Lunch* — Buckwheat sesame noodles, sea vegetable salad; *Dinner* — Vegetarian lasagna, lentil soup, red grapes; *Snacks* — Almond butter on apple slices.

- **Day 7:** *Breakfast* — Cream of whole wheat or brown rice, banana; *Lunch* — Chili, cornbread, cole slaw; *Dinner* — Roast turkey, sweet potatoes, broccoli, peach cobbler; *Snacks* — Dried figs and dates.

How much is a portion?

The Dietary Guidelines for Americans, created by the USDA, recommends a certain number of servings of different foods each day. They define a serving as follows:

- ✔ **Vegetables:** ½ cup cooked vegetables, 1 cup lettuce

- ✔ **Beans:** ½ cup cooked beans

- ✔ **Fruit:** A medium apple, ½ grapefruit, ½ cup berries, ¼ cup dried fruit

- ✔ **Bread:** 1 slice

- ✔ **Yogurt:** 1 cup

- ✔ **Meat, poultry, fish:** 3 ounces or the size of a deck of playing cards

Making Changes to Your Diet

Most people can improve their diet, even if they're eating pretty well right now. There's no time like the present to improve on the foods you eat. You'll be feeling heathier and more energetic that much sooner. Substitute a food that is healthy for one that is so-so and stick with this for a week or two. Then make another change. Give yourself six months or more for a complete overhaul of your diet.

Be a good friend to yourself as you add new foods to your meals and eliminate others. Unless you prefer radical change, it's perfectly fine to take some time with this if it helps you not revert to your old ways of eating. Even with small changes, when you look back in a few months, you may be surprised how far you've come.

1. Go step by step.

If you're like most people, big changes happen in little steps. You can still reach your goals if you're changing your diet slowly. You'll be giving your body the chance to comfortably adjust to not having certain foods. You'll also be less likely to trigger symptoms of withdrawal from potentially addictive substances such as caffeine and white sugar.

Think of the quality of food in terms of good, better, and best. Making even a partial improvement in ingredients is progress. If you never eat beans, having canned beans is great. If you eat only beans from a tin, making them from scratch is that much better. The same goes for no vegetables — canned vegetables — frozen vegetables — fresh vegetables.

2. Forgive and forget.

Don't ever say never and set yourself up to fail. Forgive yourself when you lapse into old habits and have a hotdog and french fries for lunch. Your transgressions are a chance to notice how you feel after eating such foods. Check whether they load you down and make you feel tired or edgy. You may find that old favorites are not as appealing as they once were. Taste can change once you've eaten healthier foods for a month or two.

3. Keep focused on your goals.

Be forewarned that shaping up your diet may require some rugged individualism. If you're getting harassed for eating smart, read Chapter 25, which gives you ten good reasons for eating healthy foods.

Feeding Yourself and Others

Of course, food is love! It is a gift you give yourself and others. Make a point of cooking thoughtfully. Serve your creations with kindness. Enjoy your meals in a nurturing setting and consume them with a thank you.

As you decide on what to cook, consider what foods your body especially needs, but also be sensitive to the needs of the other people you feed.

 ✔ **Begin with yourself.** Listen to what foods your body is asking for. Say it's demanding fat. See whether a salad made with extra-virgin olive oil or a handful of nuts will satisfy. If you're craving sugar, try instead eating some protein such as a piece of chicken or some hummus on pita bread. A desire for sweets can mask a need for protein. The idea is to give yourself a food of quality rather than a quick fix of fries or candy.

 ✔ **Be sensitive to the food preferences of others.** These often reflect real and differing nutritional needs. For example, you may thrive on a vegetarian diet, while someone else eating this way may tend to feel cold and tired. You may need more of a certain vitamin or mineral than the amount a family member needs. Children will have different nutritional needs than their parents. (See Chapter 19 for more on healthful foods for children.)

Eating in comfort and with good cheer

For good digestion and absorption of your food, you need to eat in peace. Set time aside and arrange a special place where you can dine, alone or with family and friends.

The nurturing and communal aspects of mealtime, as well as the enjoyment of good food, is not addressed in the standard American dietary guidelines. However, these very human aspects of eating are valued enough in other cultures that they are written into the dietary recommendations of many countries. In the United Kingdom, the guideline is "Enjoy your food." In Thailand, they say, "A happy family is when family members eat together, enjoy treasured family tastes and good home cooking." In Vietnam, they officially recommend, ". . . a healthy family meal that is delicious, wholesome, clean, and economical, and served with affection."

Having gratitude for the food you eat

Some people give thanks before a meal for what they are about to eat. If you've never tried this, I invite you to. Saying grace can bring a sense of peace and connect you to family and friends sitting at your dinner table. I wrote this with the help of my friend Paula. I invite you to make up your own!

> *Thank you for these healing foods*
> *And for the earth, air, and light from which they came.*
> *As we take these foods into our body and they*
> *Become one with us,*
> *May we be nourished, so that we may nourish others.*

Practice meal: A lunch to linger over

Have some good friend over for talk and lunch. Start with the Mediterranean Olives (Chapter 10) and the Marinated Goat Cheese (Chapter 9). Then serve these cod cakes and finish with Apple and Almond Cobbler (Chapter 19) and mint tea.

Cod Cakes with Tomato Tarragon Sauce

Codfish supplies all the B vitamins that support the health of the nervous system, but their comforting texture is what keeps us coming back asking for more.

Preparation time: 25 minutes

Cooking time: 40 minutes

Yield: 8 servings

(continued)

1 pound medium potatoes, peeled and quartered

1 pound cod

2 bay leaves

1½ cups fresh fish or chicken stock

1 tablespoon plain yogurt

2 scallions, thinly sliced

4 sprigs parsley, stems removed, leaves chopped

½ cup whole-grain bread crumbs

1 tablespoon organic unsalted butter

3 large tomatoes, chopped

3 sprigs fresh tarragon, leaves only, chopped

Lemon zest from 1 organic lemon

½ cup filtered water

2 tablespoons organic unsalted butter

Salt and freshly ground black pepper to taste

1 *To make the cod cakes:* In a medium pot, place the potatoes and cover with water. Bring to a boil and cook for 20 minutes until tender. Drain and mash.

2 Place the cod in a large skillet, along with 1 bay leaf and stock. Bring to a boil and simmer, covered, 6 to 7 minutes. Using a slotted spatula, carefully remove the fish and, with a fork, flake the cod.

3 In a large bowl, mix the potato and fish, yogurt, scallions, and parsley. Season the fish cakes with salt and pepper. Cool, cover, and chill 1 hour.

4 Sprinkle the bread crumbs on a plate. Divide the mixture into 8 portions and shape each into a patty about 3 to 4 inches in diameter. Press each fish cake into the bread crumbs.

5 In a large, nonstick sauté pan, melt the butter over medium heat. When bubbly, add the cod cakes; gently shake the pan to evenly coat them with butter. Cook for 6 minutes, turn over, and continue to cook 5 to 6 minutes, until golden. Drain on paper towels and keep warm.

6 *To prepare the tomato sauce:* In a saucepan, place the tomatoes, the remaining bay leaf, fresh tarragon, lemon zest, and filtered water. Simmer for 15 minutes, covered, until tomatoes have softened.

7 Remove the bay leaf and transfer the tomato mixture to a blender or processor and blend.

8 Put the sauce into a small pot and cook, uncovered, on medium heat, until mixture is somewhat reduced, about 10 minutes.

9 Add the butter to the sauce. Season with salt and pepper to taste.

10 Serve the cod fish cakes on heated dinner plates and top each with several tablespoon-fuls of sauce.

Chapter 22

Eating on the Run

● ●

In This Chapter

▶ Selecting healthy foods from restaurant menus

▶ Grabbing a healthy bite at the local joint

▶ Ordering healthy foods in ethnic restaurants

▶ Traveling with healing morsels

● ●

*Y*ou probably eat many of your meals out — it's estimated that 46 percent of American adults eat out at least once a day. So these days, it's just as important to know your way around a restaurant menu as it is to know how to cook.

Yes, you *can* eat healthy foods in restaurants. Granted, restaurants serve plenty of dishes made with lots of easy-to-like fats and sugar because they're in the business of giving you a good time, not extending your life. But this doesn't mean you should never eat out. This chapter helps you make smart choices even when you're not the person preparing the food.

Dining Out

The local steakhouse, the main dining room of the fancy hotel in town, and the country club restaurant are all places that serve standard American dishes. Many foods, such as those that follow, fit right into a healthy diet.

✔ **Order the soup or salad.** If you opt for the salad, ask for it with bleu cheese dressing, not vinaigrette, which is probably made with refined oil, or request some extra-virgin olive oil on the side and vinegar or a wedge of lemon and sprinkle these over your salad to make your own dressing.

- ✔ **Order lean, broiled chicken, which is cooked at higher temperatures than you use at home, sealing in the juices.** Grilled fish is also a good choice.

- ✔ **Enjoy a baked potato, with toppings if you like, but in modest amounts.**

- ✔ **If you're vegetarian, order *off the menu.*** The cook or chef will usually put together a special plate of all the vegetable side dishes on the menu that day. Sometimes you hit the jackpot!

- ✔ **Vary your diet by ordering foods you don't cook at home.** Order the duck, even if it's a little more expensive. Have oysters to start. Or let the chef cook you lobster!

Don't be shy. You can ask your waiter how a dish is prepared.

Grabbing a Bite When You're Out and About

As of yet, there's no chain of drive-through health-food restaurants serving organic ingredients. But healthy food is out there — you just have to look for it. Search out local restaurants and when you suddenly realize that you're starving, you can head for those places rather than having a donut just because you're parked in front of a store that sells them.

Here's what to buy when you're looking for a quick bite:

- ✔ **At coffee shops:** Hot oatmeal, poached eggs, Greek salads, fresh-made soups, rye bread, roast turkey with trimmings, fruit compote, and herbal teas

- ✔ **At salad bars:** Bean salads, a variety of raw vegetables, a variety of salad greens, sprouts, and raw seeds and nuts

- ✔ **At delicatessens:** Fresh-made chicken soup, smoked salmon and white fish, whole-grain bagels, cole slaw, tomato and cucumber salad, fruit salad, Swiss cheese, borscht, kasha with mushroom gravy, stuffed cabbage, olives, and sauerkraut

- ✔ **At gas stations:** Bottled water, V-8 juice, bottled orange and apple juices, and fresh fruit (when you can find it), but not much else!

Stay away from the usually rancid roasted nuts and seeds sold in little cellophane packets!

Eating Ethnic Foods

When eating out, walk yourself into an ethnic restaurant to feast on the variety of nutritious and natural whole-foods ingredients featured in these cuisines. Smaller ethnic restaurants usually offer food that's well priced, and you can be sure that healthy dishes will be featured on the menu.

Table 22-1 lists some common ethnic restaurants and the healthy foods to try in each of them.

Table 22-1 Ethnic Restaurants and the Healthy Foods They Offer

Ethnic Restaurant	Healthy Foods to Try
Asian	Miso soup, vegetable and tofu stir-fry, soba noodles, brown rice, sukiyaki, steamed whole fish
Indian	Curries (which are made with medicinally active spices), cauliflower, okra, eggplant, potatoes, lentil dal, mango lassi
Mexican	Stewed pinto beans (not refried), guacamole, corn tortillas, grilled fish and poultry, slow-cooked pork (carnitas), cactus salad (nopales)
Middle Eastern	Chickpea hummus, Greek salad with feta and olives, stuffed grape leaves, lentil soup, grilled lamb kebabs
Thai	Salads made with a variety of vegetables and herbs and topped with a small portion of meat, seafood and chicken, spicy chicken-coconut soups, such as Tom Ka Gai

Packing Foods for Traveling

Traveling can present a special challenge to healthful eating. You may be tempted to grab quick, empty-calorie snacks and indulge in whatever local dishes are made available to you (which may or may not be good for you). But be conscious of what you're putting into your mouth, and you'll find yourself with more energy to enjoy the sights. Here are some foods to pack for your trip:

✔ **Bottled filtered water** for when you really want to quench your thirst, especially when you're in an airplane, which is a dehydrating environment

✔ **Bananas** for when you need quick energy in a tidy package

✔ **Trail mix** (such as the recipe for Magnesium Munchies in Chapter 10) for when you want a nourishing snack

✔ **A bag of homemade organic popcorn** for a crunchy late-afternoon, wake-up snack that's light to carry — the bagful can function as packaging when you need to cushion fragile items in your luggage

✔ **Your favorite herbal teas,** because they may not be available where you're going

✔ **Organic dried fruit,** such as apple slices and peaches from a natural-food store

✔ **Instant cereal in a cup** to eat in your hotel room (plus an electric coil to heat the water) so that you can be sharp-witted at your breakfast meeting

✔ **Instant soup in a cup** for a quick and cheap little lunch back in your hotel room

✔ **Tasty whole-grain crackers** for when you need a crunchy little nibble

✔ **Small cans of top-quality tuna, sardines, or salmon** to make a meal by adding instant soup and crackers, for when you arrive late and room service is closed

Part V
The Part of Tens

The 5th Wave   By Rich Tennant

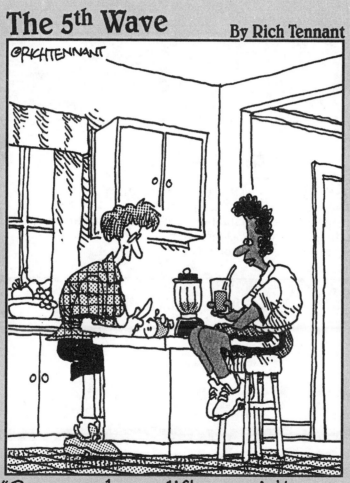

"Bananas always lift my spirits.
Especially when I hide the over ripe
hunks in my husband's running shoes."

In this part . . .

Every ...*For Dummies* book ends with top-ten lists, and this one is no exception. Take a look at these chapters — ten beautiful ways to serve healing foods, ten eating strategies for elders, and ten reasons to begin eating healing foods today.

Chapter 23

Ten Beautiful Ways to Serve Healing Foods

● ●

Recipes in This Chapter

↻ Boston Lettuce Crudite

▶ Caviar for Company

🍴 🥄 🍶 🌶 🥕

● ●

The days of funny-looking health food are long gone. Healing foods are beautiful foods. The healthiest fruits and vegetables display a dazzling array of color because many nutrients are also pigments. Beta-carotene, the flavonoids, and chlorophyll tint foods with pinks, oranges, fire-engine red, purple, and emerald. The wonderful vitality and freshness of healing foods is also a delight to the eye.

When you cook with healthy ingredients, making the most of their good looks is even good for your health. As soon as you see a food that looks appetizing, the digestive processes begin, even before the food goes into your mouth! Good digestion helps you absorb food so you can benefit from the vitamins and minerals it contains. In this chapter, I give you ways to show off your healthy creations.

Flaunt Your Colors

When you cook, you have the chance to be an artist. Use colorful foods like an artist uses colorful paint and create a picture.

> ✔ Say that you have a dessert sauce made of raspberry puree that you plan to pour over some fruit and a little slice of cake. Instead, spoon the sauce onto a plate, covering all or just a part. Next place the fruit and the cake slice on top of the sauce to make the most of its color and give your dessert a pretty backdrop.

- ✔ Enjoy extra-virgin olive oil on your bread instead of using butter. Display its lovely translucent greens by serving the oil in a small glass bowl.

- ✔ To show off a food's color, serve it on a plate of contrasting color: red on green, green on yellow, pale green on purple, and yellow on turquoise. It may be the same old recipe, but they'll think you cooked something special.

- ✔ If you overcook your veggies, you won't have much color to show off. To keep vegetables such as spinach from turning muddy green, cook them without a lid and don't overcook. Adding baking soda also is a way to retain the green, but doing this destroys vitamins, especially vitamin B1 and vitamin C.

- ✔ Create meals that provide foods of various colors, and you'll be eating a greater variety of nutrients. Include something orange and something green, and you'll be sure to have some beta-carotene and magnesium. Beta-carotene is an orange pigment, and magnesium is part of green chlorophyll.

Frame Your Creations

Using attractive serving plates adds to a food's appeal, as does a little garnish.

- ✔ Select dinner plates with a border pattern — frames for your picture-perfect foods.

- ✔ Garnish with a sprig of fresh, healing dill, tarragon, rosemary, or sage. Clip three stems of chive and arrange them in a fan.

- ✔ Use a sprinkling of nuts and seeds as a garnish for all sorts of dishes and benefit from these nutritious foods everyday.

Think Shapes

Health food used to show up as formless mounds of beans and grains, but these days it's taken a tip from the gourmet world and comes with shape.

- ✔ When you're slicing something, consider what shapes you want to end up with. If you're cutting strawberries or mushrooms, slice them vertically to show off their unique shapes. Cut green peppers crosswise to create little scallops.

- ✔ Give your whole grains some shape instead of serving them in a little pile on your plate. Once they are cooked, spoon them into a mold, lightly pressing them into this form, and then turn them out onto a plate. Use a larger gelatin mold or individual custard cups to make single servings.

Beautiful food is party food. These two recipes for hors d'oeuvres both make use of the elegant shape of endive.

Boston Lettuce Crudite

This is a gorgeous way to serve raw vegetables that I learned in my catering days. Just be sure to tell people they're really allowed to eat it — people stay away thinking it is a centerpiece! You'll keep your arrangement looking very well designed and sophisticated if you use only white and green vegetables. Stay away from radishes and carrot sticks!

Preparation time: *30 minutes, including prepping vegetables*

Cooking time: *None*

Yield: *10 hors d'oeuvres servings*

1 head Boston lettuce with outside leaves intact

1 head endive, leaves separated

1 large cucumber, peeled, seeded, and cut into sticks

20 spears thin asparagus, trimmed and blanched (or blanched string beans)

1 turnip, peeled, thinly sliced, and cut into half-moon shapes

1 Very gently open the leaves of the head of lettuce, as if you were opening a flower. Be especially careful with the leaves in the center. Place the head of lettuce in the middle of a large round serving platter.

2 Insert leaves of endive between the leaves of lettuce to help hold the lettuce leaves open. Distribute endive evenly.

3 Continue to add the cucumber, asparagus, and turnip to the arrangement, creating an attractive composition as you proceed. (Note)

4 Serve immediately or keep refrigerated until serving time and sprinkle with cold water to refresh. Accompany with a sauce for dipping served in a silver bowl or in the cup of a halved acorn squash, cut horizontally and seeds removed.

Note: *Besides these vegetables, you can also add small florets of green broccoli and white cauliflower.*

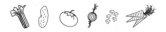

Caviar for Company

Caviar is rich in omega-3 essential fatty acids, which are great for the heart and also reduce inflammation associated with many medical problems, including allergies. Endive stimulates the functioning of the liver and gallbladder to help cleanse the system. The sour cream is simply delicious. This is uptown health food.

Preparation time: *10 minutes*

Cooking time: *None*

Yield: *6 hors d'oeuvres servings*

1 head endive

1 cup sour cream

1 small jar red caviar

1 Cut the head of endive at the base and separate endive spears. Place 1 or 2 paper towels on a work surface and arrange spears, edges upward, in several rows.

2 Using a teaspoon, daub a small amount of sour cream on the wide end of each spear, which serves as a cup. With another spoon, scoop out several beads of caviar and place on top of the sour cream. Repeat until all endive spears are filled

3 Use a dramatically colored serving plate such as a black ceramic platter or a round silver tray and arrange the spears, tips outward, like the petals of a flower. Serve with white cocktail napkins. (Your guests will think you hired a caterer.)

Chapter 24

Ten Eating Strategies for Elders

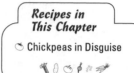

Recipes in This Chapter

♻ Chickpeas in Disguise

*A*merica is growing older. As baby boomers age, the number of people over 65 is increasing, expected to reach 39 million in the near future. By 2030, 1 out of 5 Americans, or 66 million people, will have had their 65th birthday! Good nutrition is as important for these elders as it is for children, pregnant women, and athletes. While much of the nutrition advice that applies to younger people is also true for older folks, elders also have their special needs. Whether you are older, or to some degree responsible for aging parents, you can benefit from being savvy about nutritional needs in later life.

Adding Antioxidants to Every Meal

Now more than ever your body requires *antioxidants,* nutrients that prevent your body from, in effect, rusting away! Antioxidants such as beta-carotene, vitamin C, vitamin E, and selenium quench *free radicals,* molecules that can harm body tissues and lead to such medical conditions as arthritis, cataracts, atherosclerosis, deterioration of memory, and many other conditions. The antioxidants beta-carotene, vitamin C, vitamin E, and selenium can help stop this process of decay before it begins. Seafood, whole grains, unrefined vegetable oils, raw seeds and nuts, and fruits and vegetables are excellent sources. (Read more about antioxidants in Chapter 6.)

Buying a Little of a Lot

Just like when you were younger, you still need to eat a variety of foods. Starting in the produce section, grab about eight or ten of those filmy plastic bags to make it as easy as possible to buy a variety of stuff. Put just one or two of a particular fruit or vegetable into each bag. Resist buying three pounds of pears just because they're on sale. Do the same at the meat counter. Also take advantage of natural-food stores, which sell food in bulk, so that you can measure out just the amount you need of such items as cereals, beans, nuts, seeds, and dried fruit.

Getting Fresh and Eating Raw

With age, your ability to digest food easily may decline. To improve your digestive function, add living enzymes to your meals, supplied by fresh and *raw* fruits and vegetables. Enzymes break down food and, in your stomach, join forces with your body's own digestive enzymes, which diminish as the body ages. Heat destroys enzymes, so be sure to eat a little salad, sliced fruit, or a garnish of raw vegetable at each meal to have the benefit of these digestive allies.

Fresh pineapple and fresh papaya are particularly rich in enzymes (bromelain and papain respectively) and deserve to be staples in your kitchen. These two fruits are absolutely delicious pureed together and served slushy, like applesauce. Bromelain and papain are also sold as supplements.

Spice Up Healing Foods

If you think of healthy foods as bland and unappealing, you can always spike the flavors with spices, garlic, onions, and hot sauce, in themselves healing ingredients. Serve peppery salad dressings and substantial condiments such as Red Onions with Vinegar and Chilies in Chapter 16. Or have a go with this recipe made with good-for-you chickpeas.

Chickpeas in Disguise

Pureed chickpeas mixed with sesame seed paste is known as *hummus* in the Middle East, where it is a very common food. This recipe adds exotic spices to the normally pale flavorings. Use this spread on sandwiches and enjoy its smoothness as a dip, along with crunchy raw vegetables.

Preparation time: *10 minutes*

Cooking time: *1 minute*

Yield: *2 cups*

1 15-ounce can chickpeas, drained	*¼ teaspoon ground turmeric*
Juice of 1 lemon	*¼ teaspoon ground cardamom*
4 tablespoons tahini sesame paste	*1 pinch cinnamon*
1 clove garlic	*Salt and freshly ground black pepper to taste*
1½ teaspoons ground cumin	

1 Put the chickpeas, lemon juice, tahini, and garlic in a food processor fitted with a blade. Blend together until smooth, about 2 minutes.

2 Put the cumin, turmeric, cardamom, and cinnamon in a small skillet and warm over low heat until spices begin to darken slightly and become aromatic, about 30 seconds.

3 Add the toasted spices to the chickpea mixture. Blend for 1 minute. Season with salt and pepper and blend again briefly. Scoop into a colorful bowl and serve as a starter course, with whole-grain pita bread, radishes, scallions, watercress, and olives.

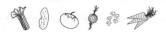

Trimming Your Weight

As you age, maintaining a normal, healthy weight can help protect you from heart disease, the No. 1 killer in the United States today. But I am not suggesting you go on a crash diet of any sort and do without food. Subsisting on nonfat diet products is also not the answer. Eating the wide range of natural unprocessed foods recommended throughout this book should help you attain your natural weight if you eat moderate portions.

You need some protein and fat at each meal. If you just eat sweets or starch alone, your body tends to convert this food into fat.

Giving Your Body Water

Make a habit of drinking a generous amount of filtered water throughout the day. If you have a cup of coffee, a diuretic, drink twice that amount of water. Drinking sufficient water can clear the mind, give you energy, and even smooth out fine wrinkles. (Read more about the benefits of water in Chapter 12.)

Eating to Keep Going

Constipation is not inevitable in old age. Eating high-fiber foods such as whole grains, vegetables, and fruits, drinking plenty of fluids, and making sure to regularly exercise can go a long way to help prevent this condition. Older individuals in other countries where natural, high-fiber foods are the norm are much less likely to be troubled by this problem.

If you do take laxatives to relieve your constipation, be aware that they can lead to a loss of minerals, such as potassium, and a loss of fluids. Mineral oil interferes with the absorption of the fat-soluble vitamins A, D, E, and K.

Eat Dinner Foods for Breakfast

Have leftovers from last night's dinner for breakfast. Refrigerator treasures such as filet of sole and cooked potatoes can be quickly reheated to provide a nutritious break from the same old, same old breakfast foods. Wholesome leftovers are far healthier than toaster tarts and sugar-coated breakfast cereal.

Making Meals with Medications in Mind

About half of everyone over 65 takes between two and five medications a day. If you're on any form of medication, you need to have your physician or the nutritionist who works with your doctor fully explain how the drugs you are taking may affect or interfere with what you eat. Some medications can reduce absorption and metabolism of certain nutrients and decrease appetite, especially if several are taken together. Taking a diuretic can leave you low in potassium. Antibiotics can result in deficiencies of folate and vitamin K. Be sure to add foods to your diet that replenish lost nutrients.

Filling Your Fridge

Is there a lonely head of lettuce, a loaf of bread, maybe some jam, and a little butter in your refrigerator and nothing much more? Many seniors, especially those who live alone, tend to be lax about giving themselves good food and enough of it. Take a quick inventory right now of what you have in your refrigerator and on your shelves. Are the foods that you find those you would serve an honored guest? Guess what. That's you!

Take the time and use the energy to do some really thoughtful shopping and plan some interesting meals for *yourself*. Buy that luscious-looking persimmon, the fresh asparagus in season, some pork chops, and a gourmet loaf of fresh-baked bread. As you eat more nutritious — and face it, more appetizing — foods, you can look forward to having more energy and generally better health.

Chapter 25

Ten Reasons to Begin Eating Healing Foods Today

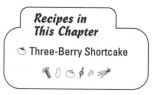

Recipes in This Chapter

☽ Three-Berry Shortcake

W hat you eat affects all aspects of your life. Your food choices even have an effect on the world around you. Start eating healthy foods from this moment on to begin reaping the rewards.

Save Money

Better to spend on groceries now than pay medical bills later. Whatever the price of fresh pineapple and free-range chicken, quality food is cheaper than health care. You also save the collective wealth when you support your health by simple means. Consider this: Arthritis costs the country 65 billion dollars annually. The direct and indirect costs of cardiovascular disease are 286.5 billion dollars per year in health expenditures and lost productivity.

Have More Energy

Nutritious natural foods are high-octane fuel. They provide vitamins, minerals, and special phytonutrients that make it possible for hundreds of body functions to occur. Nutrients such as B vitamins and magnesium allow your body to convert food into energy.

Get More Done

If you're a slow starter in the morning and wade through a major midafternoon low, you don't have much of the day left to get something done! But just think of what you could accomplish in a day if you were blessed with more stamina.

Play More

If you currently have just enough energy to keep you going 9 to 5, try changing what you eat. Begin to eat eggs, fruits, and whole grains for breakfast and fish, soups, fresh vegetables, salads, and tasty traditional dishes for your other meals. I predict that in a few weeks you'll begin to have more energy for your away-from-work life!

Be in a Better Mood

Nutrient deficiencies, highs and lows of blood sugar, and caffeine jitters can all affect your mood. On the other hand, unrefined, unprocessed foods, nourish the nervous system and the adrenal glands in charge of managing stress. Such foods can help you stay calm, even-tempered, and cheerful. Others may notice the difference, and you're likely to enjoy your own company more as well!

Reach a Healthy Weight

The standard American diet has plumped up the population. Current estimates are that 20 to 30 percent of adults and at least 25 to 30 percent of children are obese. The body is designed to demand food until it receives sufficient nourishment, not just calories. Starve it of nutrients, and you're likely to have vague cravings that keep you eating.

Become More Attractive

If your system is brimming with vitamins, minerals, phytonutrients, and healthy oils, your skin and hair will show it. No, you can't eat just one food or supplement with a particular nutrient and expect to be gorgeous. But eating a nutrient-rich, natural foods diet can help you look healthy and vital, both very attractive qualities. Eating clean food, free of pesticides and added chemicals, can also add to your aura of good health.

Protect the Environment

Eating organic produce is one way to do your part in putting a dent in the tonnage of pesticides and other chemicals ladled on growing plants and the land. By purchasing organic foods, you also support the farmers who have committed their futures to producing such food and the stores, which have taken a stand to sell it. When you buy organic produce, you help to keep organic foods an option in the marketplace and available to others.

Have a Youthful Old Age

What if you could live your 70s, 80s, and 90s in health rather than encumbered by disease? The risk of health problems such as arthritis, diabetes, and cardiovascular disease can often be significantly reduced by eating foods that heal rather than foods that harm.

Enjoy the Pleasures of the Table

By eating healing foods, you have good reason to look forward to mealtime and relish what you eat. Natural, fresh foods are full of taste and unique flavors. Take these foods into your body without fear — and fire the food police! Wholesome, nutritious creations, like good old-fashioned shortcake, are dishes to savor.

Three-Berry Shortcake

This version of strawberry shortcake uses an extravagant mix of berries full of healing flavonoids and biscuits made from spelt, an ancient grain. (For more on spelt, see Appendix B.)

Preparation time: 25 minutes

Cooking time: 18 minutes

Yield: 8 servings

(continued)

1 pint strawberries, preferably organic

½ pint blackberries, preferably organic

½ pint raspberries, preferably organic

¼ cup maple syrup

½ cup whipping cream (or 1 cup plain active-culture yogurt to turn this dessert into a luscious breakfast)

1 teaspoon vanilla extract

Butter for coating baking sheet

1⅓ cups finely ground spelt flour

2 teaspoons aluminumfree baking powder

1 pinch sea salt

⅔ cup milk, residuefree and preferably organic

1 Gently rinse berries. Remove strawberry stems and slice strawberries vertically.

2 In a medium bowl, partially mash strawberry slices. Add the blackberries, raspberries, and maple syrup and gently mix together. Set aside.

3 In a small bowl, combine the whipping cream and vanilla. Using an electric beater, whip the cream mixture. Cover and refrigerate.

4 Preheat oven to 425°. Butter the 12-by-15-inch baking sheet and set aside.

5 In a medium bowl, thoroughly combine the spelt flour, baking powder, and salt.

6 Gradually add the milk to the flour mixture, stirring just enough to wet dry ingredients.

7 Using a large soup spoon, scoop a generous spoonful of batter and drop onto baking sheet to form 8 to 10 biscuits. *Bake until brown, about 15 to 18 minutes.

8 Using a spatula, transfer biscuits to a cooling rack. Allow them to cool slightly and then split them in half. Arrange biscuit halves on individual serving plates or bowls. Spoon the berry mixture over the warm biscuits and top with whipping cream or yogurt. Dig in.

*If batter forms a peak, use the back of the spoon to press down peak so that the final biscuit will lay flat on plate.

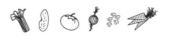

Appendix A

A to Z Guide to Ailments and Healing Foods

•••

*U*se this appendix to look up certain common ailments and find out the recommended diet for each. Under the listing for each ailment or disease, I include what foods are best to eat, which foods you should stay away from, and the special nutrients and medicinal herbs that may be helpful. Of course, this information is not meant to replace a physician's diagnosis or recommendations for your particular needs. A condition may require additional treatment beyond diet, but in general, the following information can give you a good starting point for using healing foods for prevention and recovery.

Acne: Eat whole grains, legumes, poultry, game, fresh fruits and vegetables, and high-fiber foods to promote normal bowel movements, and healthy fats including extra-virgin olive oil, unrefined vegetable oils, and flaxseed oil. Avoid sugar, refined white flour, unhealthy fats like margarine, refined and hydrogenated oils, fried foods, and milk and dairy products. Special nutrients: Vitamin A, antioxidants, B complex and especially vitamin B6, zinc, chromium, and essential fatty acids. Medicinal herbs: Dandelion, milk thistle, and goldenseal.

Age-related macular degeneration: Eat eggs, spinach, collard greens, and kale. Special nutrients: The carotenoids — lutein and zeaxanthin.

Anemia (iron deficiency): Eat iron-rich red meat and also dried beans, blackstrap molasses, dried fruit such as apricots, shellfish, plus vitamin C foods like citrus and sweet peppers. Avoid coffee and tea. Special nutrients: Iron and vitamin C.

Anxiety: Eat a piece of bread with an all-fruit preserve, alone and not with protein or fat. Best bites for tryptophan: Bananas, almonds, cashews, eggs, beef, and pork. Special nutrients: B complex, especially niacin and vitamin B6, vitamin C, calcium, chromium, magnesium, zinc. Medicinal herbs: Chamomile and valerian.

Arthritis: Eat a whole-foods diet that supplies complex carbohydrates, fiber, and antioxidants in whole grains, fruits, and vegetables. Select foods that can normalize weight. Avoid unhealthy fats including refined and hydrogenated oils and transfatty acids. Best bites: Sweet potatoes, cherries, blueberries, blackberries, citrus, millet, shrimp, almonds, spinach, chicken, walnuts, unrefined vegetable oils, and flaxseed oil. Avoid if you find these foods worsen symptoms: Tomatoes, eggplant, peppers, and potatoes. Special nutrients: Vitamin A, vitamins B5 and B6, vitamin C, vitamin E, copper, zinc, and essential fatty acids.

Asthma: To rule out dietary causes, avoid common allergens such as eggs, fish, shellfish, nuts and peanuts, milk, chocolate, wheat, citrus, and food colorings and preservatives. Best bites: Papaya, pineapple, garlic, onions, chili pepper, lima beans, brown rice, and dark green vegetables such as kale. Special nutrients: Magnesium, vitamin B6, vitamin B12, vitamin C, carotenes, vitamin E, and selenium. Medicinal herbs: Licorice and black and green tea.

Bad breath (halitosis): Nibble on parsley, swish your mouth with a solution of baking powder and water or allspice and water. Avoid onions and garlic. Take digestive enzymes including amylase, protease, and lipase. Brush your tongue. Have your dentist check for tooth decay.

Bladder infection (cystitis): Sip cranberry juice concentrate diluted in water (or take a cranberry capsule) or eat blueberries. Other best bites: Garlic, parsley, and celery root. Avoid caffeine, alcoholic beverages, including beer, and chocolate. Special nutrients: Vitamin C, bioflavonoids, vitamin A, beta-carotene, and zinc. Medicinal herbs: Uva ursi.

Brain fog: Drink plenty of filtered water. Have breakfast. Include in each meal some starch, protein, and fat. Avoid fatty meals, sugar, caffeinated beverages, and alcohol. Special nutrients: B complex including choline, folic acid, and vitamin B12. Medicinal herbs: Milk thistle. Check for sensitivities to foods such as wheat.

Bronchitis: Follow diet recommendations for treating colds. Enjoy chilies and spicy foods. Special nutrients: Zinc, vitamin C, bioflavonoids, vitamin A, and beta-carotene. Medicinal herbs: Comfrey, ginger, cayenne, echinacea, goldenseal, and licorice.

Burns (minor): Immediately put cold water (not a fat such as butter or oil) on affected area. Drink plenty of fluid.

Increase intake of foods that supply protein. Best bites: Meat, organic liver, green leafy vegetables, whole grains, oysters and shellfish, sweet potatoes, and sunflower and pumpkin seeds. Eat papaya and pineapple to reduce inflammation. Special nutrients: Vitamin A, vitamin C, folic acid, vitamin E, potassium, zinc, and essential fatty acids. Medicinal herbs used topically: Aloe vera, comfrey, St. John's wort, and marigold.

Carpal tunnel syndrome: Best bites: Turkey, fish, avocado, sweet potatoes, banana, lima beans, spinach, and navy beans. Avoid red meat. For inflammation: Eat turmeric, which contains curcumin, papaya, and pineapple. To increase circulation: Eat garlic, onion, and cayenne. Special nutrients: B complex, including vitamin B6.

Cataracts: Increase intake of foods that supply antioxidants, including leafy green vegetables, orange fruits and vegetables such as apricots and carrots, citrus, sweet peppers, and unrefined vegetable oils. Best bites: Organic liver, peas, avocado, berries, nuts, seeds, and yogurt. Don't smoke. Special nutrients: Zinc, selenium, vitamin A, vitamin C, vitamin E, riboflavin, flavanoids, and calcium. Medicinal herbs: Gingko biloba.

Cellulite: Eat whole-grain complex carbohydrates and high-fiber foods such as beans and lentils. Eat green and orange vegetables. Have healthy unrefined vegetable oils. Drink plenty of water. Avoid refined and hydrogenated oils, and transfatty acids, fried foods, and sugar. Limit salt and alcohol. Special nutrients: Vitamin A, beta-carotene, vitamin C, B complex, and essential fatty acids.

Cholesterol (elevated): Limit saturated fat and avoid sugar. Avoid excessive amounts of animal foods, which contain cholesterol. Increase intake of soluble fiber in foods, like oats and pears. Special nutrients: Antioxidants — beta-carotene, vitamin C, vitamin E, selenium, and essential

fatty acids. Nutrients that support the metabolization of cholesterol — B complex, vitamins C and E, magnesium, manganese, zinc, and lecithin.

Chronic fatigue syndrome: Eat a wholefoods diet that supplies ample protein, nutrients, and healthy fats, including butter, extra-virgin olive oil, and flaxseed oil. Best bites: Fish, poultry, beans, whole grains, vegetables. Avoid refined and processed foods, high intake of unhealthy refined and hydrogenated oils and transfatty acids, refined sugar, caffeine, and alcohol. Special nutrients: B complex vitamins, especially thiamin, pantothenic acid, vitamin B6, folate, and vitamin B12, betacarotene, vitamin C, vitamin E, and the minerals iron, magnesium, manganese, molybdenum, and selenium, and essential fatty acids.

Cold sores: Follow a vegetarian diet. Best bites: Cooked vegetables such as winter squash, carrots, bell peppers, broccoli, beans, pureed fruit, cantaloupe juice, wellcooked brown rice and oats, garlic, onion, and plain yogurt. Avoid fried foods, sugar, coffee and black tea, spices, chocolate, alcohol, and crunchy foods that can irritate tissues. Special nutrients: Vitamin A, vitamin B complex, vitamin C, vitamin E, and zinc. Medicinal herbs: Lemon balm, echinacea, siberian ginseng, nettle, and goldenseal.

Colds: Drink plenty of fluids such as filtered water, vegetable juice, herbal tea, and chicken broth, especially beverages that are hot. Eat mostly plant foods: Fruits, vegetables, beans and lentils, nuts, and seeds rather than meat. Best bites: Winter acorn and hubbard squash, watercress, lamb, whole grains, sea vegetables, melons, tropical fruit, garlic, onions, chili peppers, ginger, and fennel. Avoid sugar, eggs, grains, dairy products, and starchy root vegetables such as potatoes. Special nutrients: Vitamin A, vitamin C, zinc, and the amino acid lysine. Medicinal herbs: Echinacea and goldenseal.

Constipation: Best bites: Whole grains such as whole wheat and oats, legumes, fresh fruits such as figs and prunes, vegetables, nuts, and seeds. Avoid processed and refined foods including white flour and sugar. Herbal laxatives: Senna, aloe vera, cascara sagrada, and psyllium seed husks.

Cystitis: See Bladder infection.

Dandruff: Follow a nutritious whole-foods diet with an emphasis on raw foods. Include high-fiber foods for digestive health and healthy fats such as unrefined vegetable oils, butter, and flaxseed oil. Drink plenty of water and avoid food additives to rid the body of toxins. Reduce intake of poor quality fats such as refined and hydrogenated oils and transfatty acids, and avoid all fried foods. Avoid sugar and reduce dairy products. If diagnosed as a yeast problem, follow the recommendations under Yeast infection. Special nutrients: B complex, biotin, zinc, essential fatty acids.

Depression: Avoid refined flour, sugar, caffeine, and alcohol. Follow the diet for low blood sugar included in this appendix and also monitor for food sensitivities and exposure to environmental toxins and heavy metals. Special nutrients: B vitamins including thiamin, niacin, vitamin B6, folic acid, and also lecithin, vitamin C, calcium, and zinc. Medicinal herbs: St. John's wort and lemon balm.

Dermatitis: Try eliminating grains with glutens (wheat, oats, rye, and barley) and avoid dairy products. Enjoy green vegetables such as broccoli and kale, whole grains, and fatty fish like salmon and tuna. Best Bite: Yogurt with live cultures. Take digestive enzymes. Special nutrients: B complex including vitamin B6, magnesium, zinc, and essential fatty acids.

Diabetes: Have three moderate-sized meals a day, plus between meal snacks, including one at bedtime. Avoid all concentrated sweets including white sugar, maple syrup, honey, and fruit juice. Include some protein and fat in each meal and snack. Eat whole grains rather than refined. Limit fat intake to 20 percent to 25 percent of calories: Enjoy lowfat sources of protein such as beans. Increase fiber. Special foods: Nopales cactus, flaxseeds, dandelion, juniper berries, and fenugreek. Special nutrients: Chromium and manganese in particular, plus niacin, vitamin B6, biotin, vitamin C, vitamin E, magnesium, potassium, selenium, and zinc.

Diarrhea: Drink plenty of fluids such as filtered water, diluted vegetable and fruit juices, and broths. Avoid all solid food in the acute stage and then begin with soups, stewed fruit, and steamed rice, adding a little salt. Best bites: As diet advances, add bananas, live culture yogurt, whole grains, legumes, apples, beets, carrots, and potatoes.

Earache, ear infection: Increase intake of fruits and vegetables. Reduce fat intake. Best bites: Anti-inflammatory foods like pineapple, papaya, ginger, onion, garlic, walnuts, and flaxseed oil. Avoid refined sugar and foods that trigger inflammation, such as red meat and dairy products. Special nutrients: Vitamin A, vitamin C, and zinc.

Eczema (chronic, itching, inflammatory skin condition): Drink plenty of filtered water and follow a whole-foods diet, which provides plenty of fruits and vegetables (especially dark leafy greens, winter squash, onions, berries, and citrus), nuts, and pumpkin seeds and enjoy fish and legumes for protein. Rule out food sensitivity to dairy foods and grains that contain gluten. Special nutrients: Zinc, essential fatty acids, vitamin A, beta-carotene, vitamin C, bioflavonoids, vitamin E, and selenium. Healing supplements: Evening primrose oil, licorice root, and goldenseal.

Enlarged prostate (benign prostatic hyperplasia): Eat a diet high in plant foods with smaller amounts of animal protein, especially fish. Consume only organic, hormonefree ingredients. Best bites: Pumpkin seeds, sardines, organic liver, lean beef, and Brazil nuts. Lower intake of saturated fatty acids and avoid refined and hydrogenated oils. Avoid sugar. Maintain a normal weight. Special nutrients: Zinc, vitamin B5, vitamin B6, vitamin E, selenium, and essential fatty acids (the equivalent of 1 teaspoon a day). Medicinal herbs: Saw palmetto, pygeum, flower pollen, and ginseng.

Fatigue: Drink several glasses of filtered water over five minutes. Take a ten-minute walk outdoors. Breathe fresh air. Rest. Avoid caffeinated coffee, tea, colas, and chocolate. Notice whether you have more or less energy after eating meat and other animal foods and and if you do feel tired after such a meal, follow a more vegetarian diet. Special nutrients: B complex, vitamin C, vitamin E, iron, magnesium, potassium, zinc, and essential fatty acids.

Fibrocystic breast disease: Avoid caffeine in coffee, tea, and chocolate. Best bites: Avocado, unrefined vegetable oils such as extra-virgin olive oil, raw nuts, seeds, and dark green and orange vegetables. Follow a basically vegetarian diet with some fish and poultry. Select organic meats, poultry, and produce to avoid added hormones and pesticides. Eat high-fiber foods and active-culture yogurt for bowel health. Special nutrients: Beta-carotene and vitamin E.

Flu: For prevention: Eat a varied, nutritious whole-foods diet that includes whole grains, salads, vegetables, meats, poultry, fish, citrus, and seeds and nuts, such as pumpkin and Brazil nuts. Avoid refined and processed foods, white sugar and flour, and processed fats. Best bites for treatment: Melon, papaya, mango, pineapple, cinnamon, ginger, garlic, honey, and herbal tea. Limit starchy foods and dairy products. Special nutrients: Vitamin C, bioflavonoids, vitamin A, beta-carotene, and zinc.

Fluid retention (edema): Decrease sodium intake and increase foods that contain potassium, like potatoes, green leafy vegetables, parsley, meats, nuts (unsalted), sunflower seeds, and blackstrap molasses. Drink sufficient filtered water. Best bites: Asparagus, artichoke, black currants, celery, cucumbers, parsley, blueberries, blackberries, cherries, and citrus. Check for food allergies. Special nutrients: Vitamin B6 and the amino acid taurine.

Food sensitivity: You may need to avoid one or more of the following: Grains that include gluten (wheat, rye, oats, and barley), sulfites in fruit, processed meats, wine, beer, restaurant foods such as avocado dip, salads, and potatoes. Other common sensitivities: Milk, chocolate, wheat, citrus, berries, soy products, foods that contain salicylates, and additives such as MSG, food coloring, sulfites, and preservatives.

Gas: Foods that tend to cause gas: Milk, dried beans and peas, onion, broccoli, caulifower, turnips, foods that contain soluble fiber such as oats and apples, and all starch including potatoes, bread, and pasta. Rice is the least likely to cause problems. Best bites: Garlic, ginger, fennel, dill, caraway, cinnamon, and cardamon added to foods as they cook. Medicinal herbs: Peppermint and chamomile.

Gout: Omit foods that contain purines: Meat, organ meats, shellfish, brewer's and baker's yeast, sardines, herring, mackerel, anchovies, spinach, and soybeans. Keep refined flour and saturated fat to a minimum. Avoid refined sugar. Keep protein intake low. Eliminate all alcohol. Best bites: Cherries, blueberries, blackberries, celery, parsley, onions, leeks, and apples. Special nutrients: Essential fatty acids, niacin, vitamin B5, folate, vitamin C, vitamin E, and selenium. Special supplements: Bromelain and quercetin.

Gum, infected (gingivitis): Eat high-fiber foods such as whole grains and raw vegetables. Avoid refined and processed soft foods. Best bites: Carrots, winter squash, avocados, citrus, seafood, pumpkin seeds. Special nutrients: Vitamin A, folic acid, vitamin C, flavonoids, zinc, and co-enzyme Q10. Floss your teeth daily.

Hair and scalp (dry): Eat natural foods high in B vitamins, antioxidants and essential fatty acids. Best bites: Whole grains, orange and green vegetables, fish, butter, unrefined vegetable oil including extra-virgin olive oil, walnuts, and flaxseed oil. Special nutrients: Vitamin A, B complex, vitamin E, beta-carotene, biotin, vitamin C, vitamin D, selenium, zinc, iron, and essential fatty acids.

Hay fever: Best bites: Garlic, onions, papaya, pineapple, flaxseeds, and flaxseed oil, walnuts, fatty fish, horseradish, cloves, cinnamon, ginger, rosemary, thyme, licorice, and raw honey and honeycomb. Increase foods high in fiber. Avoid red meats, coffee, sugar, white flour, foods that worsen mucus, including potatoes, white flour, and dairy foods. Special nutrients: Vitamin C, omega-3 essential fatty acids, and quercetin. Medicinal herbs: Echinacea, elderflower, hyssop, and nettle.

Headaches: For a common headache, try eating something salty such as olives cured in brine or Japanese preserved Umeboshi plums. If this does not produce relief in a few minutes, try quickly drinking several glasses of cool water or have a glass of cool apple juice. Avoid common triggers such as MSG, aspartame, and certain processed, preserved, and fermented foods (these include processed ham, wine, and pickles), which may contain nitrites, sulfites, tyramine, or artificial food coloring. Medicinal herbs: Feverfew.

Heart disease: Prevention: Eat heart-protective foods, such as fish, fruits and vegetables, whole grains, legumes, nuts such as almonds and walnuts, seeds, olive oil, garlic, and onions. Include foods with soluble fiber, such as oats and legumes. Reduce intake of saturated fat and cut out regular consumption of sugar and sweets. Avoid all processed and hydrogenated oils. Special nutrients: B complex, antioxidants, chromium, magnesium, manganese, zinc, lecithin, and omega-3 fatty acids.

Heartburn: Avoid fried, fatty, and very acidic foods, especially eaten in combination, such as a corned beef sandwich, french fries, and coffee. Avoid peppermint tea. Medicinal herbs: Ginger, licorice, and aloe vera.

Hemorrhoids: See a physician. Follow a whole-foods diet with an emphasis on raw fruits and vegetables. Increase high-fiber foods such as dried figs and whole grains to avoid constipation. Have 1 tablespoon a day of unrefined vegetable oil. Best bites: Cherries, blueberries, blackberries, currants, and citrus including the rind and pulp. Drink plenty of filtered water. If severe, may require a soft and liquid diet.

Herpes: Foods that contain the amino acid lysine (fish, seafood, chicken, turkey, and eggs) can inhibit the recurrence of herpes. Avoid chocolate, nuts, seeds, and coconut. Special nutrients: Vitamin C, zinc, and L-lysine. Medicinal herbs: Echinacea and, for external use in salves, aloe, goldenseal, lavender, and licorice root.

High blood pressure: Reduce sodium and increase potassium intake. Consume adequate magnesium and calcium in such foods as broccoli and figs. Avoid sugar. Special nutrients: Potassium, magnesium, calcium, and the amino acid taurine.

Hot flashes: Best bites: Flax seeds and flaxseed oil, green vegetables, unrefined vegetable oils, plant foods, and soybeans to supply phytohormones. Drink plenty of filtered water. Avoid common triggers such as coffee and caffeine, alcohol, sugar, and spices. Special nutrients: Phytohormones, vitamin E, and magnesium to help prevent hot flashes and sodium, potassium, and magnesium to replenish minerals lost in perspiration. Medicinal herbs: Dong quai and black cohosh.

Hypothyroidism: Eat seafood and seaweed. Drink filtered tap water. Limit eating certain foods if they are raw — broccoli, cauliflower, spinach, turnips, cabbage, pears, and millet. Special nutrients: Iodine, vitamin A, riboflavin, niacin, vitamin B6, vitamin C, vitamin E, manganese, zinc, and the amino acid tyrosine.

Impotence (erectile dysfunction): Follow a heart-healthy diet and eat organic foods free of added hormones. Limit alcohol and caffeine. Don't smoke. Special nutrients: Zinc, vitamin E, B complex, Vitamin B6, PABA (para-aminobenzoic acid), magnesium, manganese, and selenium.

Indigestion: Best bites: Celery, asparagus, papaya, pineapple, oats, parsley, horseradish, fennel, ginger, and cinnamon. Eat fruit, especially melon, separate from other foods. Limit meat and dairy products. Avoid fried foods and fatty meats. Special nutrients: Digestive enzymes including amylase, protease, and lipase. Medicinal teas: Peppermint and chamomile.

Infection: Follow a basically vegetarian diet with some fish or poultry. Avoid refined sugar and limit whole fruit and fruit juice, including orange juice, which contain fruit sugar. Enjoy broths and herbal teas. Special nutrients: Vitamin A, beta-carotene, vitamin C, flavonoids, zinc, vitamin B6, and iron. Medicinal herbs: Echinacea, goldenseal, and licorice.

Injury (minor trauma or damage to some part of the body): Eat a nourishing wholefoods diet. Best bites for inflammation: Tuna, salmon, sardines, pineapple, papaya, apples, black currants, ginger, onion, garlic, sage, hot chili peppers, walnuts, and flaxseed oil. Avoid refined sugar and foods that trigger inflammation, such as red meat and dairy products. Special nutrients:

Vitamin C, B complex, vitamin A, and zinc. Medicinal herbs: Comfrey applied as an ointment. Tip: Immediately after injury, apply ice to bruises and swollen area, 15 minutes on and 15 minutes off. Use heat only after a few days if injury persists.

Insomnia: Avoid all caffeine in coffee, tea, and chocolate. Before retiring, eat a small portion of a starchy food, such as a piece of whole-wheat toast with all-fruit preserve, alone and not with protein or fat. Special nutrients: B vitamins including vitamin B6, vitamin B12, and inositol, vitamin C, calcium, magnesium, and potassium. Medicinal herbs: Chamomile and valerian.

Jet lag: Have one glass of filtered water every hour while you're in the plane. During the flight, snack on mineral-rich raw nuts, seeds, and fruits such as bananas and dried figs. Avoid caffeine and alcohol before and during the flight. Catch some direct sunshine (best in the late afternoon) once you arrive and don't wear sunglasses! Special nutrients: Melatonin.

Joint pain: Follow the diet for Arthritis, earlier in this appendix.

Kidney stones: Requires a physician's attention for analysis of composition of stones to customize diet. May require reducing consumption of red meat, following a vegetarian diet, limiting sodium intake, eating adequate but not excessive calcium, and avoiding foods that contain oxalic acid, especially spinach, beet greens, Swiss chard, and rhubarb. Drink adequate water. Special nutrients: Magnesium, vitamin B6, vitamin A, thiamin, vitamin D, and potassium if deficient.

Laryngitis: Sip vegetable broths and enjoy melon. Best bites: Papaya, pineapple, ginger, garlic, onion, cardamom, and nutmeg. Avoid sugar, white flour, fried foods, coffee, and black tea. Special nutrients: Vitamin A, vitamin C, and zinc (in the form of zinc lozenges.). Medicinal herbs: Spearmint, licorice, thyme, and rosemary.

Low blood sugar (hypoglycemia): Best bites: Eat some protein and fat for each meal and snack, eat whole grains rather than refined, and eat small meals more frequently. Avoid sugar and concentrated sweets, including maple syrup, honey, and fruit juice. Special nutrients: Chromium, manganese, zinc, essential fatty acids, and co-enzyme Q10.

Lower back pain: Follow a diet low in saturated fat and high in fiber. Try having a small serving of complex carbohydrates, such as oatmeal, alone, without fat or protein. Avoid sugar and other concentrated sweets, including fruit juice, maple syrup, and honey, and avoid fried foods and all processed fats and hydrogenated oils. Don't smoke.

Memory: Enjoy a nutritious, natural-foods diet and avoid refined and processed foods. Best bites: Shellfish, meat, organic liver, chicken, legumes, whole grains, mushrooms, dark leafy greens, dates, figs, apricots, citrus, almonds, pumpkin seeds, and whole grains. Special nutrients: Thiamin, riboflavin, choline, inositol, beta-carotene, vitamin C, iron, zinc, and phytohormones in flax seeds, buckwheat, and soybeans as well as many other plant foods. Medicinal herbs: Gingko biloba.

Menopause: Follow a whole-foods diet and avoid refined and processed foods. Enjoy organic ingredients and avoid added hormones in meat. Eat plenty of plant foods, which supply phytohormones, including buckwheat, currants, soybeans, flax seed, and unrefined oils. Special nutrients: Phytohormones, flavonoids (including ipriflavone supplements), B complex, vitamin C, vitamin E, and magnesium. Medicinal herbs: Black cohosh and dong quai.

Menstrual cramps: Avoid red meat and dairy foods. Try chicken and turkey or eat vegetarian for a few days and eat beans and whole grains for protein. Increase foods that supply fiber. Avoid processed cheese and other high sodium foods. Avoid sugar

and sweets. Special nutrients: Magnesium, calcium, and essential fatty acids.

Migraine headache: Avoid common triggers (dairy products, chocolate, eggs, citrus, meat, poultry, fish, wheat, nuts, peanuts, tomatoes, onions, corn, apples, and bananas) and any foods to which you are sensitive. Also avoid caffeine, alcohol, MSG, aspartame, sulfites, and nitrites in preserved meats. Best bites: Organic foods, including organic meats without added hormones and organic residuefree poultry. Special nutrients: Vitamin A, magnesium, and calcium.

Mood swings: Include in each meal or snack a source of complex carbohydrate, protein, and fat, avoid all refined sugar, natural sweeteners, and fruit juice. Eat three meals a day and, if needed, snack between meals and at bedtime. Eat organic foods and avoid hormones in animal products. Increase intake of seafood for fish oils. Eat more plant foods, which supply phytohormones, such as soybeans, buckwheat, and currants. Avoid added hormones in animal products. Don't smoke.

Morning sickness: Drink ginger tea on waking. Eat a bedtime snack of nuts, dried, fruit, seeds, crackers, or a healthy cookie, plus filtered water.

Muscle cramps and spasm: Follow a whole-foods diet rather than refined and processed. Special nutrients: Calcium, magnesium, and vitamin E. Special herbs: St. John's wort, valerian, skullcap, peppermint, and chamomile.

Muscle strain: Anti-inflammatory foods such as seafood, pineapple, papaya, apples, black currants, ginger, onion, garlic, sage, hot chili peppers, walnuts, and flaxseed oil. Avoid refined sugar and foods that trigger inflammation, such as red meat and dairy products. Supplement with papain and bromelain enzymes.

Nausea: Best bites: Ginger and peppermint and chamomile teas to start and, as nausea subsides and solid food is resumed, bananas, rice, dry toast, and active culture plain yogurt. Avoid acidic citrus fruit juices, coffee, and black tea. For motion sickness: Eat ginger and avoid fatty foods.

Osteoporosis: Avoid or limit your intake of acidifying foods that promote bone loss, including red meat, white flour and sugar, carbonated beverages, coffee, black tea, caffeine, and salt. Best bites: Consume moderate amounts of fish, shellfish, poultry and chicken broth made with the bones, as well as fruit, vegetables, whole grains, legumes, nuts, and seeds. Special nutrients: Calcium (supplemented in the form of calcium citrate or microcrystalline hydroxyapatite), magnesium, boron, copper, manganese, silicon, strontium, zinc, vitamin B6, folic acid, vitamin C, vitamin D, and vitamin K.

Premenstrual syndrome: Eat whole foods rather than refined and processed. Also eat plant foods that supply phytohormones, such as buckwheat, soybeans, currants, and unrefined oils including essential fatty acids. Enjoy organic foods and avoid added hormones in meats. Avoid refined sugar, excess salt, caffeine, and alcohol.

Psoriasis (skin rash or plaques): Eat high-fiber foods such as beans, peas, apples, and cauliflower as well as fish, flax seed, and walnuts. Give yourself ten to 15 minutes a day of morning or afternoon sunshine. Avoid or limit red meat and dairy products, alcohol, sugar, and chemical additives. Try eliminating wheat, rye, oats, and barley, the grains with gluten. Special foods: Fish, walnuts, unrefined vegetable oils. Special nutrients: Zinc, chromium, vitamin E, selenium, folic acid, vitamin C, B-complex, and essential fatty acids. Medicinal herbs: Milk thistle (silymarin is the active ingredient) and goldenseal.

Rheumatoid arthritis: Eat a natural foods diet rather than one that is refined and processed. Best bites: Antioxidant-rich foods, such as green and orange vegetables, and anti-inflammatory foods like tuna, salmon, sardines, pineapple, papaya, apples, black currants, ginger, onion, garlic, sage, hot chili peppers, walnuts, and flaxseed oil. Avoid refined sugar and foods that trigger inflammation, such as red meat and dairy products. Be tested for food allergies to rule out this cause.

Sexuality, lack of desire: Increase intake of zinc-rich foods, such as fish and shellfish, especially oysters, pumpkin seeds, sunflower seeds, mushrooms, meats, and cheese. Avoid sugar and caffeine. Special nutrients: B complex, vitamin C, vitamin E, and essential fatty acids.

Shingles: Enjoy papaya, apricots, sweet peppers, orange vegetables, purple grapes, liver, eggs, chicken, fish, active-culture yogurt, and unrefined vegetable oil such as extra-virgin olive oil. Avoid sugar and alcohol and limit salt. Special nutrients: Vitamin B12, vitamin C, vitamin E, flavonoids, and antioxidants.

Sinusitis: Follow diet recommendations for treating colds. Medicinal herbs: Comfrey and ginger.

Sore throat: Eat lightly and go vegetarian. Best bites: Tropical fruit, melon, whole grains, legumes, orange and green vegetables, and garlic. Avoid all refined and natural sweeteners, coffee, and teas except for herbal. Special nutrients: Zinc (in the form of zinc lozenges). Medicinal herbs: Slippery elm and chamomile.

Stress: Eat a varied, natural foods diet. Avoid refined sugar and flours and caffeine. Special nutrients: Vitamin C, zinc, magnesium, potassium, and B-complex, especially vitamin B5 (pantothenic acid). Medicinal herbs: Ginseng, chamomile, rose hips, valerian root, skullcap, passionflower, and pau d'arco.

Sunburn: See Burns.

Surgery: Increase protein foods, including fish and legumes. Include whole grains such as kasha, legumes, spinach and beets for iron, and citrus for vitamin C. Eat anti-inflammatory foods like tuna, salmon, sardines, pineapple, papaya, apples, black currants, ginger, onion, garlic, sage, hot chili peppers, walnuts, and flax seed oil. Avoid refined sugar and foods that trigger inflammation, such as red meat and dairy products. Special nutrients: Vitamin A, B complex including B6, vitamin C, flavonoids, and zinc.

Tooth decay: Avoid sugary foods and minimize natural sweeteners. After eating sweets and drinking fruit juice, swish your mouth with water. Brush your teeth after eating sweet foods such as currants and other dried fruit, which cling to teeth. Chew your food well. Floss once a day. Brush after breakfast. Best bites: Green tea rather than coffee or black tea. If supplementing with chewable vitamin C, after taking this, swish your mouth with water.

Toothache: Rub oil of clove directly on the affected area for immediate, short-term relief. Eat papaya and pineapple. Take supplements of bromelain and papain, along with the homeopathic remedy, arnica.

Ulcers: Best nutrients for prevention: Vitamin A, vitamin E, zinc, found in winter squash, unrefined vegetable oil, seafood, plus essential fatty acids and high-fiber foods like whole grains. Avoid beer, tobacco, coffee (caffeinated and decaffeinated), and foods that may trigger an allergic reaction. Best bites for treatment: Bananas, plantains, cabbage juice, New Zealand manuka honey, and licorice. Avoid milk and dairy products and black pepper but not other spices. Medicinal herbs: Aloe vera (taken as a juice), chamomile, goldenseal, sage, and slippery elm.

Vaginal infection: See Infection for treatment. Best bite: Yogurt with active cultures. Special nutrients: Vitamin A, vitamin C, zinc, and acidophilus. Medicinal herbs: Pau d'arco.

Varicose veins: Enjoy foods that supply flavonoids — all berries, buckwheat, currants, citrus including the pulp and membranes, along with foods that supply vitamin C including citrus, sweet peppers, cantaloupe, broccoli, and tomatoes. Special nutrients: Flavonoids, vitamin C, vitamin E, and zinc.

Yeast infection (Candida albicans): Best bites: All vegetables but limit starchy ones such as potatoes, corn, and parsnip. Protein foods, including meat, poultry, fish, legumes, and whole grains. Limit fruit intake to berries, including blueberries, cherries, apples, and pears, and have 2 cups of raw fruit daily. Eliminate all refined sugar as well as fruit sugars except for fruit just listed, maple syrup, and honey. Avoid foods that contain yeast or mold (cheese, dried fruit, melon, peanuts, and alcoholic beverages). Avoid milk and dairy products, which contain milk sugar and traces of antibiotics. Eliminate all food allergens. Special nutrients: Iron, zinc, and selenium. Medicinal spices and herbs: Garlic, ginger, cinnamon, thyme, rosemary, chamomile, pau d'arco, and barberry. Supplements: L. acidophilus, pancreatic enzymes, psyllium seeds, caprilic acid, and grapefruit seed extract.

Appendix B
A to Z Guide to Healing Foods

• •

*E*ach food in this guide is followed by a list of the nutrients it contains, with the most abundant toward the front and those present in smaller amounts toward the end, plus the names of featured phytochemicals. Next come various health benefits and then pertinent tips on such topics as buying, storing, cooking, and eating. At the end of each section are the names of some of the recipes in this book that include the particular ingredient. There's no lack of healthy foods and seemingly no limit to the health benefits they can provide!

Apples: *Nutrients:* Beta-carotene, B-complex, potassium, boron, soluble fiber, and pectin. *Health benefits:* Aids digestion of fatty foods, promotes elimination, supports good circulation and heart health, detoxifying, helps prevent osteoporosis, cancer, and strokes, recommended for arthritis, rheumatism, and gout. *Tips:* Enjoy raw or cooked, preferably organic. *Recipes:* Apple and Almond Cobbler (Chapter 19).

Apricots: *Nutrients:* Beta-carotene and potassium. *Health benefits:* Slows aging process and protects against high blood pressure. *Tips:* Eat fresh and dried apricots and buy dark orange, not bright orange, dried apricots, which are treated with sulfur dioxide. *Recipes:* Hot Flash Fruit Compote (Chapter 17) and North African Roast Chicken with Almonds and Dried Fruits (Chapter 11).

Artichokes: *Nutrients:* B vitamins, especially folic acid, potassium, iron, and fiber. *Health benefits:* Aids digestion, reduces fluid retention, supports liver function, and lowers cholesterol and risk of heart disease. *Tips:* Store in a dark, cool, dry place and wrap individually. *Recipes:* Artichokes with Mediterranean Garlic Sauce (Chapter 17).

Asparagus: *Nutrients:* Beta-carotene, B complex, vitamin C, and potassium. *Health benefits:* Diuretic, good for cystitis, constipation, arthritis, and rheumatism, and helps prevent heart disease and cancer. *Tips:* Cook quickly in a little water, uncovered, to prevent asparagus from turning a drab olive green. *Recipes:* None.

Avocado: *Nutrients:* Folic acid; vitamins A, D, and E, potassium; magnesium; calcium; and monounsaturated fats. *Health benefits:* Protects against heart disease and birth defects, lowers blood pressure, and helps prevent cancer and osteoporosis. *Tips:* Drizzle with lemon juice to prevent turning brown. *Recipes:* White Chili (Chapter 19).

Bananas, plantains: *Nutrients:* Potassium, magnesium, vitamin B6, and vitamin C. *Health benefits:* Soothing and promotes a sense of well-being, lowers high blood pressure. Less ripened bananas are good for constipation. Plantains traditionally used to help prevent and treat stomach ulcers. *Tips:* Enjoy raw or cooked. *Recipes:* Banana from Havana (Chapter 20).

Barley: *Nutrients:* Calcium, iron, potassium, phosphorus, protein, and fiber. *Health benefits:* Low in gluten, helps remove toxins from the body by stimulating the liver and lymphatic system, good food for convalescing, and helps manage levels of cholesterol and fat in the body. *Tips:* Use whole barley, which is highest in nutrients, rather than pearled barley. *Recipes:* None.

Beans: *Nutrients:* Lowfat source of quality protein and minerals, including calcium, magnesium, iron, and potassium. *Health benefits:* Good for heart and bone health, and weight loss. *Tips:* Store beans in a container that is air-tight and moisture-proof, and keep in a cool, dark place; add salt *after* cooking so beans don't toughen. *Recipes:* Sunday Supper White Bean Soup (Chapter 5).

Beef: *Nutrients:* Protein, zinc, potassium, iron, niacin, vitamin B6, and other B vitamins. *Health benefits:* Strengthens immunity, promotes tissue healing after injury and surgery, aids in the delivery of oxygen to the cells and energizes, and maintains healthy muscle tissue. *Tips:* Ground beef, refrigerated, stays fresh only 1 to 2 days, while other cuts last 3 to 5 days. *Recipes:* Broiled Steak Salad with Roasted Red Peppers (Chapter 7).

Beer: *Nutrients:* Niacin and other B vitamins and small amounts of minerals. *Health benefits:* Counteracts general fatigue, helps alleviate fluid retention, and increases level of desirable cholesterol. *Tips:* Up to a half pint a day is a medicinal dose. Cook in glass or enamel to avoid discoloring. *Recipes:* Milwaukee Pork Chops with Cabbage (Chapter 7).

Beets: *Nutrients:* Iron, folic acid, potassium (beet greens are very high in beta-carotene), calcium, and phosphorus. *Health benefits:* Beets strengthen blood and help prevent birth defects; beet greens lower risk of degenerative diseases. *Tips:* Cook for maximum nutrients and flavor, serve immediately to reduce generation of carcinogenic nitrites, may turn urine and feces red in individuals genetically unable to break down beet pigments. *Recipes:* None.

Berries (strawberry, blueberry, blackberry, raspberry): *Nutrients:* Flavonoids and vitamin C. *Health benefits:* Help prevent capillary fragility and associated menstrual cramping, varicose veins, and increased risk of heart disease, help balance hormones, and boost immunity. *Tips:* Short shelf life, eat fresh. *Recipes:* Three-Berry Shortcake (Chapter 25).

Blackstrap molasses: *Nutrients:* High in iron, calcium, and potassium. *Health benefits:* Sweetener, which provides energy as well as nutrients; helps prevent anemia and high blood pressure and strengthens bones. *Tips:* Medium, mild-tasting molasses provides fewer nutrients. *Recipes:* Apple and Almond Cobbler (Chapter 19).

Blueberries: *Nutrients:* Potassium, niacin, and other B vitamins. *Health benefits:* Antibacterial properties, useful for intestinal infections due to *E coli,* an effective treatment for cystitis. *Tips:* Enjoy fresh and in season. *Recipes:* Fruity Flavonoid Syrup (Chapter 20).

Broccoli: *Nutrients:* Beta-carotene, vitamin C, folic acid, calcium, magnesium, iron, and indoles. *Health benefits:* Helps protect against cancers of the digestive tract and supports general good health. *Tips:* To activate cancer-protective indoles, cut and lightly cook, but avoid overcooking. *Recipes:* Boston Lettuce Crudite (Chapter 23).

Brown rice, rice syrup: *Nutrients:* Magnesium, selenium, manganese, niacin and other B vitamins, and fiber; rice syrup is 50 percent slow-burning complex carbohydrates. *Health benefits:* Glutenfree, helps control blood sugar, strengthens bones, and helps maintain production of sex hormones. *Tips:* Retains nutritional value for several days after cooking. *Recipes:* None.

Buckwheat (kasha and buckwheat flour): *Nutrients:* A cereal plant, not a grain, which supplies potassium, rutin, phosphorus, calcium, vitamin E, vitamin B6, and phytoestrogens. *Health benefits:* Helps reduce symptoms of PMS and perimenopause, strengthens and tones walls of blood vessels, and helps prevent hardening of the arteries. *Tips:* Has a short cooking time, about 10 to 12 minutes. *Recipes:* Turkish Buckwheat Salad (Chapter 17).

Bulgur wheat: *Nutrients:* Steamed, dried, and crushed whole wheat high in niacin, plus other B vitamins, iron, calcium, protein, and fiber. *Health benefits:* Lowers risk of diverticulitis and certain cancers, fuels energy production, and supports transport of oxygen to the cells. *Tips:* Sold in natural-food stores, quick-cooking. *Recipes:* Turkish Buckwheat Salad (Chapter 17) can be made with bulgur wheat.

Butter: *Nutrients:* Vitamin A, vitamin E, traces of minerals including calcium and selenium, saturated fat. *Health benefits:* Source of energy, easy to digest for patients with liver and digestive ailments, saturated fatty acids nourish friendly intestinal flora and inhibit yeast growth, form vital part of cell membranes, can be converted into sex hormones. *Tips:* Buy unsalted and organic, suitable for cooking at high temperatures. *Recipes:* Cod Cakes with Tomato Tarragon Sauce (Chapter 25).

Cabbage: *Nutrients:* Potassium, vitamin C, calcium, folic acid, phytoestrogens, and indoles. *Health benefits:* Juice is a tonic for ulcers, helps in reducing high blood pressure, strengthens bones, and helps balance hormones. Indoles protect against stomach cancer. *Tips:* Slice and lightly cook to activate the cancer-fighting chemicals. *Recipes:* Milwaukee Pork Chops with Cabbage (Chapter 7).

Cactus (nopales): *Nutrients:* High in calcium and fiber. *Health benefits:* Promotes regularity, relieves constipation, reduces stomach acidity helping to prevent gastritis and gastric ulcers, reduces cholesterol, and lowers blood sugar levels for treatment of type 2 diabetes mellitus. *Tips:* Available fresh and canned in markets serving Latin customers. *Recipes:* None.

Carrot: *Nutrients:* Beta-carotene, lycopenes, and fiber. *Health benefits:* Ensures night vision, boosts immunity, good for health of the skin, lining of the digestive tract, and heart, and functions as an antioxidant to fight arthritis and some forms of cancer. *Tips:* Eat both raw for the fiber and cooked for the beta-carotene, which heating makes more available. *Recipes:* Antioxidant Cocktail (Chapter 16), Savory Baked Vegetables (Chapter 6), and Beta-Carotene Carrots — Three Ways (Chapter 15).

Cauliflower: *Nutrients:* Niacin, folic acid, vitamin C, potassium and indoles. *Health benefits:* Enhances immunity and energy production, supports the production of red blood cells, and protects against cancer. *Tips:* Steam to preserve most of the vitamin C and activate cancer-protective indoles. *Recipes:* Boston Lettuce Crudite (Chapter 23).

Caviar: *Nutrients:* Sodium, calcium, iron, and omega-3 essential fatty acids. *Health benefits:* Protects against heart disease by helping to prevent blood clots and lowering triglycerides, and anti-inflammatory action lessens swelling and pain associated with PMS and the symptoms of hay fever and inflammatory joint disease. *Tips:* Relish raw, used as a garnish. *Recipes:* Caviar for Company (Chapter 23).

Cayenne: *Nutrients:* Prepared from ground red chilies, hot principle is capsaicin. *Health benefits:* Improves digestion, increases circulation, warms the body easing cold symptoms, lowers blood cholesterol and triglycerides, and promotes normal metabolism of fat by the liver. *Tips:* Pain reliever used topically in creams, in nasal sprays to treat chronic rhinitis. *Recipes:* Tropical Tamer for Congestion (Chapter 12).

Celery and celery seed: *Nutrients:* Potassium, magnesium, and fiber. *Health benefits:* Diuretic, tonic for digestion and gout, lowers elevated blood pressure, anticancer properties, seeds traditionally used to calm nerves. *Tips:* Eat raw for fiber and add seeds to salad dressings. *Recipes:* None.

Cherries: *Nutrients:* Potassium, vitamin C and A, flavonoids, and ellagic acid (an anticancer phytonutrient). *Health benefits:* Tonic for gout, black cherries show antibacterial activity for reducing dental plaque, help fight cancer, traditionally used to reduce phlegm, and for kidney stones and gallbladder problems. *Tips:* Enjoy sweet cherries raw, whole and juiced, cook sour cherries, short shelf life, and seeds are poisonous. *Recipes:* None.

Chicken, chicken soup: *Nutrients:* Protein, breast meat high in vitamin B6, dark meat high in iron and zinc; both have some B complex vitamins. *Health benefits:* Broth is tonic for colds. White meat supports hormonal health, and dark meat sustains the body's biochemistry. *Tips:* Buy chicken free of antibiotics, free-range, and organically fed. *Recipes:* North African Roast Chicken with Almonds and Dried Fruits (Chapter 11), Curried Chicken with Healing Spices (Chapter 20), Simmered Chicken with Citrus (Chapter 16), and Chicken Salad Pick-Me-Up (Chapter 14).

Chickpeas: *Nutrients:* Calcium, iron, potassium, and vitamin A. *Health benefits:* Help deliver oxygen to the cells, strengthen bone, and maintain healthy skin. *Tips:* Cook slowly to retain shape. *Recipes:* Chickpeas in Disguise (Chapter 24).

Chili peppers: *Nutrients:* High in beta-carotene, vitamin C, and capsaicin. *Health benefits:* Clear congestion, aid digestion, stimulate circulation, and help prevent blood clots; many uses in traditional medicine. *Tips:* Fiery compounds are in the seeds, membranes, and core. *Recipes:* Tender Poached Eggs (Chapter 9), Flounder with Flavor (Chapter 8), and Simmered Chicken with Citrus (Chapter 16).

Cinnamon: *Nutrients:* Cinnamic acids. *Health benefits:* Therapeutic stimulant, a mild sedative and painkiller for backache and arthritis, cinnamic acids have anti-cancer properties, traditionally used as an expectorant for congestion. *Tips:* Breathe the steam for congestion. *Recipes:* Magnesium Munchies (Chapter 10).

Citrus (orange, lemon, lime, grapefruit, and tangerine): *Nutrients:* Vitamin C, flavonoids, calcium, folic acid, lycopenes, and hesperidine and limonene in peel. *Health benefits:* Boost immunity, slow aging, segment membranes and pith contain flavonoids, which help strengthen blood vessels to help prevent varicose veins and heart disease; peel aids bronchitis; and citrus supports the liver in detoxifying carcinogens. *Tips:* Eat fresh and raw as vitamin C is destroyed by heat and oxygen, if using peel in cooking buy organic citrus. *Recipes:* California Sunrise (Chapter 12), Greek Lemon Lamb (Chapter 7), and Simmered Chicken with Citrus (Chapter 16).

Cloves: *Nutrients:* Potassium and calcium. *Health benefits:* Digestive aid, relieves nausea, powerful antiseptic and warming stimulant for the circulation, and soothes bronchitis. *Tips:* Chew as a breath freshener after meals, oil of clove dulls toothache. *Recipes:* Pears Poached in Red Wine (Chapter 15).

Coconut: *Nutrients:* Potassium, iron, zinc, fiber, and saturated fat. *Health benefits:* In small amounts, supplies needed saturated fats that are essential for hormone production. *Tips:* Can be heated to high temperatures as fats are relatively stable. *Recipes:* Orange-Scented Coconut Macaroons (Chapter 20).

Cod: *Nutrients:* Protein, potassium, selenium, phosphorus, iron, and niacin. *Health benefits:* Makes a good addition to a weight loss diet, helps preserve tissue elasticity and skin quality, counteracts fatigue, and contributes to bone strength. *Tips:* If using salt cod, remove salt by soaking cod for three to six hours, changing the water two or three times. *Recipes:* Cod Cakes with Tomato Tarragon Sauce (Chapter 21).

Corn: *Nutrients:* Magnesium, potassium, zinc, B vitamins, beta-carotene, protein, and fiber. *Health benefits:* Helps prevent osteoporosis, fuels body metabolism, and protects cholesterol from oxidizing. *Tips:* Buy cornmeal with added lysine, which makes the grain a better source of high-quality protein. *Recipes:* Wild Western Corn Bread (Chapter 19).

Cranberry: *Nutrients:* Vitamin C, beta-carotene, and some B complex. *Health benefits:* Remedy for cystitis, supports immunity and health of the nervous system. *Tips:* As a tonic, use sugarfree concentrated cranberry juice found in natural-food stores. *Recipes:* None.

Cucumber: *Nutrients:* Some potassium and small amounts of other nutrients. *Health benefits:* Watery summer food good for replenishing fluids, provides crunch for healthy teeth and gums, only 14 calories per cup. *Tips:* Buy unwaxed or peel waxed skin and enjoy raw and cooked. *Recipes:* Poached Salmon and Cucumbers (Chapter 2).

Currants, black: *Nutrients:* Vitamin C, iron, potassium, some B vitamins, phytoestrogens, and fiber. *Health benefits:* Help prevent anemia and help reduce symptoms of menopause by promoting hormone balance. *Tips:* Scrub teeth after eating as currant sugars are sticky and can lead to tooth decay. *Recipes:* North African Roast Chicken with Almonds and Dried Fruits (Chapter 11).

Dairy foods (milk, cheese, and butter): *Nutrients:* Protein, calcium, vitamin E, and fortified with vitamin A and D. *Health benefits:* Strengthen bones, provide a source of energy, and supply raw materials for building body tissues. *Tips:* Only buy diary products free of added growth hormones and antibiotics, go out of your way to buy organic milk and especially organic butter; may be difficult to digest due to lactose deficiency, avoid highly processed "cheese foods." *Recipes:* Marinated Goat Cheese (Chapter 9) and Warm Bruschetta with Fresh Basil (Chapter 11).

Dark leafy greens (kale, collard greens): *Nutrients:* High in calcium, beta-carotene, fiber, and indoles. *Health benefits:* Help prevent osteoporosis, protect against heart disease and cancer, help in recovery from stroke, and may prevent cataracts. *Tips:* Most beneficial when cooked. *Recipes:* Leafy Greens with Garlic (Chapter 6).

Dates and date sugar: *Nutrients:* Potassium, boron, niacin, and calcium. *Health benefits:* Replace potassium lost due to diarrhea and due to diuretic medication and help prevent chronic fatigue and osteoporosis. *Tips:* Use date sugar rich in minerals and complex carbohydrates, substitute for brown sugar, and buy dates not treated with sulfites to avoid an allergic reaction. *Recipes:* Hot Flash Fruit Compote (Chapter 17), Breakfast Wake Up Muffins (Chapter 13).

Eggs: *Nutrients:* Complete and balanced protein, B complex, vitamins D, selenium, zinc, high in cholesterol, and low in saturated fat. *Health benefits:* Easily digestible food for convalescing, help build body tissues, and play a role in cell metabolism and energy production. *Tips:* Poach eggs to minimize effects of cholesterol on heart disease and never cook scrambled. *Recipes:* Tender Poached Eggs (Chapter 9).

Endive: *Nutrients:* Beta-carotene, folic acid, calcium, and terpenoids. *Health benefits:* Stimulates gallbladder and liver, thereby detoxifying and cleansing the system, and promotes healthy skin; traditionally used as a diuretic. *Tips:* Eat raw or cooked. *Recipes:* Caviar for Company (Chapter 23).

Fennel, bulb and seeds: *Nutrients:* Potassium, calcium, and volatile oils such as limonine. *Health benefits:* Functions as a diuretic, and seeds aid digestion and reduce gas. *Tips:* Enjoy raw, steamed, or braised. *Recipes:* Busy-Day Bouillabaisse (Chapter 13).

Figs: *Nutrients:* Potassium, calcium, magnesium, iron, zinc, and fiber. *Health benefits:* Home remedy for constipation, excellent for building bones, and a traditional treatment for cancer. *Tips:* Fresh figs spoil quickly; dried figs store for months. Avoid figs treated with sulfites if allergic. *Recipes:* North African Roast Chicken with Almonds and Dried Fruits (Chapter 11) and Magnesium Munchies (Chapter 10).

Fish: *Nutrients:* Protein, omega-3 essential fatty acids, wide range of minerals including iodine, selenium, phosphorus, potassium, iron, and calcium, B vitamins, and oil-soluble vitamins A and D in fish oil. *Health benefits:* Supports normal thyroid function, mineral balance, absorption of calcium, lowers undesirable form of cholesterol and increases beneficial cholesterol, helps maintain the health of the nervous system and the ability to withstand stress, and has anti-inflammatory benefits. *Tips:* Cook thoroughly (10 minutes per inch of thickness) to kill all toxic organisms and parasites; eat the soft bones of canned salmon, mackerel, and sardines for a dose of calcium; always buy quality. *Recipes:* Flounder with Flavor (Chapter 8) Sardine Tapenade (Chapter 8), and Cod Cakes with Tomato Tarragon Sauce (Chapter 21).

Flax seed, flaxseed oil: *Nutrients:* Omega-3 essential fatty acids, phytoestrogens, and lignans. *Health benefits:* Promotes hormonal health in women and helps prevent symptoms of PMS and perimenopause, lowers cholesterol and reduces risk of heart disease, anticancer properties, aids digestion, and good for brittle hair and dry skin. *Tips:* To avoid generating toxic byproducts, *never* heat flaxseed oil. Use at room temperature or add to a dish once it is cooked. *Recipes:* Green Beans with Sautéed Shallots (Chapter 3).

Game: *Nutrients:* Usually higher in protein and lower in fat and cholesterol than common cuts of meat and may supply essential omega-3 fatty acids, especially if fed a diet of wild foods. *Health benefits:* Nourishes the nerves, supports energy production and helps keep skin and hair in good condition. *Tips:* Buy game at gourmet markets, farmers' markets, and specialty meat stores. Look for White Pekin duck, which is low in fat and supplies iron, zinc, and B vitamins. Remember to order game when you are dining out. *Recipes:* None.

Garlic: *Nutrients:* Small amounts of potassium and phosphorus. *Health benefits:* Antibacterial and antiviral properties for fighting infection including AIDS, reduces inflammation, promotes heart health and good circulation, lowers the risk of stroke, lowers elevated blood sugar levels, and inhibits formation of tumors. *Tips:* Raw garlic, as well as cooked, picked, and aged garlic, and garlic extracts are beneficial; to activate the healing allium compounds, first crush garlic and set aside for 15 minutes before eating; baked whole garlic bulb of little benefit. *Recipes:* Garlic Shrimp (Chapter 16) and Garlic Soup Remedy (Chapter 20).

Ginger: *Nutrients:* Gingerol. *Health benefits:* Antidote for nausea, digestive aid, subtle energizer, anti-inflammatory action of use in arthritis, expectorant for colds and flu, helps prevent blood clots, and stimulates circulation. *Tips:* Enjoy raw, cooked, and prepared as a tea. *Recipes:* Ginger-Pear Cooler (Chapter 12), Motion Potion (Chapter 20), Mango Salsa Cha Cha Cha (Chapter 6), and Breakfast Wake Up Muffins (Chapter 13).

Grapes, raisins: *Nutrients:* Potassium, vitamins A and C, chromium, boron, quercetin, and polyphenols in grape skins, and cancer-protective tannins, ellagic acid, and pycnogenol in seeds. *Health benefits:* Compounds in red grape skin protect against oxidation of LDL cholesterol and heart disease; ellagic acid in Concord grapes blocks the growth of cancer cells; antiviral activity. Grape seed oil is a powerful antioxidant known to protect capillary walls and useful for the prevention of such ailments as varicose veins and diabetic retinopathy. *Tips:* Enjoy fresh and uncooked. *Recipes:* None.

Green beans: *Nutrients:* Vitamin C, beta-carotene, and fiber. *Health benefits:* Support immunity and promote digestive and heart health. *Tips:* To retain bright green color, steam briefly or cook uncovered; heat diminishes vitamin C but not beta-carotene. *Recipes:* Green Beans with Sautéed Shallots (Chapter 3).

Honey: *Nutrients:* Small amounts of magnesium and potassium and trace amounts of copper, manganese, zinc, and some B vitamins, several antioxidant compounds. *Health benefits:* Readily absorbed for quick energy, aid for upset stomach, antibacterial properties traditionally used to heal infections of the respiratory and digestive tract, especially raw manuka honey, which can reduce ulcer pain. Pollen in honeycomb may reduce pollen allergies. Darker honeys such as buckwheat and tupelo have greater antioxidant activity. *Tips:* Use raw honey and honeycomb for maximum benefits. *Recipes:* Motion Potion (Chapter 20).

Kiwi: *Nutrients:* High in vitamin C, plus potassium, mucilage, and the enzyme actinidin. *Health benefits:* Strengthens immunity, maintains supporting structure of skin, and is a gentle laxative and digestive aid. *Tips:* Whole fruit stores well in refrigerator and retains vitamin C. Best eaten raw. Added to gelatin, it prevents gelling. *Recipes:* None.

Lamb: *Nutrients:* Protein, B vitamins, iron, and zinc. *Health benefits:* Provides raw material for building muscle, helps prevent anemia and facilitates transport of oxygen to the tissues, boosts immunity, helps maintain the production of energy within the cells, and nourishes the nervous system. *Tips:* Shop for naturally raised Australian and New Zealand lamb. Leanest meat is spring lamb and leg of lamb. *Recipes:* Braised Lamb Shanks and Lentils (Chapter 5) and Greek Lemon Lamb (Chapter 7).

Lentils: *Nutrients:* High in potassium, plus calcium, folic acid, iron, protein, and fiber. *Health benefits:* Help lower high blood pressure and cholesterol, stabilize blood sugar levels in diabetes, good for weight loss, and an antidote for stress and nervous conditions. *Tips:* Lowfat, high-protein meat substitute. *Recipes:* Braised Lamb Shanks and Lentils (Chapter 5) and Lentils and Leftovers (Chapter 15).

Lettuce: *Nutrients:* Beta-carotene, potassium, folic acid, magnesium, iron, vitamin C, and vitamin E. *Health benefits:* Good for the liver and nervous disorders, aids digestion, helps prevent heart disease, stroke, and cancer. *Tips:* The darker the green, the more nutritious the leaf (romaine is especially beneficial). *Recipes:* Broiled Steak Salad with Roasted Red Peppers (Chapter 7).

Licorice: *Nutrients:* Glycyrrhizing, flavonoids, coumarins, triterpenoids, sterols, and other natural compounds. *Health benefits:* Activates immune system to inhibit bacteria and viruses such as herpes simplex and has been used to treat hepatitis. Supports gastrointestinal health and eases symptoms of PMS and menopause. Prescribed in traditional

medicine to treat asthma, allergies, diphtheria, and tetanus. *Tips:* Licorice can promote sodium retention and increase blood pressure in sensitive persons. Imported licorice candy contains actual licorice while common "licorice" candy is usually flavored with anise. *Recipes:* None.

Lima beans: *Nutrients:* Copper, folic acid, iron, magnesium, potassium, and zinc. *Health benefits:* Healing food for recovering from colds and the flu, is a bone builder, and helps form red blood cells. *Tips:* Fresh lima beans available June to September. *Recipes:* Puree of Green Soybean Soup (Chapter 17).

Liver (beef): *Nutrients:* Loaded with B vitamins, iron, zinc, copper, selenium, potassium, phosphorus, and some vitamin E. *Health benefits:* Tonic for fatigue, restorative food while convalescing, strengthens the nervous system, and increases immunity. *Tips:* Only eat liver that is organic, at home or in restaurants. *Recipes:* None.

Mango: *Nutrients:* Beta-carotene, vitamin C, vitamin E, niacin, potassium, and fiber. *Health benefits:* Slows the aging process, protects against heart disease, produces energy, and is a digestive aid. *Tips:* Enjoy raw and in season. *Recipes:* Mango Salsa Cha Cha Cha (Chapter 6) and Tropical Tamer for Congestion (Chapter 20).

Maple syrup, maple sugar: *Nutrients:* Potassium and calcium. *Health benefits:* Provides some nourishment and quick energy and raises blood sugar levels less than refined white sugar. *Tips:* Grade C is dark brown and highest in mineral content, must be labeled "pure" maple syrup, or it may have been mixed with corn syrup. Avoid "pancake syrup." *Recipes:* Orange-Scented Coconut Macaroons (Chapter 10).

Melon: *Nutrients:* Potassium, calcium, magnesium, iron, some manganese and copper, and lycopenes. *Health benefits:* Replenishes system with fluids, increases the body's store of minerals, which helps to prevent the development of disease in general, reduces free-radical damage, tea from seeds traditionally used to treat bladder and kidney problems. *Tips:* Melon is easier to digest if eaten alone and not with other foods. *Recipes:* Tropical Tamer for Congestion (Chapter 20) and California Sunrise (Chapter 10).

Millet: *Nutrients:* Protein, iron, niacin, thiamin, magnesium, potassium, lecithin, choline, and fiber. *Health benefits:* Helps maintain normal fat metabolism and the health of the liver, gallbladder, kidneys, and the nervous system. Good for ulcers and colitis. *Tips:* An exceptionally nutritious ancient grain that deserves to be included in more meals and not just used as birdseed. *Recipes:* None.

Mushrooms: *Nutrients:* Fiber and depending upon the variety, phosphorus, potassium, some B vitamins including B12, chromium, and copper. *Health benefits:* Lentinan in skiitake mushrooms is antiviral and anticancer. Maitake mushrooms lower blood pressure and stop tumor growth in animals. *Tips:* Cooking makes nutrients more available and removes naturally occurring carcinogens. Avoid common button mushrooms, which contain carcinogens, even when cooked, as well as unusually high levels of pesticides. Other edible varieties include portabella, oyster, and commercial wild mushrooms, such as chanterelle, morels, porcini or cèpes, and wood ear. *Recipes:* None.

Mustard: *Nutrients:* Active ingredients are the enzyme, myrosin, and a glycoside, sinallein. *Health benefits:* Laxative, used by herbalists as a gargle for sore throat and a treatment for bronchitis and hypothermia. Mustard plaster relieves inflammation and congestion. *Tips:* Powdered seeds release heat when mixed with water. To avoid blistering skin when using externally, put mustard plaster on fabric and place fabric on skin. *Recipes:* None.

Nutmeg: *Nutrients:* Trace of potassium, phosphorus, magnesium, calcium, and myristicin. *Health benefits:* Traditionally used as a digestive aid and to ease pain, myristicin, which is similar to the psychedelic drug mescaline, in large doses far beyond culinary amounts can produce hallucinations and euphoria. *Tips:* Use whole nutmegs and grate fresh for best flavor. *Recipes:* None.

Nuts: *Nutrients:* Excellent source of minerals, healthy fats, and fiber, as well as some B vitamins. *Health benefits:* Almonds, Brazil nuts, cashews, pecans, and pistachios a good source of potassium, magnesium, and zinc. Almonds and hazelnuts provide vitamin E. Brazil nuts exceptionally high in selenium, which increases the effectiveness of vitamin E and protects against skin cancer. Peanuts high in niacin. Macadamia, hazelnuts, pistachios, and almonds especially high in monounsaturated fat, which protects against heart disease, walnuts high in omega-3 fatty acids, which benefit female health. *Tips:* Eat raw for maximum benefits. Avoid salted, roasted, and sugar-coated nuts. Store in refrigerator and discard immediately when oils smell rancid. *Recipes:* Magnesium Munchies (Chapter 10), Walnut Pesto Pasta (Chapter 10), North African Roast Chicken with Almonds and Dried Fruits (Chapter 11), and Ali Baba's Toasted Sesame/Nut Rub (Chapter 10).

Oats: *Nutrients:* B vitamins, zinc, magnesium, and fiber. *Health benefits:* Counteract fatigue and stress, contribute to enzymatic reactions that support life, and help lower cholesterol. *Tips:* Choose steel-cut, rolled, and oat groats over flakes and instant oats. Buy whole oats, not instant-cooking oat flakes. *Recipes:* None.

Okra: *Nutrients:* Fiber, beta-carotene, vitamin C, potassium, and calcium. *Health benefits:* Gums and pectins reduce levels of cholesterol in the blood and protect against intestinal disorders and stomach ulcers. *Tips:* Cook with young, tender green pods 3 to 4 inches long. *Recipes:* Quick and Easy Cajun Okra (Chapter 18).

Olives and olive oil: *Nutrients:* Sodium, beta-carotene, iron, and monounsaturated fatty acids. *Health benefits:* Lower LDL cholesterol and associated with a lower incidence of heart disease. *Tips:* Enjoy whole olives and extra-virgin olive oil, which is minimally processed. Black olives have the least sodium, while Greek and Italian olives are salt-cured. *Recipes:* Mediterranean Olives (Chapter 10).

Onion (also leek, shallot, scallion, chive): *Nutrients:* Vitamin C, some B vitamins and minerals, quercetin, and adenosine. *Health benefits:* Diuretic helpful for rheumatism and gout. Fights infection for treatment of sore throats and cold sores. Lowers blood pressure, reduces cholesterol, lowers risk of stomach and colon cancer, helps steady blood sugar levels to treat diabetes. Reduces risk of stroke. Anti-inflammatory compounds help prevent hay fever and asthma attacks. *Tips:* Quercetin and adenosine not destroyed in cooking, but raw onions most beneficial. When slicing onions, keep root end intact to keep eyes from tearing. *Recipes:* Red Onions with Vinegar and Chili Peppers (Chapter 16) and Savory Baked Vegetables (Chapter 6).

Oysters: *Nutrients:* Exceptionally high in zinc, plus selenium, iron, calcium, phosphorus, and B vitamins. *Health benefits:* Traditionally used as an aphrodisiac, zinc is a component of male reproductive fluid. Counteract fatigue, enhance immune function, reduce the risk of macular degeneration, and protect against cancer of the skin, esophagus, and prostate. *Tips:* Cook only fresh live oysters with closed shells and only eat oysters in shells that have opened after cooking. *Recipes:* Don Juan's Oyster Stew (Chapter 18).

Papaya: *Nutrients:* High in vitamin A, C, and potassium, calcium, and living enzymes. *Health benefits:* Digestive aid, powerful anti-inflammatory action, promotes healing of damaged tissue, and protects against degenerative disease. *Tips:* For anti-inflammatory benefits, eat raw. *Recipes:* Tropical Tamer for Congestion (Chapter 20).

Parsley: *Nutrients:* Vitamin C, beta-carotene, iron, magnesium, and calcium. *Health benefits:* Relieves indigestion, breath freshener, helps to heal gums, boosts immunity, helps prevent anemia, and helps with bone strength. *Tips:* Nibble raw or cooked. *Recipes:* Turkish Buckwheat Salad (Chapter 17).

Peaches: *Nutrients:* Beta-carotene, some potassium, boron, and fiber. *Health benefits:* Gentle laxative. Prevent tissue damage by free radicals, help lower blood pressure, and contribute to bone structure and strength. *Tips:* Enjoy fresh, not canned in heavy sugar syrup. *Recipes:* None.

Pears: *Nutrients:* Potassium, boron, magnesium, copper, and iron. *Health benefits:* Help maintain mineral balance within the system, contribute to bone structure and strength. Laxative, traditionally used as a remedy for arthritis and gout and the treatment of disorders of the gallbladder. *Tips:* Enjoy raw or cooked. *Recipes:* Pears Poached in Red Wine (Chapter 15).

Peas: *Nutrients:* High in thiamin, folic acid, iron, vitamin C, zinc, magnesium, and protein. *Health benefits:* Help stabilize blood sugar, reduce risk of heart disease, and lower blood cholesterol. *Tips:* Beneficial fresh or frozen. *Recipes:* None.

Pineapple: *Nutrients:* Vitamin C and living enzymes. *Health benefits:* Digestive aid, powerful anti-inflammatory action, which helps reduce swollen gums after dental work and the chronic inflammation associated with arthritis. *Tips:* Eat raw for anti-inflammatory benefits. *Recipes:* None.

Pomegranate: *Nutrients:* Potassium, some phosphorus, sodium, B vitamins, and phytoestrogens. *Health benefits:* Helps nourish and balance the hormonal system, traditionally used in the sweltering Middle East to replenish fluids lost from perspiration, and to treat diarrhea. Given to patients with fever, juice taken as a gargle. *Tips:* Buy those heavy for their weight, which indicates juiciness. Store refrigerated and use within the week. *Recipes:* Fizzy Fruit Cocktail (Chapter 12).

Pork: *Nutrients:* Protein, thiamin, niacin, riboflavin, zinc, vitamin B6, phosphorus, and iron. *Health benefits:* Supports energy production within the cells of the body, protects against heart disease, and helps prevent anemia. *Tips:* Shop for naturally raised pork and uncured bacon free of nitrites. Select the leaner cuts labeled "loin." *Recipes:* Milwaukee Pork Chops with Cabbage (Chapter 7).

Potatoes: *Nutrients:* Potassium, magnesium, some iron, copper, zinc, B vitamins, and vitamin C. *Health benefits:* Lower high blood pressure, compounds in raw white potatoes and especially potato skin block viruses and carcinogens. *Tips:* People with diabetes need to limit intake. If areas of potato have turned green, do not eat. Have baked rather than fried. *Recipes:* Cod Cakes with Tomato Tarragon Sauce (Chapter 21).

Prunes: *Nutrients:* Fiber, iron, potassium, and benzoic acid. *Health benefits:* Gentle laxative effect, help eliminate parasites, lower blood cholesterol, benzoic acid used to treat blood poisoning, kidney disorders, and liver disease. *Tips:* To benefit from the fiber, have the whole prune, not the juice. *Recipes:* None.

Pumpkin seeds: *Nutrients:* High in zinc, iron, niacin, phosphorus, and fiber. *Health benefits:* Promote health of the prostate, strengthen immune system, good for impotency, block viruses and carcinogens from becoming active in the intestinal tract. *Tips:* Chew thoroughly for maximum benefits. *Recipes:* Magnesium Munchies (Chapter 10).

Radishes (and horseradish, daikon): *Nutrients:* Vitamin C, iron, and potassium. *Health benefits:* Stimulate appetite and act as a diuretic. Traditionally used to relieve symptoms of cold and flu. *Tips:* Hotter when sliced. Enjoy raw, cooked, or pickled. *Recipes:* None.

Raspberries: *Nutrients:* Vitamin C, flavonoids, potassium, and some vitamin A and C. *Health benefits:* Natural astringency helps counteract gum disease and intestinal problems. Herbalists use raspberries for their cooling effect to treat fever. Red raspberry leaves are a female tonic. *Tips:* Enjoy fresh and raw. *Recipes:* Three-Berry Shortcake (Chapter 25).

Salmon: *Nutrients:* Protein, high in omega-3 essential fatty acids, niacin, vitamin B12 and other B vitamins, and potassium. *Health benefits:* Energizes and counteracts fatigue, lowers undesirable form of cholesterol and increases beneficial cholesterol, anti-inflammatory benefits, and helps maintain the health of the nervous system and the ability to withstand stress. *Tips:* Enjoy poached and baked. *Recipes:* Poached Salmon and Cucumbers (Chapter 3).

Seaweed: *Nutrients:* Magnesium, potassium, phosphorus, iron, sodium, iodine, and B vitamins, including vitamin B12. *Health benefits:* Promotes general good health, nourishes bones and nervous system. Iodine may help counteract exposure to radiation. *Tips:* Soak arame and use in soups and salads. Toast nori over a flame to use as a sushi wrap. Spike flavors with powdered dulse. *Recipes:* None.

Sesame seeds: *Nutrients:* Zinc, calcium, magnesium, B vitamins such as niacin and folate, copper, gums, and mucilages. *Health benefits:* Help maintain steady blood sugar levels, reduce cholesterol, cleanse the system and remove toxins, and contribute to bone structure. *Tips:* Nutrients are more available in sesame paste known in the Middle East as tahini. *Recipes:* Ali Baba's Toasted Sesame/Nut Rub (Chapter 10).

Shrimp: *Nutrients:* Selenium, zinc, iron, niacin, and other B vitamins. *Health benefits:* Helps maintain tissue elasticity and enhances the benefits of vitamin E, which functions as an antioxidant. Plays a role in the conversion of food to energy, counteracts fatigue, and prevents anemia. *Tips:* Remove shells, clean thoroughly before cooking and eating. *Recipes:* Garlic Shrimp (Chapter 16).

Spinach: *Nutrients:* Beta-carotene, vitamin C and E, potassium, lutein, zeaxanthin, and fiber. *Health benefits:* Protects against cancer, supports colon health, and lowers risk of macular degeneration. *Tips:* Eat cooked and well drained to reduce oxalic acid that binds with minerals, making them unavailable. *Recipes:* None.

Soybeans, whole: *Nutrients:* Protein, iron, potassium, calcium, and phytoestrogens (genistein, daidzein). *Health benefits:* Help balance hormones and reduce symptoms of PMS and perimenopause, lowfat source of protein for weight management, and help reduce risk of hormone-related cancers of the breast, cervix, and uterus. *Tips:* Phytoestrogens most concentrated in soybeans, tempeh, and miso. *Recipes:* Puree of Green Soybean Soup (Chapter 17).

Spelt: *Nutrients:* A complete protein with all eight amino acids, B vitamins, phytochemicals, and fiber. *Health benefits:* Helps fight cancer, enhances immunity, and reduces the risk of blood clots. *Tips:* Can be successfully substituted for wheat in baking. *Recipes:* Three-Berry Shortcake (Chapter 25).

Squash, summer (zucchini, pattypans, and yellow crooknecks): *Nutrients:* Potassium, beta-carotene, magnesium, folic acid, calcium, iron, and fiber. *Health benefits:* Low-calorie diet food, juicy and rehydrating on summer nights. Promotes heart health. *Tips:* Enjoy raw with dips or cooked on the grill. *Recipes:* None.

Squash, winter (acorn, butternut, hubbard): *Nutrients:* High in beta-carotene, plus vitamin C, potassium, calcium, iron, and fiber. *Health benefits:* Helps reduce risk of some cancers of the stomach, colon, and lungs, and promotes normal blood pressure. *Tips:* Enjoy baked. *Recipes:* Wintry Squash Soup (Chapter 2).

Strawberries: *Nutrients:* Vitamin C, pantothenic acid, manganese, ellagic acid, P-coumaric, and chlorogenic acids. *Health benefits:* Boost immunity, promote energy, help manage blood sugar levels and stress, and possess anticancer properties. *Tips:* To preserve vitamin C, wash berries just before eating, never freeze them, and eat them uncooked. *Recipes:* Three-Berry Shortcake (Chapter 25).

Stevia: *Nutrients:* Stevioside. *Health benefits:* Herb that is 250 to 300 times sweeter than sugar and is noncaloric. *Tips:* Sold as a dietary supplement, no known harmful effects. Use only a few drops for sweetness; more can taste bitter. *Recipes:* Uncoffee Cappuccino (Chapter 12).

Sunflower seeds: *Nutrients:* Good amounts of potassium, iron, calcium, zinc, thiamin, vitamin B6, niacin, copper, phosphorus, and essential fatty acids. *Health benefits:* Strengthen bones, help prevent angina and heart disease, slow the aging process, and protect against cataracts and cancer. *Tips:* Hull before eating and buy organic. *Recipes:* None.

Sweet peppers: *Nutrients:* Beta-carotene (higher in red peppers), vitamin C, niacin, and vitamin E. *Health benefits:* Therapeutic for skin problems and health of mucous membranes and beneficial for night and color vision, immune booster, and anticancer activity. *Tips:* In shopping, look for firm peppers that are thick and fleshy with brightly colored skins. *Recipes:* Antioxidant Cocktail (Chapter 12) and Tender Poached Eggs (Chapter 9).

Sweet potato: *Nutrients:* Exceptionally high in beta-carotene, plus vitamin C. *Health benefits:* Antioxidants slow aging process. One variety has pale yellow flesh; another variety with vivid orange flesh is often called a yam but is not. Both yellow and orange sweet potatoes have insignificant estrogenic activity and do not help balance hormones. (True yams are rare in American markets. The wild Mexican yam, which is inedible, is a rich source of diosgenin, an estrogenic compound, which tastes soapy and bitter.) *Tips:* Buy sweet potatoes that are heavy for their size and free of bruises and mold, which can indicate contamination with toxins. *Recipes:* Curried Golden Sweet Potatoes (Chapter 2) and North African Roast Chicken with Almonds and Dried Fruits (Chapter 11).

Tea: *Nutrients:* Caffeine, polyphenols (green tea contains more polyphenol than black tea, and oolong ranks in the middle). *Health benefits:* Lowers levels of the undesirable form of cholesterol and helps lower elevated blood pressure, inhibits blood clots, helps prevent tooth decay, antiviral, and polyphenols protect against cancer *Tips:* Herbal teas offer a caffeine-free alternative. *Recipes:* Icy Pear Cooler (Chapter 12).

Tomato: *Nutrients:* Vitamin C, beta-carotene, potassium, fiber, lycopene, P-coumaric acid, and chlorogenic acid. *Health benefits:* Promotes a healthy digestive tract, helps lower blood pressure, protects against colon and bladder cancer, and slows aging. *Tips:* Active compounds more available when tomato is eaten cooked and with a little fat, may aggravate symptoms of arthritis, possible allergen, especially green tomatoes. *Recipes:* Busy-Day Bouillabaisse (Chapter 13) and English Breakfast Broiled Tomatoes (Chapter 6).

Tuna: *Nutrients:* Protein, high in omega-3 essential fatty acids, niacin, iron, potassium phosphorus, folic acid, and magnesium. *Health benefits:* Helps maintain health of the digestive system, skin, and tongue, energizes and reduces fatigue, helps prevent anemia, and promotes heart health. *Tips:* Buy tuna canned in water, not oil if using canned, and also treat yourself to fresh tuna! *Recipes:* Two-Fisted Tuna Sandwich (Chapter 18).

Turkey: *Nutrients:* Protein, high in omega-3 essential fatty acids, niacin, selenium, zinc (especially in dark meat), iron, potassium, and B vitamins. *Health benefits:* Lowfat meat alternative to beef for heart health, helps manage stress and reduce fatigue, supports the many chemical reactions that sustain life. *Tips:* Not the reason you get sleepy at the end of a Thanksgiving dinner (it's because of all the starchy side dishes). *Recipes:* White Chili (Chapter 18).

Turnips, turnip greens: *Nutrients:* Potassium, calcium, vitamin C, fiber, and indoles. *Health benefits:* Lowers risk of cancer, heart disease, and stroke. May help prevent cataracts and helps regulate blood pressure. *Tips:* Cutting and lightly cooking turnips helps to activate anti-cancer properties. Overcooking turnips destroys many of their healing components. *Recipes:* Savory Baked Vegetables (Chapter 6).

Turmeric: *Nutrients:* Curcumin. *Health benefits:* Powerful antioxidant that protects against heart disease and inhibits tumor growth at each stage of the cancer process, anti-inflammatory treatment for respiratory conditions, muscle injuries, arthritis, and stimulates the flow of bile helping to cleanse the system. *Tips:* Heating develops its ginger-pepper flavor. *Recipes:* Curried Chicken with Healing Spices (Chapter 20).

Watercress: *Nutrients:* Substantial amounts of B vitamins including folic acid, potassium, carotenes, calcium, iron, vitamin C, and vitamin E. *Health benefits:* Supports normal liver function, helps reduce risk of heart disease and cancer, counters anemia, antibacterial activity, fights infection, and treatment for eczema.

Tips: Not recommended in cases of stomach and intestinal ulcers because watercress contains irritating mustard oils. *Recipes:* None.

Wine, red: *Nutrients:* Red grape juice: quercetin, reservatrol, anthocyanin pigments in red grape skins (purple grape juice has lower amounts of protective compounds). *Health benefits:* Increases HDL cholesterol, prevents the oxidation of LDL cholesterol and blood clots, helps dispel brain fog, and arrests cancer at all three stages in animals. *Tips:* One glass a day is the maximum necessary to produce benefits; more can begin to interfere with health. *Recipes:* Pears Poached in Red Wine (Chapter 15).

Whole wheat: *Nutrients:* B vitamins, folic acid, vitamin E, iron, magnesium, potassium, selenium, zinc, and calcium. *Health benefits:* Sustains the health of the nerves, strengthens immunity, increases endurance and stamina, and supports normal heart function. *Tips:* Look for newly marketed whole-wheat baked goods such as whole-wheat English muffins and bagels. *Recipes:* Orange-Scented Coconut Macaroons (Chapter 10) and Breakfast Wake-Up Muffins (Chapter 13).

Yogurt: *Nutrients:* Calcium and niacin. *Health benefits:* Helps prevent gastrointestinal and urinary tract infections and yeast infections, aids in the recovery from diarrhea, and helps prevent ulcers. Good food for convalescing. *Tips:* Buy brands that state on the label "live cultures," or "active cultures." If taking to counteract intestinal upset due to antibiotics, eat two hours after taking antibiotics. *Recipes:* Yogurt Cream (Chapter 9).

Appendix C

Mail-Order Sources for Good Foods and Supplies

● ●

*T*his list of mail-order resources for quality foods and related health products is meant to give you options if you don't have a store near you that sells these items or you prefer to shop by phone. I list several sources of organic meats, which can be especially difficult to find. By ordering from these companies, and others like them, you support the marketing of quality products and help make them available to others.

Foods

American Health & Nutrition, Donna Lyman, 3900 Varsity Dr., Ann Arbor, MI 48108; 734-677-5570, ext. 18; ahn@organictrading.com. Beans, grains, seeds, and rice.

Artesian Acres Natural Foods, Rural Route #3, Lancombe, Alberta, Canada, ISO; 888-400-2842; art@agt.net. Green kamut, rice, grains, potatoes, quinoa, and barley.

Diamond Organics, P.O. Box 2159, Freedom, CA 95019; 888-ORGANIC, or 674-2642; Diamondorganics.com. Fruits, vegetables, greens, herbs, mushrooms, grains, breads, pastas, flowers, and oils. Farm organic-grown "samplers" available to introduce products. Full-service, year-round. Federal Express delivery available.

Gold Mine Natural Food Company, 7805 Arjones Dr., San Diego, CA 92126-4368; 800-475-3663; goldmine@ix.netcom.com. Organic grains, rice, and macrobiotic foods. Sole importer of Ohsawa macrobiotic products.

Good Eats, Box 756, Richboro, PA 18954; 800-490-0044; Goodeats@voicenet.com. Organic, kosher, macrobiotic, unique and environmentally friendly, crueltyfree products. Send $3 (refundable with first order) for catalogue featuring 2,000 products.

Hills Foods Ltd., Suite 109, 3650 Bonneville Place, Burnaby, British Columbia V3N 4T7, Canada; 604-421-3100; sales@hillsfoods.com. Top-quality wild game meats. Vegetables also.

Hoven Farms, RR #3, Eckville, Alberta, Canada TOM OXO; 800-311-2333; www.hovenfarms.com. Family-owned and operated certified organic farm grown homestead beef, pasteurized chicken, eggs, turkey, and pork.

Jody Maroni Sausage Kingdom, 808 South Hindry, Unit G, Inglewood, CA 90301; 800-Hautdog or 428-8364; www.maroni.com. Natural, gourmet chicken, pork, beef, and lamb sausages. Their sausages contain 60 to 80 percent less fat than other brands.

Lakewinds Natural Foods, 17523 Minnetonka Blvd., Minnetonka, MN 55345; 612-473-0292; Lakewinds.coop@minn.net. Full-service natural-foods grocery store supplying all-natural meats, poultry, fish, frozen deli meats without additives, wide selection of produce, organic or rBGHfree cheeses and dairy products, wheat/gluten/yeastfree breads and pastries, coffee, homeopathic herbal remedies, housewares, and so much more!

Mercantile Food Company, Box SS, Philmont, NY 12565; 518-672-0190; info@mercantilefood.com, www.mercantilefood.com. Organic bulk grains, flours, beans, seeds, and tropicals, such as medium macarooned coconut and cocoa powder. Hot and cold cereals, all-purpose baking mixes, and ready-to-serve canned beans.

Natural Lifestyle Supplies, 16 Lookout Dr., Asheville, NC 28804; 800-752-2775; www.natural-lifestyle.com. Grains, nuts, beans, seeds, oils, teas, and herbs. Personal hygiene products. Healthy cooking cookware. Clothing.

Omega Nutrition, 1924 Franklin St., Vancouver, British Columbia, V5L 1KZ, Canada; 800-661-FLAX; omegaflow.com. Unrefined organic oils, including essential fatty acid oils, culinary and massage oils, formulas, pet supplies, glutenfree products, and children's products.

Piper Ranch Organic Beef, RR #1, Box 2180, Buckfield, ME 04220; 207-336-2325; www.lpbeef.com. Finest quality organically grown beef.

Timber Crest Farms, 4791 Dry Creek Rd., Healdsburg, CA 95448; 707-433-8251; tcf@timbercrest.com. Dried apples, cherries, apricots, prunes, tomatoes, and other fruits. Almonds and pistachios.

Van Wie Natural Foods, 6798 Route 9, Hudson, NY 12534; 518-828-0533; Smirensky@aol.com. Natural pork, beef, chicken, buffalo, seafood, yogurt, and cheese. Member USDA certified natural growers.

Vine-Maple Farm, Norman Billesberger, 10620 277 St., Maple Ridge, British Columbia, Canada V2W 1M7; 604-462-7539; Norman_B@BC.sympatico.ca.

Range-fed emus, chicken, and meats are available as well as oils. If the product is to be shipped to the United States, allow ten days for delivery.

Walnut Acres Organic Farms, Penns Creek, PA 17862; 800-433-3998; www.walnutacres.com. Organic baking essentials, granola, canned goods, jams and preserves, peanut butter, vitamins, and select meats.

Whole Foods Market, 601 North Lamar, Austin, TX 78703; 512-477-4455; Wholefoods.com. Complete online store featuring natural and organic produce, seafood, namebrand canned goods, pastas, baby foods, soups, dried fruits, and vegetables. Wide assortment of vitamins, minerals, herbs, and homeopathic and other medicinal products. Gifts, flowers, clothing. Save up to 40 percent of what you would pay elsewhere.

Health Supplies

Discount Natural Foods and Vitamin Warehouse, 3990 New Court Rd., Syracuse, NY 13206; 800-541-1121; Order@juicenet.com. Vitamin supplements, juicers, teas, and herbs. "If you find a cheaper price on any of our juicers, we'll match it." Free shipping.

Natural Goodness — The Natural Health & Wellness Shop, Box 307, Chatsworth, Ontario, Canada NOH 160; 519-794-3043; www.natural-goodness.com. Comprehensive online natural supplement source. Herbs, vitamins, minerals, homeopathy, aromatherapy, and formulas for men, women, and children. Beauty aids and books.

Peaches & Green Natural Foods, 1561 Bayview Ave., Toronto, Ontario, Canada M46 3B5; 416-488-6321; peachesandgreen.com. Supplies unusual supplements and range of vitamins. Enzyme therapy, herbal extractions, Swiss herbal remedy, and up-to-date health-oriented news.

Information

Organic Materials Review Institute, Box 11558, Eugene, OR 97440-3758; 541-343-7600; info@omri.org. Nonprofit organization created to benefit organic consumers and general public. Publishes information about producing, processing, and handling organic foods.

Organic Trading Center; www.organicfood.com. International informational Web site for consumers and producers of organic foods.

Index

• *B* •

• C •

• S •

• Z •

Notes

Notes

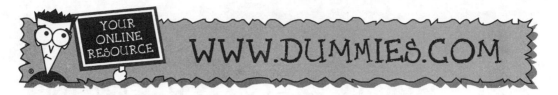

Discover Dummies Online!

The Dummies Web Site is your fun and friendly online resource for the latest information about ...For Dummies® books and your favorite topics. The Web site is the place to communicate with us, exchange ideas with other ...For Dummies readers, chat with authors, and have fun!

Ten Fun and Useful Things You Can Do at www.dummies.com

1. Win free ...For Dummies books and more!
2. Register your book and be entered in a prize drawing.
3. Meet your favorite authors through the IDG Books Author Chat Series.
4. Exchange helpful information with other ...For Dummies readers.
5. Discover other great ...For Dummies books you must have!
6. Purchase Dummieswear™ exclusively from our Web site.
7. Buy ...For Dummies books online.
8. Talk to us. Make comments, ask questions, get answers!
9. Download free software.
10. Find additional useful resources from authors.

Link directly to these ten fun and useful things at **http://www.dummies.com/10useful**

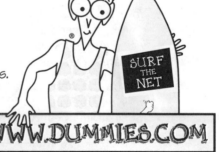

For other technology titles from IDG Books Worldwide, go to **www.idgbooks.com**

Not on the Web yet? It's easy to get started with *Dummies 101*®: *The Internet For Windows*®*98* or *The Internet For Dummies*®, 6th Edition, at local retailers everywhere.

Find other ...For Dummies books on these topics:
Business • Career • Databases • Food & Beverage • Games • Gardening • Graphics • Hardware
Health & Fitness • Internet and the World Wide Web • Networking • Office Suites
Operating Systems • Personal Finance • Pets • Programming • Recreation • Sports
Spreadsheets • Teacher Resources • Test Prep • Word Processing

IDG BOOKS WORLDWIDE BOOK REGISTRATION

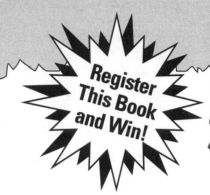

Register This Book and Win!

We want to hear from you!

Visit **http://my2cents.dummies.com** to register this book and tell us how you liked it!

- ✔ Get entered in our monthly prize giveaway.
- ✔ Give us feedback about this book — tell us what you like best, what you like least, or maybe what you'd like to ask the author and us to change!
- ✔ Let us know any other ...*For Dummies*® topics that interest you.

Your feedback helps us determine what books to publish, tells us what coverage to add as we revise our books, and lets us know whether we're meeting your needs as a ...*For Dummies* reader. You're our most valuable resource, and what you have to say is important to us!

Not on the Web yet? It's easy to get started with *Dummies 101*®: *The Internet For Windows*® *98* or *The Internet For Dummies*, 6th Edition, at local retailers everywhere.

Or let us know what you think by sending us a letter at the following address:

...*For Dummies* Book Registration
Dummies Press
7260 Shadeland Station, Suite 100
Indianapolis, IN 46256-3917
Fax 317-596-5498

™

FOR DUMMIES

BESTSELLING
BOOK SERIES